Disease: Identification, Prevention, and Control

Disease: Identification, Prevention, and Control

Barbara P. Hamann, Ph.D.
University of Wisconsin-Superior

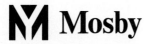 Mosby

St. Louis Baltimore Berlin Boston Carlsbad Chicago London Madrid
Naples New York Philadelphia Sydney Tokyo Toronto

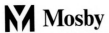

Mosby

Dedicated to Publishing Excellence

Editor-in-chief: James M. Smith
Editor: Robert J. Callanan
Senior Developmental Editor: Jean Babrick
Project Manager: Barbara Bowes Merritt
Design, Editing and Production: York Production Services
Book Designer: York Production Services
Cover concept, unit openers, and computer art: Elizabeth Rohne Rudder/Pagecrafters
Cover images:
Left: Mummy of Egyptian pharaoh Ramses, showing smallpox lesions along jaw. Courtesy WHO.
Right: T-lymphocyte and cancer cell. © B.S.I.P/Custom Medical Stock Photo.

Printed in the United States of America

Composition by Graphic World, Inc.
Printing/binding by Maple Vail-Binghamton

Mosby–Year Book, Inc.
11830 Westline Industrial Drive
St. Louis, Missouri 63146

Library of Congress Cataloging in Publication Data
Hamann, Barbara P.
  Disease : identification, prevention, and control / Barbara P. Hamann.
      p.   cm.
  Includes bibliographical references and index.
  ISBN 0-8016-6364-4
  1. Diseases.   I. Title.
  [DNLM: 1. Disease.   QZ 40 H198d 1994]
  RC46.H225 1994
  616—dc20
  DNLM/DLC
  for Library of Congress   93-43192
                                                                CIP

93 94 95 96 97 / 9 8 7 6 5 4 3 2 1

PREFACE

For the past twenty-five years I have taught about disease to health education students in introductory and community health courses. During that time, the field of health education has grown steadily. Today, with the burgeoning interest in holistic health and fitness, it is expanding even more rapidly, and the need for a course in disease designed for health educators has become urgent. The topic of "Disease: Prevention and Control" has been identified by health methods texts and curriculum committees as one of the ten core content areas in health. National certification in health has become an important career goal for health educators working in schools, corporations, and communities. Certification guidelines for such organizations as The National Commission for Health Education Credentialing (NCHEC) and The American College of Sports Medicine (ACSM) either imply or require knowledge of diseases. The ACSM's emphasis on the need for knowledge of noninfectious diseases such as heart disease and arthritis suggests a need for knowledge about infectious diseases, such as Lyme disease or strep throat, that can lead to chronic disease in later life.

When I began teaching a course specifically concerned with disease ten years ago, my research revealed that no appropriate text existed for my class. The texts available were written for pre-med students, nurses, and allied health personnel. These texts were more technical and clinical than necessary for preparing students who will be health educators in schools, corporations, or community agencies. This text has been written for these students, although it could also serve as an introductory course in disease for those entering allied health fields. The text assumes that students have had a class or classes in anatomy and physiology.

ORGANIZATION

Unit 1 of the text presents a brief history of disease (Chapter 1), discusses the principles of disease occurrence (Chapter 2), and explains the body's defenses (Chapter 3).

Unit 2 of the text organizes infectious diseases in a somewhat different format than other texts. Diseases are grouped by disease agent, rather than by body system; this has the advantage of keeping information on a specific agent in one chapter, rather than scattered among several different chapters. In each chapter, general characteristics, transmission, symptoms, treatment, prevention, and control are discussed for each disease covered. Time and space did not allow for coverage of all infectious diseases; discussed in this text are infectious diseases common in the United States, as well as some (such as smallpox and leprosy) that have historical significance.

Unit 3 begins by discussing the two major noninfectious diseases: cardiovascular disease (Chapter 12) and cancer (Chapters 13 and 14), followed by other noninfectious diseases (Chapters 15-17). (In this text, the word "chronic" will be used as an adjective meaning long-lasting; it may be used for either infectious or noninfectious disease.) In each of these chapters, general characteristics, predisposing factors, symptoms, prevention, and treatment of selected diseases are discussed. Again, diseases discussed are those prevalent in the United States. The final chapter of this part, Chapter 18, deals with genetic and pediatric diseases.

PEDAGOGY

Brief opening discussions for each part are designed to arouse interest. Behavioral objectives and an outline at the start of each chapter will prepare the student for an organized approach to chapter content. A summary table of diseases discussed and review questions at the end of each chapter will reinforce that content. Each chapter concludes with up-to-date suggestions for further reading.

ILLUSTRATION PROGRAM

Timelines in the opening chapter put the history of disease and the accomplishments of the last two centuries into perspective for the student. Throughout, illustrations (both line drawings and photographs) have been chosen or created for their effectiveness in depicting relevant disease states or explaining disease processes.

AIDS FOR THE INSTRUCTOR

I have written an Instructor's Manual, incorporating a chapter outline, objectives, and hints on how to teach difficult concepts. Also included in the Instructor's Manual is a test bank, composed of class-tested questions developed in my years of teaching a course in disease.

ACKNOWLEDGMENTS

I would like to express my appreciation for the help I have received in writing this text. First, I thank the many instructors in health who responded to an extensive survey on what a text like this should include. Their response validated my belief that this text was needed. In addition to the invaluable panel of formal reviewers, listed below, selected chapters have been reviewed and suggestions made by Dr. Philip Hamann, organic chemist, Dawn Hamann, RN, and John Hamann, biologist. The rest of my family, friends and colleagues at the university, have supported and helped me in this endeavor, enabling me to spend the time and make the effort needed to research and write such a text. I want to thank my students for their suggestions and help, and my secretary, Beverly Penney, for being there when I needed her typing and computer skills. Finally, I would like to thank my physician, Dr. Douglas Newman, whose caring and expertise have helped me to continue my work even though I "sampled" a number of the diseases described in this text.

REVIEWERS

Jaqueline Balon, Henry Ford Hospital
Danny Gonsalves, Southern Connecticut State University
James A. Herauf, Northwest Missouri State University
Gerald Hyner, Purdue University
Dawn Larsen, Mankato State University
Karen Porter, Lorain County Community College
Jane Rosenblatt, California State University/Northridge
Frank E. Schabel, Iowa State University
Gerry Silverstein, University of Vermont
Sherman Sowby, California State University/Fresno

CONTENTS

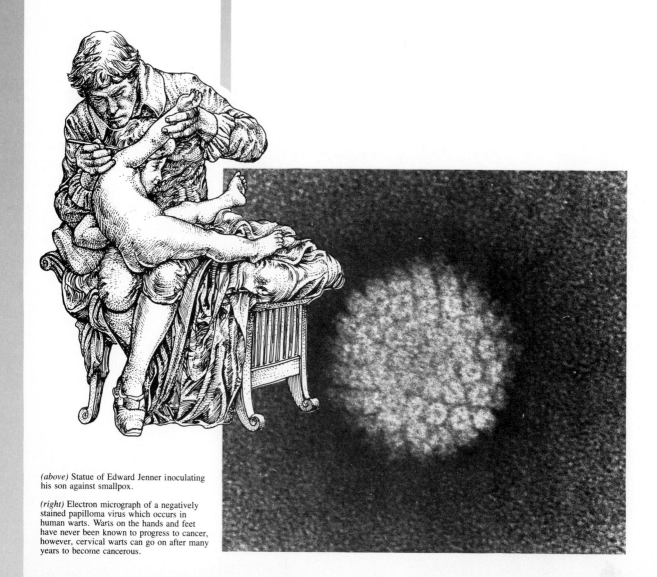

Unit

1 Introduction

(above) Statue of Edward Jenner inoculating his son against smallpox.

(right) Electron micrograph of a negatively stained papilloma virus which occurs in human warts. Warts on the hands and feet have never been known to progress to cancer, however, cervical warts can go on after many years to become cancerous.

Some of the earliest traces of community life have included signs of infectious or noninfectious disease (see Figure 1-1). The efforts of early people to understand why disease happened and then to prevent it met with little success. In fact, not until the revolutionary scientific discoveries of the 19th and 20th centuries could humanity begin to make significant headway against one of its oldest enemies. However, the benefits of those discoveries have not yet reached many of the people in the developing countries.

The heartrending picture of a young boy, squatting on stick-thin legs and too weak to use his equally thin arms to brush away the flies and other insects surrounding him, has been used in televised appeals for help for children in developing countries. This boy shows the effects of too little food, little or no medical treatment, and other factors, such as poverty and poor sanitation. These factors combine to make such children, as well as their elders, vulnerable to the attack of disease.

Poverty, ignorance, and often politics have kept information on human anatomy and physiology, infectious and noninfectious disease, drugs and treatment procedures from many in the developing countries. Defense against disease there often is limited to folk medicine, religious ritual, and cultural practices.

In an attempt to change conditions in developing nations and globally, the World Health Organization (WHO) has developed "A Global Strategy for Health for All by the Year 2000." Among the strategies intended to prevent disease and promote health are safe water and adequate sanitary facilities within homes or no more than 15 minutes' walking distance away; adequate nutrition for children; medically trained personnel to assist with pregnancy, childbirth, and care of the newborn; local health care; availability of at least 20 essential drugs within one hour's travel; and immunization against many infectious diseases.

In the developed countries, the discoveries of the last 200 years have led to an understanding of the necessity for clean water supplies and sanitation, a decrease in the incidence of most infectious diseases, lower disease and death rates, and (in the last 25 years) emphasis on preventive medicine.

Ironically, however, progress against infectious disease means that more people are living longer and are suffering from more chronic noninfectious diseases. At a 1991 forum conducted by WHO, reported in the *Journal of American Medicine,* one conclusion was that "As people live longer and survive threats such as starvation, malnutrition, and infectious diseases, they increasingly fall prey to hazards of industrialization, urbanization, and lifestyle."

The eradication of smallpox through WHO's efforts, along with the understanding of how to prevent or control most other infectious diseases, is a great accomplishment. However, the advent of aquired immune deficiency syndrome (AIDS), continuing problems involved in establishing and delivering adequate health care to all, and the need to convince all the world's citizens to take responsibility for their own health pose continuing challenges.

Chapter 1, The History of Disease, is a look backward in time, a brief review of humanity's triumphs and failures in the ongoing fight against disease. Chapter 2 explains the epidemiologic model of disease, now used by public health workers as they study the causes of disease. This model proposes the interaction of disease agent, host, and environment as the key to disease occurrence. The chain of infection, or means of disease transmission, and the stages of disease are also discussed in this chapter.

The final chapter in this part of the text deals with the body's defenses against disease, and a few of the disorders that occur because, at times, these defenses are mistakenly turned inward.

The History of Disease

O B J E C T I V E S

1 State important events in the understanding and treatment of disease through the ages.

2 Explain the theories that have been held concerning the cause of disease from the earliest times to the present.

3 Identify the contributions of key individuals to advances in medicine through the ages.

4 Identify highlights in the history of disease prevention and control.

5 Describe the development of the major methods used to prevent and control infectious and noninfectious diseases today.

6 Explain the reasons for the change in focus from prevention and control of disease to health promotion.

7 Identify new technologies and techniques used to diagnose and treat disease today.

THE PREHISTORY OF DISEASE

The seeds of disease were present long before recorded history began. Bacteria are among the earliest forms of plant life on earth, and evidence of their ability to infect humans and animals has been found in fossils from prehistoric times. These fossil remains show signs of a number of diseases, including osteomyelitis, tuberculosis, arthritis, rickets, and bone tumors. The well-preserved remains of Egyptian mummies, along with the papyri upon which the Egyptians inscribed case histories of polio, tuberculosis, pneumonia, leprosy, and kidney stones, provide additional evidence of assaults upon the body by disease agents. Lesions on the head of the

FIGURE 1-1 Mummified head of Pharaoh Ramses V, showing smallpox lesions.

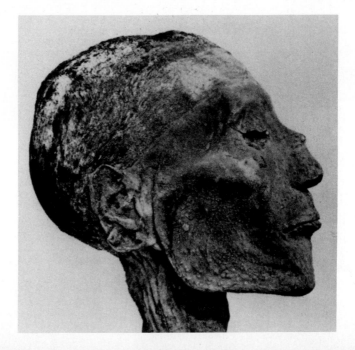

3

mummy shown in Figure 1-1 indicate that smallpox may also have been present in early times. Physical discomfort, sickness, and death from "unnatural" causes have been unwanted companions of the human race since its beginning. The information in this chapter will give you a brief glimpse of the progress made in identifying and learning to prevent and control disease from the time of the early Egyptians to the present. The timeline on this and succeeding pages show this progress.

ANCIENT CIVILIZATIONS: THEORIES OF DISEASE CAUSATION

EGYPTIAN MEDICINE

The early Egyptians (4000 to 1000 BC) had many remedies for illness. Spells, incantations, and magic were integral parts of their medicine. Among early races, illness and death were attributed to actions of the gods and demonic possession. (The concept is present today among some isolated races and individuals.) Despite the Egyptians' lack of scientific knowledge, some of the treatments they used were effective and are still used, and the Egyptians are recognized as the first to treat disease systematically.

Egyptian physicians recognized that weather and the ingestion of "noxious" substances affected the body. They used drugs such as castor oil, olive oil, opium,

HIGHLIGHTS IN DISEASE IDENTIFICATION, PREVENTION, AND CONTROL

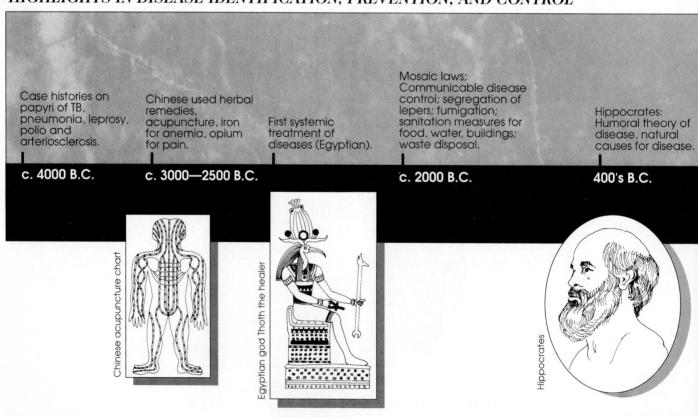

Case histories on papyri of TB, pneumonia, leprosy, polio and arteriosclerosis.

c. 4000 B.C.

Chinese used herbal remedies, acupuncture, iron for anemia, opium for pain.

c. 3000—2500 B.C.

First systemic treatment of diseases (Egyptian).

Mosaic laws; Communicable disease control; segregation of lepers; fumigation; sanitation measures for food, water, buildings; waste disposal.

c. 2000 B.C.

Hippocrates: Humoral theory of disease, natural causes for disease.

400's B.C.

Chinese acupuncture chart

Egyptian god Thoth the healer

Hippocrates

and saffron. Pulses were taken, body temperature noted, the heart was regarded as the vital organ, and respiration was considered the most important function. There were severe penalties for letting a patient die, and for this reason no one was accepted for treatment who appeared to have a fatal condition. Unfortunately, one of the conditions looked upon as fatal was a compound fracture.

Egypt was regarded as the medical center of the ancient world, and physicians there were sought after by foreign rulers. Prescriptions for diet and cleanliness were part of the religion. Records also indicate that physicians specialized. Some treated only diseases of the eye, others diseases of the head, others diseases of the intestines, and so on.

The treatments the early Egyptian doctors used were based on what they perceived as the cause of the disease, and medical science still uses this principle today.

CHINESE MEDICINE

Chinese medicine of the same period also contributed to the remedies in use today. An early Chinese emperor is credited with identifying over 100 herbal remedies and also inventing the technique of acupuncture (see the acupuncture diagram in the timeline). As with the Egyptians, magic and superstition played a part in the development of medicine in China, yet some Chinese prescriptions were also effective in treating disease. Among these were the use of iron to treat anemia and the use of opium as a narcotic.

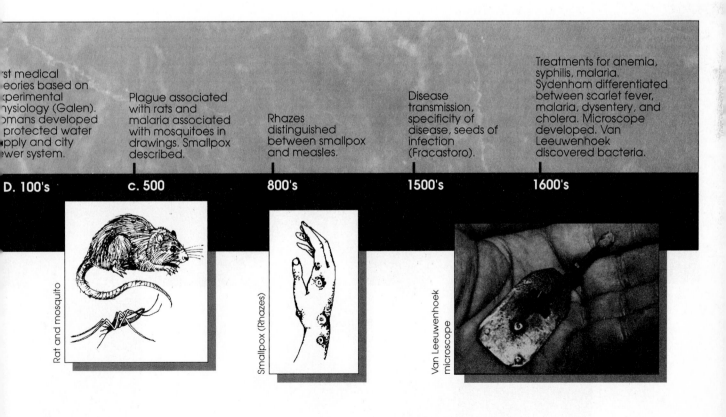

rst medical
eories based on
xperimental
hysiology (Galen).
omans developed
protected water
pply and city
ewer system.

Plague associated with rats and malaria associated with mosquitoes in drawings. Smallpox described.

Rhazes distinguished between smallpox and measles.

Disease transmission, specificity of disease, seeds of infection (Fracastoro).

Treatments for anemia, syphilis, malaria. Sydenham differentiated between scarlet fever, malaria, dysentery, and cholera. Microscope developed. Van Leeuwenhoek discovered bacteria.

D. 100's   c. 500   800's   1500's   1600's

Rat and mosquito

Smallpox (Rhazes)

Van Leeuwenhoek microscope

THE BIBLE AND MEDICINE

In biblical times and earlier, treatments that were effective in helping people with disease were developed and used without any understanding on the part of the practitioners as to why they worked. And we have no indication that there was any concerted effort to discover the cause of most diseases, probably because disease was generally thought of as coming from gods who controlled human events. But glimmerings of the understanding of disease can be found in the Bible. For example, the story of plague among the Philistines in the Old Testament indicates recognition of a relationship between rats and the disease, and the segregation of lepers, indicates some understanding of preventive medicine. The Mosaic law or code, in addition to providing for the segregation of lepers, also prescribed the control of communicable diseases, fumigation, decontamination of buildings, protection of water supplies, disposal of wastes, protection of food, and sanitation of campsites.

GREECE: THE TEACHINGS OF HIPPOCRATES

The writings of Hippocrates (460 to 377 BC) show that by his time interest in determining the cause of and treatment for disease was widespread. Hippocrates, known as the Father of Medicine, believed that each individual contained four *humors,* or fluids: blood, phlegm, yellow bile, and black bile. Disease occurred when these humors were not in balance and could be treated by removing any excess. The practice of bloodletting (Figure 1-2), which persisted well into the nineteenth century, was based on this theory.

HIGHLIGHTS IN DISEASE IDENTIFICATION, PREVENTION, AND CONTROL (continued)

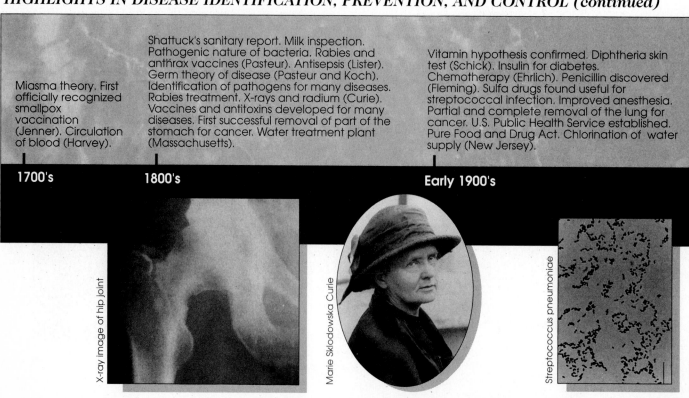

Miasma theory. First officially recognized smallpox vaccination (Jenner). Circulation of blood (Harvey).

Shattuck's sanitary report. Milk inspection. Pathogenic nature of bacteria. Rabies and anthrax vaccines (Pasteur). Antisepsis (Lister). Germ theory of disease (Pasteur and Koch). Identification of pathogens for many diseases. Rabies treatment. X-rays and radium (Curie). Vaccines and antitoxins developed for many diseases. First successful removal of part of the stomach for cancer. Water treatment plant (Massachusetts).

Vitamin hypothesis confirmed. Diphtheria skin test (Schick). Insulin for diabetes. Chemotherapy (Ehrlich). Penicillin discovered (Fleming). Sulfa drugs found useful for streptococcal infection. Improved anesthesia. Partial and complete removal of the lung for cancer. U.S. Public Health Service established. Pure Food and Drug Act. Chlorination of water supply (New Jersey).

1700's

1800's

Early 1900's

X-ray image of hip joint

Marie Sklodowska Curie

Streptococcus pneumoniae

Hippocrates also believed in the healing power of nature, taught that disease developed from natural causes, and prescribed diets, rest, fresh air, massage, and baths as treatments. Although it would be centuries before the first pathogenic organism was identified, Hippocrates's logical approach to disease and clinical observation were first steps on the way to the prevention and control of disease.

We are not sure how many of the books credited to Hippocrates were actually written by him, but we do know that the ideas those books contained were revolutionary in the practice of medicine. Among them was the first known work on physiotherapy; a description of the symptoms that precede death; and 42 case histories presented in a style close to modern scientific form for case histories.

ROME: THE CONCEPT OF PUBLIC HEALTH

Roman civilization adopted many Greek ideals, including respect for the search for scientific knowledge and an appreciation of physical health and beauty. As Roman power grew, public health measures were adopted. Aqueducts were built to carry pure water to the cities (Figure 1-3). Sewers prevented the spread of epidemics, and street cleaning was required. Public and private baths were available everywhere. Physicians were educated at public expense, and their services were made available to the poor. One Roman, Marcus Terentius Varro (116 to 21 BC), described "small

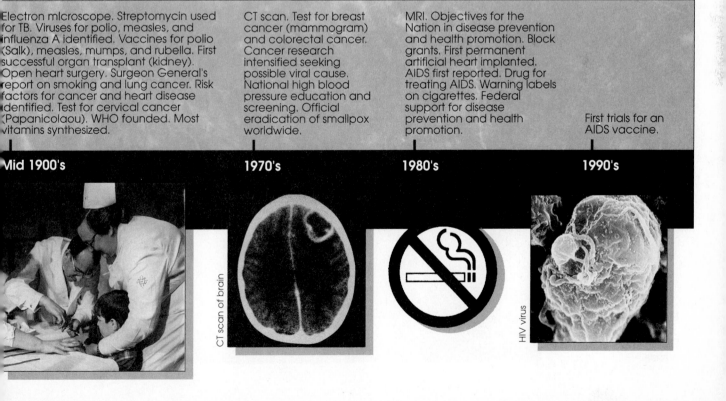

Electron microscope. Streptomycin used for TB. Viruses for polio, measles, and influenza A identified. Vaccines for polio (Salk), measles, mumps, and rubella. First successful organ transplant (kidney). Open heart surgery. Surgeon General's report on smoking and lung cancer. Risk factors for cancer and heart disease identified. Test for cervical cancer (Papanicolaou). WHO founded. Most vitamins synthesized.

CT scan. Test for breast cancer (mammogram) and colorectal cancer. Cancer research intensified seeking possible viral cause. National high blood pressure education and screening. Official eradication of smallpox worldwide.

MRI. Objectives for the Nation in disease prevention and health promotion. Block grants. First permanent artificial heart implanted. AIDS first reported. Drug for treating AIDS. Warning labels on cigarettes. Federal support for disease prevention and health promotion.

First trials for an AIDS vaccine.

Mid 1900's   **1970's**   **1980's**   **1990's**

CT scan of brain

HIV virus

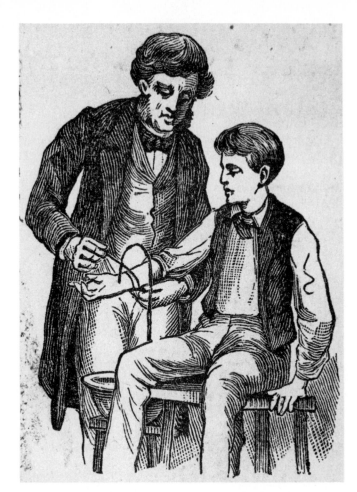

FIGURE 1-2 Bloodletting, a practice that derived from the concept of humors in the body, which must be kept in balance to prevent disease. This practice continued into the early nineteenth century.

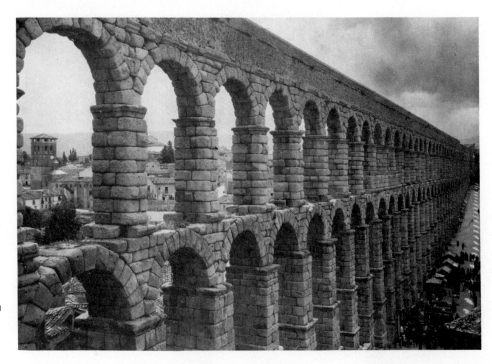

FIGURE 1-3 A Roman aqueduct at Pont du Gard, Nimes, in France.

creatures, invisible to the eye." These creatures, according to Varro, filled the air, were breathed in, and caused dangerous diseases. The microscope, enabling researchers to actually see pathogenic organisms, would be invented centuries later.

THE TEACHINGS OF GALEN

Galen (AD 130 to 200), a native of Asia Minor, was the imperial physician of the Roman Empire (Figure 1-4). Regarded as the founder of experimental physiology, he dissected animals and wrote extensively on the anatomy of the brain and other organs. However, the religious beliefs of the time forbade human dissection. This limited Galen's investigations, and he reached some incorrect conclusions about the structure and function of the human body. Because of his position, he was accepted as the final authority by the early church. His influence persisted for centuries, delaying advances in understanding the human body.

THE MIDDLE AGES: WAR, RELIGION, AND DISEASE

After the fall of Rome (AD 476) political chaos and the rise of new religions affected the search for scientific knowledge. Those same factors also influenced the spread of disease. The collapse of centralized government led to the collapse of the Romans' aqueducts and sewer systems. New cities arose, but the kind of public engineering known under the Romans had been lost.

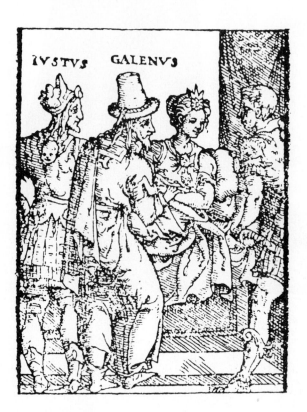

FIGURE 1-4 Galen, considered the first physiologist, is shown here in a medieval woodcut.

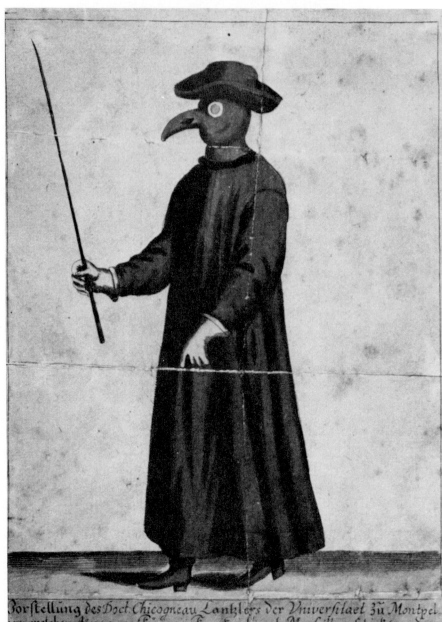

FIGURE 1-5 Protective clothing worn by physicians when treating plague victims.

CHRISTIANITY, ISLAM, AND CONTAGION

In Europe, early Christians reacted against the Greco-Roman emphasis on physical health and beauty. This seemed to them to glorify the body at the expense of the spirit. A healthy mind in a healthy body was no longer the ideal. The body became something shameful, to be ignored in the pursuit of spiritual perfection. This reaction softened somewhat as the Middle Ages progressed, but the Greco-Roman ideal was lost.

The rise of another religion, Islam, in the seventh century also contributed to the spread of disease. Followers of Islam, called Moslems, were required to make a pilgrimage to the holy city of Mecca in what is now Saudi Arabia. Because this faith had spread from southern Europe to India, large numbers of pilgrims traveled long distances to reach Mecca, carrying and transmitting infectious diseases as they went. Among these diseases was cholera, which became pandemic after each hajj, or pilgrimage.

Christian reaction to Islam also contributed to the spread of disease. From the eleventh to the thirteenth centuries, crusades against the "infidels," as Moslems were called, swept thousands of Europeans into the Middle East. Returning crusaders sometimes brought back treasures; they also brought back diseases. Cholera was one of these diseases; leprosy was probably another.

The most deadly of all pandemics, however, were the waves of disease caused by bubonic plague (the "Black Death"). Figure 1-5 shows the protective clothing worn to treat victims of this deadly disease. Twenty percent of the population of Europe perished from a combination of the plague and pulmonary anthrax (Figure 1-6). In England, 2 million died, approximately half of the population. London alone had 100,000 of these deaths. Another "killing" disease, syphilis, spread rapidly throughout Europe and the Near East shortly after the return of Columbus from America. It is thought to have been carried back to Europe by Columbus and his men. Other diseases known to exist during this period, although little mention of them is made in history books, include typhoid, typhus, diphtheria, streptococcal infections, and dysenteries.

During all this time there was little understanding of the ways by which disease was spread. Isolation and quarantine, as with the lepers, were the only control methods, and they were practiced unevenly, depending upon the recognition of symptoms that were thought to be dangerous.

THE RENAISSANCE: DA VINCI, VESALIUS, GALILEO, AND THE MICROSCOPE

It took the intellectual revolution and stimulation of the Renaissance to once more release the spirit of scientific inquiry. As this "rebirth" swept through all areas of human knowledge, among those who contributed to advances in medicine were Leonardo da Vinci (1452-1519) and Andreas Vesalius (1514-1564). Each produced anatomical works based on dissection of the human body that were to show Galen's mistakes and become the foundation for modern anatomy. Figure 1-7 shows an illustration from a page from one of their works. As was mentioned earlier, syphilis appeared in Europe in 1495 (Figure 1-8). It was named by Girolamo Fracastoro

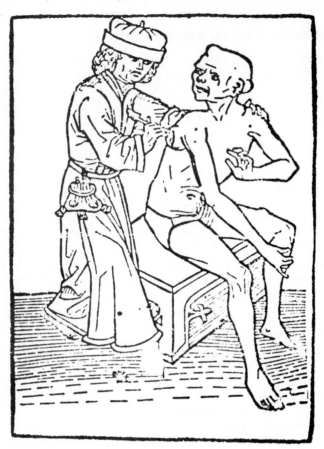

FIGURE 1-6 Medieval woodcut of a surgeon lancing a bubo, one of the manifestations of plague.

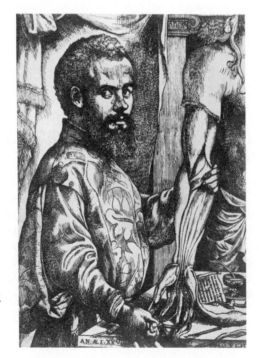

FIGURE 1-7 Page from the treatise of Andreas Vesalius on anatomy, showing the author.

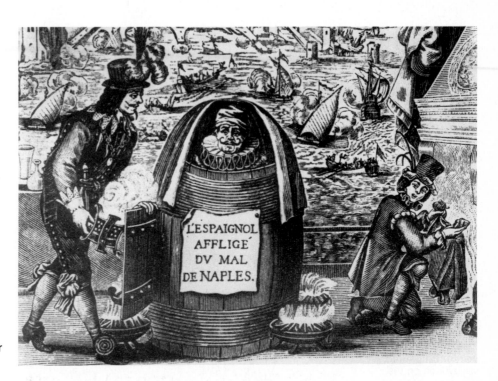

FIGURE 1-8 Spanish soldier being treated for syphilis.

(1483–1553), who also recognized typhus and the contagious nature of tuberculosis. In his writings, he spoke of "the existence of invisible seeds of infection which multiply and penetrate the organism." Fracastoro's book, *De contagione,* was convincing enough that the humoral doctrine of disease, taught by Hippocrates almost a thousand years earlier, was replaced by the idea of specific causes for specific diseases.

One of the most significant inventions of the sixteenth century was the microscope. Although the ability to magnify objects with spherical pieces of glass had been known to the ancients, it was not until the late sixteenth century that microscopes were used in scientific investigations. It is not known who first used magnifying lenses in researching disease, but Galileo (1564–1642) is given credit for actually placing a tube between two lenses to examine a specimen some time after he had constructed his first telescope in 1608.

THE SEVENTEENTH CENTURY: ADVANCES IN UNDERSTANDING DISEASE

In the seventeenth century, inductive reasoning emphasized by Francis Bacon (1561–1626) and the philosophical writings of René Descartes (1596–1650), which encouraged questioning of any former "truths", opened the way for the development of the scientific method. William Harvey described his experiments, which demonstrated the circulation of blood. Figure 1-9 shows an illustration from Harvey's book on this topic. It was not long before Anton van Leeuwenhoek described the red blood cells. Van Leeuwenhoek constructed more than 200 microscopes (Figure 1-10 shows one of them) and was the first to identify bacteria, although he did not connect them to disease. Athanasius Kircher was the first to connect the live mi-

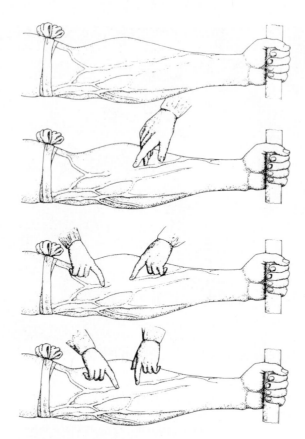

FIGURE 1-9 Illustration from William Harvey's book on the circulation of blood, showing one of his experiments.

FIGURE 1-10 Microscope made by Anton van Leeuwenhoek.

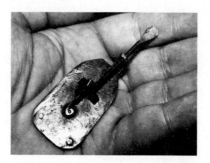

croorganisms in the blood with disease. Increasingly, as more scientists were able to use the microscope—and with more understanding of human anatomy and physiology—advances in the knowledge of disease accelerated.

ADVANCES IN DIAGNOSIS

The vitamin deficiency diseases rickets and beriberi were described, the difference between diabetes mellitus and diabetes insipidus was discovered, and the possibility of a nonvenereal route for syphilitic infection was demonstrated. Physicians learned to count the pulse with a watch. Thomas Sydenham was responsible for many advances, including differentiation between acute rheumatism and gout and between scarlet fever and measles. But it was to take over 100 years before scientists would begin to identify the organisms and causes for most diseases.

THE EIGHTEENTH CENTURY: VACCINATION

The eighteenth century was a time for nurturing the new scientific spirit that had begun in the Renaissance. Progress in the search for answers about disease continued amid the remnants of earlier times. It was a century of paradoxes: an age of enlightenment, an age of quackery; an age of rationalism, yet an age of superstition. Toward the end of this century, Edward Jenner, an English country doctor, made a discovery that was to open the doors for the relief of untold suffering and death.

JENNER'S MILESTONE

Smallpox had killed millions, and there was no indication that the number of cases was decreasing. Jenner overheard a dairymaid say that she could not catch smallpox since she had already had cowpox. Knowing that cowpox was a mild disease, he decided to experiment and vaccinated a small boy with pus from a cowpox lesion. Eight weeks later, the boy was inoculated with regular smallpox but did not get the disease. Jenner published his findings in 1798. Although Jenner was greeted with some skepticism at first (Figure 1-11), it was not long before the incidence of smallpox was greatly reduced in developed countries all over the world.

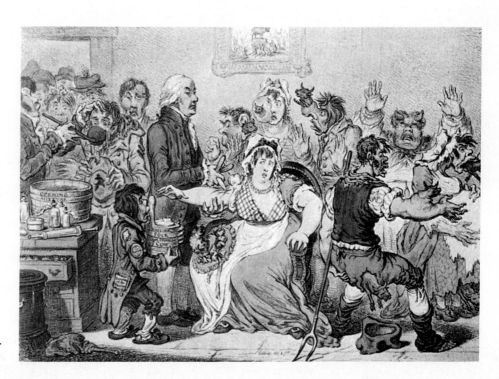

FIGURE 1-11   1700s cartoon satirizing smallpox inoculation.

THE NINETEENTH CENTURY: PASTEUR, LISTER, KOCH, AND THE GERM THEORY

Jenner's discovery of the benefits of vaccination was just the beginning of a great cascade of scientific breakthroughs in the nineteenth century. Scientists in different laboratories all over the world identified many microorganisms and the diseases they caused at such great speed that following each new discovery is beyond the scope of this text. The timeline below shows the fast pace of progress against disease in the latter half of the nineteenth century.

Many individuals made contributions to the prevention and control of disease in the nineteenth century. Claude Bernard (1813-1878), Louis Pasteur (1822-1895), and Robert Koch (1843-1910) (Figures 1-12 to 1-14) were research scientists whose work brought attention to the value of laboratory research in addition to clinical observations.

The understanding of the human body was enhanced by Bernard, who demonstrated that digestion took place in the small intestine as well as in the stomach, discovered glycogen and its manufacture by the liver, unfolded some of the mysteries of the endocrine system, and formulated the basic principles of research and experiment. Louis Pasteur was the first to show without question that microorganisms could be pathogenic to humans. He also continued Jenner's work in immunology

PROGRESS IN DISEASE IDENTIFICATION, PREVENTION, AND CONTROL 1855-1899

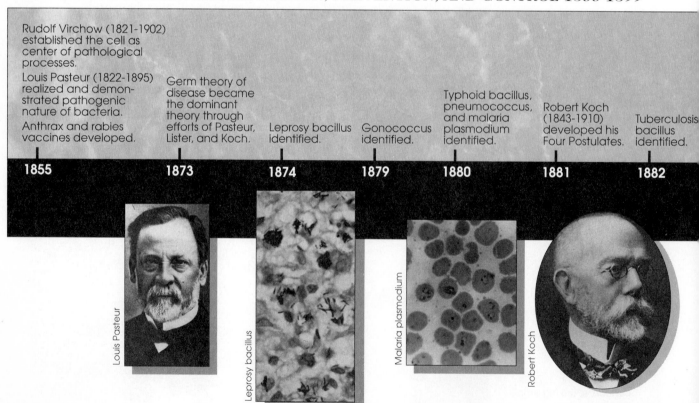

Rudolf Virchow (1821-1902) established the cell as center of pathological processes.

Louis Pasteur (1822-1895) realized and demonstrated pathogenic nature of bacteria.

Anthrax and rabies vaccines developed.

1855

Germ theory of disease became the dominant theory through efforts of Pasteur, Lister, and Koch.

1873

Leprosy bacillus identified.

1874

Gonococcus identified.

1879

Typhoid bacillus, pneumococcus, and malaria plasmodium identified.

1880

Robert Koch (1843-1910) developed his Four Postulates.

1881

Tuberculosis bacillus identified.

1882

Louis Pasteur

Leprosy bacillus

Malaria plasmodium

Robert Koch

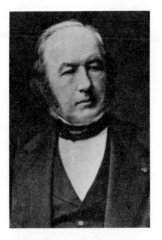

FIGURE 1-12   Claude Bernard.

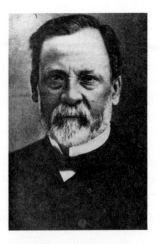

FIGURE 1-13   Louis Pasteur.

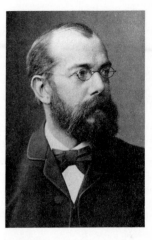

FIGURE 1-14   Robert Koch.

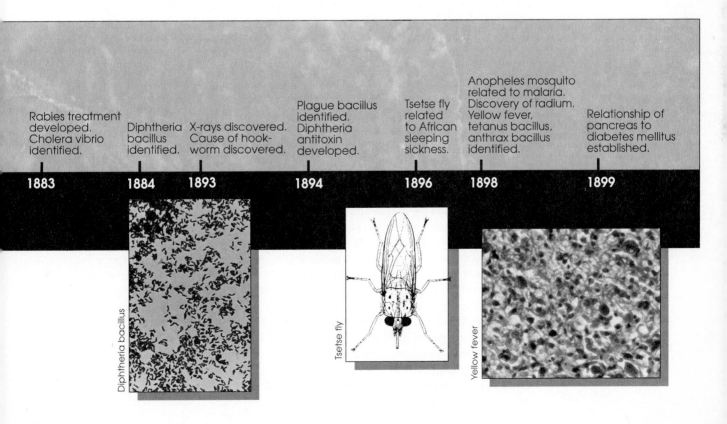

Rabies treatment developed. Cholera vibrio identified.

Diphtheria bacillus identified.

X-rays discovered. Cause of hookworm discovered.

Plague bacillus identified. Diphtheria antitoxin developed.

Tsetse fly related to African sleeping sickness.

Anopheles mosquito related to malaria. Discovery of radium. Yellow fever, tetanus bacillus, anthrax bacillus identified.

Relationship of pancreas to diabetes mellitus established.

1883   1884   1893   1894   1896   1898   1899

Diphtheria bacillus

Tsetse fly

Yellow fever

with the development of vaccines for anthrax and rabies. His procedure for destroying pathogenic organisms in milk and other liquids, pasteurization, is well known.

Building on the work of Louis Pasteur, Joseph Lister (1827-1912) applied antiseptics to surgical wounds and thus made surgery a hundred times safer. Koch developed postulates concerning disease that stated that, for an organism to be identified as the cause of a specific disease, it must (1) always be present in the disease, (2) be capable of growth in pure culture in the laboratory, (3) cause the disease when injected into a susceptible healthy animal, and (4) be recovered from the experimental animal. These postulates clearly established the germ theory of disease and are still used today. Among Koch's many other contributions was the discovery of the bacilli for anthrax, cholera, and tuberculosis.

PROGRESS IN PUBLIC HEALTH

During this century there was rapid population growth in major cities in Europe and America. Little was then known about the connection between sanitation and disease, and piles of garbage and waste accumulated because of lack of community organizations to deal with the problem. In response to this, Edwin Chadwick published a report in England (1842) concerning the poor state of health and the deplorable sanitary conditions. England then passed the British Public Health Act of 1848.

Soon after the passage of this act in England, an American, Lemuel Shattuck, published a report (1850) that was to be a guide in the field of health for many years. Shattuck (1792-1859) was chairman of the newly appointed Sanitary Commission of Massachusetts. Although many of his provisions (see box on page 19) have not yet been fulfilled, the report provided the impetus for a concerted public effort in the struggle to identify, prevent, and control disease.

At the time of these reports, the miasma theory of disease was popular. This theory ascribed disease to bad air (the term *miasma* means noxious air or vapor), and thus efforts to prevent disease were aimed at reducing the bad odors in the air.

Toward the end of the nineteenth century, the earlier work initiated by Pasteur, Koch, and other bacteriologists led to the acceptance of the germ theory of disease. One of the most important discoveries at this time was the protozoan malarial parasite in human blood and its carrier, the *Anopheles* mosquito. This discovery marked the beginning of the conquest of a tropical disease that had been responsible for the decline and devitalization of many civilizations for centuries. Malaria could finally be controlled by systematic destruction of the mosquito larvae.

In addition to the progress made in the area of infectious disease, new procedures were being developed that would help prevent and control noninfectious disease. Blood pressure readings were begun in the 1860s; inspection of the throat, especially the larynx and vocal cords, was facilitated by the construction of the laryngoscope; visualization of the esophagus was accomplished; and the bladder could be observed with a cystoscope. Roentgen discovered the X ray, and Marie and Pierre Curie discovered radium, both useful in diagnosing and treating cancer as well as other diseases. A photograph of Marie Curie is seen in Figure 1-15.

The nineteenth century, which began with more quackery and superstition than scientific knowledge, ended with an outstanding record of discoveries and achievements in the prevention and control of communicable disease. A longer, comparatively disease-free life at last seemed possible.

Lemuel Shattuck's Recommendations for Public Health (1850)

Establishment of state and local boards of health

Hiring of sanitary inspectors

Keeping of vital statistic records

Establishment of systems for data exchange

Studies of schoolchildren's health

Establishment of sanitation programs for towns

Studies of tuberculosis

Supervision of the mentally ill

Study of immigrants' problems

Building of model tenements

Establishment of public bathhouses and washhouses

Control of smoke nuisances

Control of food adulteration

Exposure of quack medicines

Preaching of health in the churches

Establishment of training schools for nurses

Teaching of sanitary science in medical schools

Inclusion of preventive medicine in clinical practice (routine physical examination, keeping records of family illnesses)

From Pickett and Hanlon, *Public Health: Administration and Practice,* 9th ed., Mosby, 1990.

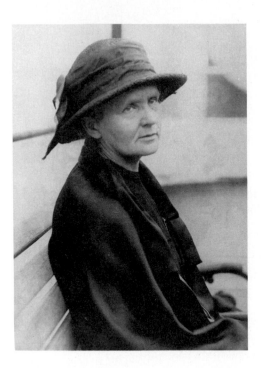

FIGURE 1-15   Marie Curie.

DID YOU KNOW?

Beginning of School and Community Health Education

In 1842, eight years before Lemuel Shattuck made his report, Horace Mann advocated health education in the schools. With Shattuck's report the value of health education for adequate human functioning was reemphasized. In a way, health education had been present since the time when a mother cleaned her children after they played in the mud or a father restricted play in favor of a good night's sleep. But formalized health education in the schools developed only bit by bit after Shattuck's report.

In 1872, the first medical inspector was employed by the New York Board of Education to control the smallpox epidemic. In 1875, because of the influence of the Women's Christian Temperance Union, 38 states passed legislation requiring alcohol education in the schools. From that time until the present, state after state has passed requirements for health education. Slowly but surely, it has

been recognized that a comprehensive health education program is needed in the schools.

Shattuck's report had its greatest effect on the development of official community health agencies in the United States. Sadly enough, Lemuel Shattuck (1793-1859) did not live to see the results of his efforts, for it was 1869 before a state board of health was established in Massachusetts, exactly as Shattuck had recommended in 1842. Today there are official public health agencies on four levels, local, state, national, and international. These health agencies provide health care services for mothers and children who would otherwise have none. They provide communicable- and chronic-disease control and medical rehabilitation services. They are also active in educating the public and provide environmental and mental health services.

THE TWENTIETH CENTURY: "WONDER" DRUGS AND NEW EPIDEMICS; TECHNOLOGY AND TECHNIQUES

In the twentieth century, studies continued with infectious diseases, and effective serums were developed for diphtheria, meningococcus meningitis, and pneumococcal pneumonia. But the most dramatic discoveries in the control and treatment of infectious diseases came with the discovery of the sulfa drugs, penicillin, and other antibiotics.

Paul Ehrlich (Figure 1-16) was the first to use a specific chemical agent against a specific organism. In 1907 he used a compound called arsphenamine, or "606," to cure syphilis. A scientist in France learned how to produce sulfanilamide in 1936, and soon after, sulfathiazole was produced and is still one of the best cures for meningococcus meningitis. But the most dramatic breakthrough in chemotherapy came with the discovery of penicillin by Alexander Fleming in 1928. Although it was to be over 10 years before the drug was ready for public use, it soon became the treatment of choice to cure many bacterial infections.

ANTIBIOTIC BREAKTHROUGHS

Streptomycin, the first antibiotic that helped in the treatment and cure of tuberculosis was isolated in 1943 and soon joined by two other drugs, paraaminosalicylic acid and isoniazid. The discovery of these three drugs led to cooperative efforts of many government agencies and other groups to determine the safety and effectiveness of administering them at the same time. Instead of individuals working alone as they

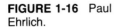

FIGURE 1-16 Paul Ehrlich.

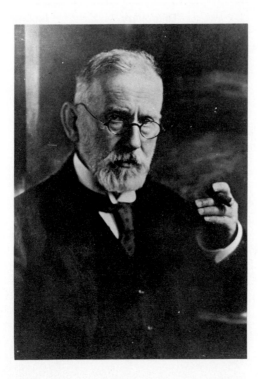

had in the nineteenth century, joint efforts now became common in the fight against disease.

VITAMIN-DEFICIENCY DISEASES

Another great advance in treating disease occurred in the early years of the twentieth century with the discovery of the cause for a number of disorders, now known as vitamin-deficiency diseases, which had afflicted humans for centuries. For years physicians had treated pellagra, rickets, and beriberi with lime juice because it seemed to help. After the germ theory of disease was accepted in the nineteenth century, most scientists believed that these diseases were due to bacteria and toxins. But evidence was gradually accumulating that some "accessory substance" to the known nutrients was necessary for health and growth.

In 1912, the experiments of an English biologist left no doubt that there were other elements vital to good nutrition, and Casimir Funk, a Polish biochemist, suggested the name "vitamine." Later, when it was realized that these substances were not amines, the name was changed to vitamin. Vitamin A was the first to actually be identified (1915), followed by vitamin D (1918), and thiamine (vitamin B_1) in 1921. By 1946 all but one of the vitamins that are known today had been identified and synthesized. Cobalamin (B_{12}) was not discovered until 1948 and was synthesized in 1973 (Table 1-1).

The availability of vitamins led to spectacular cures for the deficiency diseases and commercial mass production of vitamins as the public began using them

TABLE 1-1 Discovery, isolation, and synthesis of vitamins

	Discovery	Isolation	Synthesis
Fat-Soluble Vitamins			
Vitamin A	1915	1937	1946
Vitamin D	1918	1930	1936
Vitamin E	1922	1936	1937
Vitamin K	1934	1939	1939
Water-Soluble Vitamins			
Thiamine (B_1)	1921	1926	1936
Inositol	1928	1928	
Choline	1930	1962	
Ascorbic acid (C)	1932	1932	1933
Riboflavin (B_2)	1932	1933	1935
Pantothenic acid	1933	1938	1940
Biotin		1935	1942
Pyridoxine (B_6)	1934	1938	1939
Niacin (B_3)	1936	1936	
Folacin	1945	1945	1945
Cobalamin (B_{12})	1948	1948	1973

prophylactically, often in much larger quantities than necessary and in some cases (particularly vitamin A) with dangerous side effects.

ANTIVIRAL VACCINES

Although researchers had known since the nineteenth century that there existed disease-causing agents so small that they passed through filters capable of catching bacteria, it was not until the invention of the electron microscope in 1930 that viruses could be seen and studied. In 1955, Jonas Salk (Figure 1-17) introduced a killed-virus vaccine for poliomyelitis, one of the most feared diseases of the time because of its potential for permanent crippling and disability, if not death. Soon after, in 1956, the field test was made for a live-virus vaccine developed by Albert B. Sabin, which was so successful that it is now used most of the time for protection from polio. By 1969, vaccines were available for measles, mumps, and rubella.

LEGIONNAIRES' DISEASE AND AIDS

All through the history of disease, new infections have suddenly appeared. Two that have become a problem in the latter part of the twentieth century are Legionnaires' disease and acquired immune deficiency syndrome (AIDS). Legionnaires' disease was first documented in a 1957 outbreak. The disease had probably been around for some time but not reported since its symptoms could be so mild. However, at an American Legion convention in Philadelphia in 1976, it was the cause of 29 deaths and 182 hospitalizations. Once the disease agent was identified as a bacterium, antibiotics were found to treat it.

It was another story when the first cases of AIDS were reported in 1981. Since then, this devastating infection has been found to be caused by a virus that attacks the core of the body's defense system. More than 10 years after the appearance of

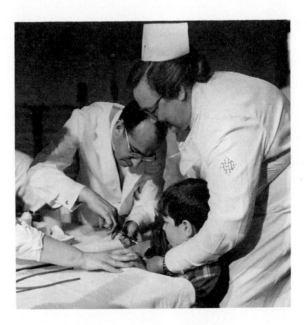

FIGURE 1-17 Jonas E. Salk inoculating a child against poliomyelitis.

AIDS there is no known cure for the immune deficiency it causes, although drugs are now in use that can slow the progress of the disease.

A NEW FOCUS: NONINFECTIOUS DISEASES

As the hope for prevention and control of infectious diseases was growing in the twentieth century, a new trend in disease became apparent. Death and suffering from infectious disease were on a downward trend in the developed countries, but the second decade saw a rise in noninfectious disease, until by 1930, deaths from noninfectious disease had surpassed those from infectious disease in the United States and other developed countries, as shown in Figure 1-18.

A number of factors led to this change and, ironically, the ability to prevent and control many communicable diseases was one of them. In countries where people were escaping death from infectious disease, they were living longer and becoming more susceptible to diseases that took a longer life span to emerge. In addition, since most noninfectious diseases do not attack with the dramatic symptoms of infectious diseases, not as much attention was given to their prevention and control until the soaring death rates from heart disease and cancer were evident.

In the United States and other developed nations, changing lifestyles and environmental influences were also involved as the accumulation of great wealth, or at least enough for a comfortable living, led to excesses in eating and drinking, a decrease in exercise, and increased physical and mental/emotional stressors, all now known as factors in the development of noninfectious disease. Table 1-2 indicates the percentage contribution of lifestyle and three other factors to the 10 leading causes of death. With a pressing need to know more about the human body and

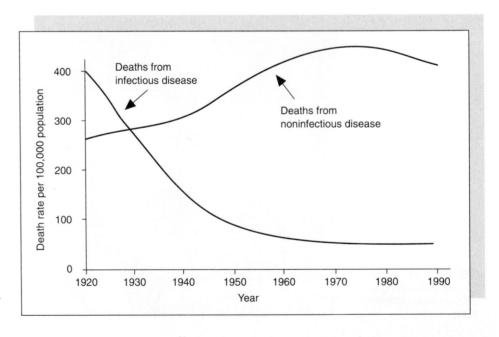

FIGURE 1-18 Trends in infectious and noninfectious disease.

which processes led to noninfectious diseases, the fight against disease became more and more research centered.

DIAGNOSTIC ADVANCES

Frederick Banting and Charles Best succeeded in producing insulin in 1922, and from their discovery came the ability to control diabetes. Cardiac catheterization, open-heart surgery, and replacement of clogged blood vessels were among the first techniques to aid in diagnosis and repair of damaged hearts. New radiologic diagnostic modalities such as computed axial tomography (CAT) scanning, magnetic resonance (MR) imaging, and positive emission tomography (PET) scanning have increased diagnostic potential.

TRANSPLANTS AND CANCER

The ability to transplant hearts, kidneys, and other organs has alleviated suffering and extended life for some, but the progress in fighting the second leading cause of death, cancer, has been disappointing, despite much time, effort, and money spent in seeking answers.

Research is continuing to determine the origin, development, and metabolism of cancer cells, and new information is leading to new possibilities for prevention and treatment of this often fatal disease. The cure rate for cancer has risen from one-third to one-half in the past 10 years, but for lung cancer and some others, chances of survival are much less. The Papanicolaou test (Pap smear) for cervical

TABLE 1-2 The importance of lifestyle in good health: estimated contribution of four factors to ten leading causes of death (expressed in percent)

Causes of Death	Factors			
	Lifestyle	Environment	Genetics	Health Care Services
Heart disease	54	9	25	12
Cancer	37	24	29	10
Stroke	50	22	21	7
Motor vehicle accidents	69	18	1	12
Other accidents	51	31	4	14
Influenza/pneumonia	23	20	39	18
Diabetes	34	0	60	6
Cirrhosis	70	9	18	3
Suicide	60	35	2	3
Homicide	63	35	2	0
All ten causes together	51	19	20	10

Source: U.S. Centers for Disease Control.

cancer has led to earlier diagnosis and improved survival rates. Chances of surviving breast and colorectal cancer have also improved with earlier detection by the use of mammography and proctoscopy.

For cancer, as for other chronic diseases, the greatest hope seems to lie in changing lifestyles. Elimination of smoking and excesses in drinking and eating, diets that meet the nutritional requirements of the body, exercise on a regular basis, and stress management are all known to be important in sustaining the resistance to disease with which everyone is born.

DISEASE PREVENTION AND HEALTH PROMOTION

By the mid-1970s, a new interest not only in disease prevention but in health promotion was stirring among the people of the United States and other developed nations. In the United States, reports from task forces, committees, and, finally, the Surgeon General were indicative of the new focus. The Surgeon General's report on health promotion and disease prevention was in two volumes, *Healthy People* (1979) and *Promoting Health, Preventing Disease: Objectives for the Nation* (1980). These objectives were adopted as policy for the nation in 1981. Objectives for 1990 were also developed, and we now have objectives for the year 2000. "Health for All by the Year 2000" was called for by the World Health Organization (WHO) in 1977. Two worldwide targets were identified: (1) the provision of a safe drinking water supply for everyone and (2) the immunization of all children in the world against major childhood infectious diseases.

Not all of the objectives for 1990 were met, nor is it probable that all of the 298 objectives for 2000 will be met. Yet progress has been made, and it is hoped that all nations and peoples will at least be able to have safe drinking water and immunizations for their children by 2000.

Scientists and physicians have achieved much in helping us survive the attacks of invading microorganisms by repairing the damage done by disease processes and easing pain and suffering. However, many diseases have regressed and even disappeared without medical intervention. McKeown has stated, "We can attribute the modern improvement in health to food, hygiene and medical intervention in that order of time and importance—but we must recognize that it is to a modification of behavior that we owe the permanence of this improvement."*

If we are to succeed in preventing and controlling disease in the twenty-first century, all men, women, and children will have to accept the responsibility for their own health and pursue lifestyles that will enable them to present the strongest possible resistance to disease. Scientists and physicians can show us the way, but only individuals can choose which behaviors they will follow.

SUMMARY

From ancient times there has been evidence of devastation of human life by disease. Although a few treatments used by early physicians are still used, no real progress was made against infectious disease until the late seventeenth century. Then the

---

*Lee, Philip R. and Carroll L. Estes. *The Nation's Health.* Boston: Jones and Bartlett Publishers, 1990. p. 11.

newly discovered microscope opened up new worlds of swarming microorganisms to scientists and physicians, and in the late eighteenth century Jenner discovered the vaccination for smallpox. These two milestone discoveries opened the way for an avalanche of identification of diseases and disease agents in the nineteenth century. With the discovery of penicillin and other "wonder drugs" in the twentieth century, more progress was made in the control of infectious disease.

The control of noninfectious disease was another story. Although advances were made in understanding the human body, an intensive effort to deal with cardiovascular disease, cancer, diabetes, and other life-threatening noninfectious diseases did not begin in earnest until the late nineteenth and early twentieth century, when the leading cause of fatal disease changed from infectious agents to noninfectious origins. The recognition of the effect of lifestyle upon the development of noninfectious diseases brought about a new focus for the twentieth century and the years beyond. At the same time, however, the appearance of the new, devastatingly destructive, and apparently always fatal infectious disease AIDS reminded all those involved in the struggle that success in preventing and controlling disease is an elusive goal, not soon to be achieved.

QUESTIONS FOR REVIEW

1. Starting with the Egyptians, what have been the highlights in disease prevention and control?
2. What different theories have been held concerning the cause of disease from early times to the present?
3. What prescriptions used by Chinese doctors in early times are still used?
4. What kind of measures were taken to guard the health of the community in early times?
5. Why were Galen's writings on anatomy flawed, and why was he believed?
6. How were the ideas about disease affected in the Middle Ages?
7. How are the terms *pandemic* and *hajj* connected in discussion about disease?
8. Where and when in history were the Black Death and pulmonary anthrax connected?
9. What developments in the seventeenth century led to an acceleration in the knowledge of disease in the nineteenth century?
10. How did Vesalius, da Vinci, and Fracastoro contribute to advances in medicine during the Renaissance?
11. What individuals are thought to be responsible for the arrival of syphilis in Europe?
12. What were some of Thomas Sydenham's accomplishments?
13. What eighteenth-century event led to the eradication of smallpox in the twentieth century?
14. What contributions were made by Bernard, Pasteur, and Lister in the nineteenth century?
15. What report was Edwin Chadwick responsible for?
16. Who was Lemuel Shattuck, and how was he important in the prevention and control of disease?
17. What new diagnostic tools were used in the nineteenth century?
18. What are Koch's postulates?

19. What important advances in the knowledge of disease were made in the nineteenth century?
20. When did chemotherapy begin, and what was one of the most dramatic discoveries in the field?
21. When were vitamins discovered? Why was this important?
22. What twentieth-century invention led to the vaccines for polio?
23. What two newly discovered infectious diseases have caused death in the twentieth century?
24. What change in focus concerning disease occurred in the 1970s? Why?
25. What new technologies and techniques are used to diagnose, treat, and control disease today?

FURTHER READING

Ackerknecht, Erwin. *A Short History of Medicine*. rev. ed. Baltimore: Johns Hopkins University Press, 1982.

Castiglioni, Arturo. *A History of Medicine*. 2nd ed. (1958 reprint) Dunmore, Pa.: J. Aronson, 1973.

Chadwick, H.D. "The Diseases of the Inhabitants of the Commonwealth." *New England Journal of Medicine,* June 10, '37, 216:8.

Garrison, Harry. *History of Medicine*. Philadelphia: Saunders, 1914.

Hanlon, John J. and George E. Pickett. *Public Health: Administration and Practice*. St. Louis: Mosby, 1990.

Hudson, Robert P. *Disease and Its Control: The Shaping of Modern Thought*. Westport, Conn.: Greenwood Press, 1983.

McGrew, Roderick. *Encyclopedia of Medical History*. New York: McGraw-Hill, 1984.

McNeill, William H. *Plagues and Peoples*. New York: Doubleday, 1976.

Ohlendorf-Moffat, Pat. "Surgery before Birth." *Discovery*. Feb. '91, 59–65.

Rhodes, P. *An Outline History of Medicine*. Stoneham, Mass.: Butterworth, 1985.

Shattuck, Lemuel et al. *Report of the Sanitary Commission of Massachusetts,* 1850, Cambridge, Mass: Harvard University Press (Originally published by Dutton & Wentworth in 1850).

Singer, Charles and E.A. Underwood. *A Short History of Medicine*. 2nd ed., New York: Oxford, 1962.

Smith, C.E. "The Broad Street Pump Revisited." *International Journal of Epidemiology,* 11:99, 1982.

Snow, J. "On the Mode of Communication of Cholera." In *Snow on Cholera*. New York: The Commonwealth Fund, 1936.

Top, F.H. *The History of American Epidemiology,* St. Louis: Mosby, 1952.

Principles of Disease Occurrence

FOUR THEORIES OF DISEASE CAUSATION

In Chapter 1, various ideas about the cause of disease were mentioned. The oldest theory of causation, dating from prehistoric times, holds that evil spirits or supernatural beings are responsible for disease. Hippocrates introduced the idea of a natural rather than supernatural explanation for disease occurrence in the fourth century BC, but it took hundreds of years for people to recognize that some diseases were contagious and could be transmitted from person to person as well as in other ways, and it took even more time to identify the disease agents that were being transmitted.

The isolation of lepers (based on biblical teachings) led to a decrease in leprosy, and the practice of quarantine arose, based on the idea that isolation might be effective against other diseases also. This second theory of causation, the theory of contagion, soon gained acceptance.

The development of the third theory of disease causation, the germ theory (explained in Chapter 1) in the 1860s and 1870s, marked the beginning of the conquest of infectious diseases. The germ theory of disease causation was accepted for many years and brought great progress in the understanding of disease, but as infectious disease began to decline and noninfectious diseases began to increase, it became evident that the idea of one cause for one disease did not answer such questions as: Why is it that some people who are exposed to a disease do not get sick? and, How can we carry disease agents on our skin and in our body without getting sick? It was also recognized that more than one factor was responsible for the development of each noninfectious disease. Thus, to explain disease occurrence in both infectious and noninfectious diseases, epidemiologists (those who study the occurrence of disease in populations), developed the modern theory of multiple causation. In this theory, the definition of disease agent is expanded to denote any factor that needs to be present (or absent) for disease to occur.

TERMINOLOGY TO DESCRIBE DISEASE OCCURRENCE

It is not possible in a text on infectious and noninfectious disease to include all epidemiologic and public health concepts. However, for better understanding of the material in this text, a few of the terms that are commonly used to describe disease occurrence will be identified.

RATES OF DISEASE OCCURRENCE

Two terms that have a special meaning for epidemiologists and others dealing with disease are *prevalence rate* and *incidence rate.*

Prevalence rate indicates the number of cases of a particular disease in a community at a specified time. It is determined by dividing the number of existing cases by the total population under study. The resulting figure is then multiplied by a power of 10. For prevalence and incidence rates, this number is usually 1000. The formula for prevalence rates follows.

$$\text{Prevalence} = \frac{\text{Number of cases of disease present in the population at a specified time}}{\text{Number of persons in the population at that specified time}} \times 1000$$

EXAMPLE: In a college with 2569 students, 18 missed classes on October 1 because of influenza. These students did not all become ill at the same time, but all were ill on the day in question. The prevalence rate on October 1 was

$$\frac{18 \text{ (existing cases)}}{2569 \text{ (total school population)}} = .0070 \times 1000 = 7.0$$

The prevalence rate for influenza at this college on October 1 was 7.0 (per thousand students).

Incidence rate is the number of *new* cases occurring during a specific time. It is determined by dividing the number of new cases of a disease at a specific time by the population at risk. The formula for incidence rate is

$$\frac{\text{Number of new cases during a specified time}}{\text{Population at risk for the disease}} \times 1000$$

EXAMPLE: If we return to the same college and find that 8 of the flu cases actually began on October 1, then the incidence for October 1 would be

$$\frac{8 \text{ (new cases)}}{2569 \text{ (population at risk)}} = .003 \times 1000 = 3.0$$

The incidence rate for influenza at this college on October 1 was 3.0 (per thousand students).

Prevalence rate and incidence rate are another way to talk about how widespread an illness is. The formulas are used in order to get away from having to deal with decimals (which we would have if simple percentages were used) when writing and talking about disease trends.

LEVELS OF PREVENTION

The prevention of disease can be described in three levels. *Primary prevention* refers to measures taken before the disease occurs to reduce susceptibility. Vaccinations are an example of primary prevention. *Secondary prevention* refers to measures taken to diagnose a disease that is already present. The Pap smear for cervical cancer is an example of secondary prevention. *Tertiary prevention* involves all the measures taken to return the individual to a "normal" state of health or to keep the person alive. Physical therapy for polio victims is a type of tertiary prevention. This text will be concerned mostly with primary and secondary prevention.

EPIDEMIOLOGIC THEORY OF DISEASE OCCURRENCE

Classic epidemiologic theory states that whether or not anyone gets a disease depends on the relationship among three factors: the *disease agent,* the *host,* and the *environment.* This relationship is shown in Figure 2-1. Although the model was developed for infectious disease, it fits noninfectious disease as well when the broader definition is used.

Although a disease agent is necessary for disease to occur, a disease agent can also be present without the occurrence of disease. Many pathogenic organisms are present on and in our bodies all the time, but if the three elements (of the epidemiologic model) are in equilibrium, that is, if the disease agent is not too virulent (powerful), if the resistance of the host is strong, and if the environment is favorable to the host, then the disease agent will not be able to cause an infection (disease), and the host will remain well. But if the disease agent becomes more virulent and/or the resistance of the host is lowered and/or the environment is unfavorable, then the host may become sick.

A vivid example of this process is found in the infection of many people with the human immunodeficiency virus (HIV), which is responsible for AIDS. A person can be infected with HIV for months or years before any symptoms of AIDS occur.

DISEASE AGENTS FOR INFECTIOUS DISEASES

The disease agents for infectious diseases are pathogenic organisms and range in size from the submicroscopic virus, composed simply of nucleic acid, to the metazoa, which are complex and sometimes grow very large, for example, intestinal worms. Pathogenic organisms can be divided into the following broad categories (see inside back cover).

VIRUSES

The smallest of the disease-causing organisms are viruses. These minute particles could not be detected until the early 1930s, when the electron microscope was first used. Viruses are composed of nucleic acids and protein. They are made up of deoxyribonucleic acid (DNA) or ribonucleic acid (RNA) but not both. They are not technically alive by themselves but are able to penetrate cells and use the cell's nucleic acid to produce more viruses. This process may take place without any change in cell structure or function. The virus may just borrow part of the cell's machinery to synthesize new viruses without disturbing the cell.

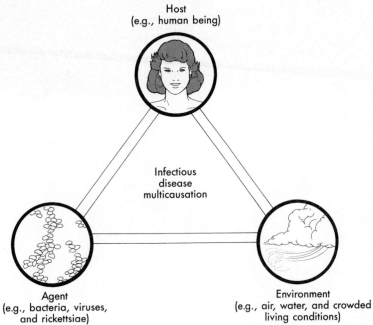

Host
(e.g., human being)

Infectious
disease
multicausation

FIGURE 2-1 Epidemi-
ologic model of disease.

Agent
(e.g., bacteria, viruses,
and rickettsiae)

Environment
(e.g., air, water, and crowded
living conditions)

DID YOU KNOW?

Some Viruses and the Diseases They Cause

Viruses contain either DNA or RNA, never both. Thus they have to find a way to replicate, and this is done by using the complete cells of hosts. Some of the viruses that are important to humans are shown below; some of the diseases they cause will be discussed later in the text.

DNA Viruses

Papillomavirus
Hepatitis B virus
Adenovirus

Herpes virus:
  I and II
  Epstein-Barr
  Varicella-zoster
Poxvirus

RNA Viruses

Paramixovirus
Orthomixovirus
Coronavirus
Rhabdovirus
Bunyavirus
Retrovirus
Rhinovirus
Togavirus
Flavivirus
Enterovirus

Human Disease Examples

Warts
Hepatitis B
Respiratory disease and diarrhea
(mostly in children)

Oral and genital herpes
Mononucleosis
Measles and shingles
Smallpox (eradicated)

Measles, mumps
Influenza
Upper respiratory infection
Rabies
California encephalitis
Acquired immunodeficiency syndrome
Colds, poliomyelitis
Rubella, Western and Eastern encephalitis
Yellow fever, St. Louis encephalitis
Hepatitis A

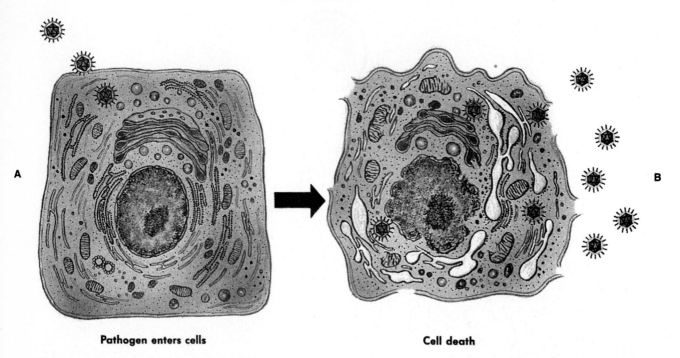

Pathogen enters cells   **Cell death**

FIGURE 2-2   A, A virus is invading a body cell. It may coexist with the cell for an indefinite time until it is "triggered" by some outside factor, takes over the cell's machinery and reproduces. **B,** At some point, the cell becomes engorged and the newly made viruses break out, causing cell death.

This peaceful coexistence may continue indefinitely. Thus the host is *infected* with the virus but does not have a *disease*. At some later time, an outside factor such as inactivity, poor nutrition, stress, hormonal imbalance, or bacterial infection may activate the virus so that it takes over all of the cell's machinery and rapidly produces more viruses. These viruses may burst out of the cell, destroying it, or the cell may simply degenerate until it can no longer function and the viruses are released as the cell dies. Then viral *disease* is present. *Viral infection* is much more common than *viral disease* (Figure 2-2).

BACTERIA

Bacteria are single-celled, plantlike organisms that are abundant in our environment—internal as well as external. Most bacteria are harmless and some beneficial, but we are concerned with those that are capable of causing disease. Although disease-causing bacteria are in the minority, there are still many different kinds that secrete toxins or enzymes that destroy cells or interfere with their function, thus causing disease in the human body.

There are three common groups of bacteria: rod-shaped or *bacilli,* round or *cocci,* and spiral or *spirilla.* For example, tuberculosis is caused by a bacillus, pneumonia by a coccus, and syphilis by a spirillum (Figure 2-3). Many bacteria "live" on the skin and in the intestinal tract of humans (see inside cover). They do so benignly unless something reduces the immune response of the host or their ecosystem is disrupted.

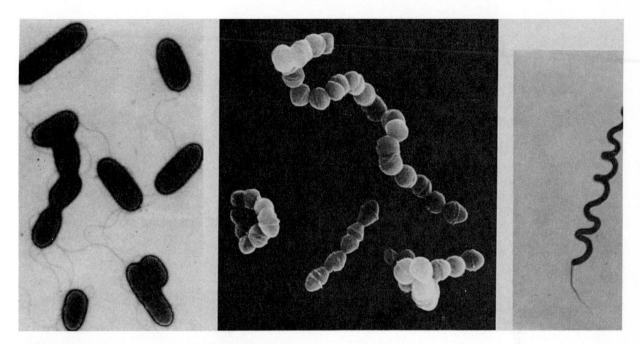

FIGURE 2-3   Three shapes of bacteria.

RICKETTSIAE

Rickettsiae are now considered to be small bacteria, although, like viruses, they are intracellular parasites. Rickettsiae are more like bacteria than like viruses, but with one exception: they are always transported by insects and other **arthropod vectors.** In the United States, Rocky Mountain spotted fever is the most common rickettsial disease.

FUNGI

Mushrooms, antibiotics, and ringworm of the scalp, groin, and feet all owe their existence to single-celled or multicelled plantlike organisms referred to as fungi (Figure 2-4). These organisms release enzymes that digest cells. Because of their constant presence in the air, they may find a favorable climate for reproduction on food or anywhere that there is high humidity, warmth, and oxygen supply (such as between human toes not adequately dried after a shower). The use of antibiotics, which destroy some of the friendly bacteria that normally restrain fungal growth, has caused an increase in fungal infections.

PROTOZOA

These microscopic single-celled parasitic animals are responsible for some of the most important diseases of humanity. They are common in temperate and

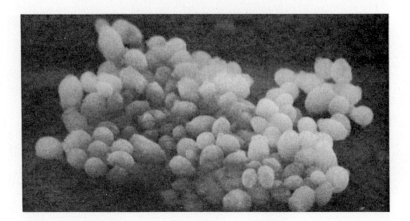

FIGURE 2-4 Fungi.

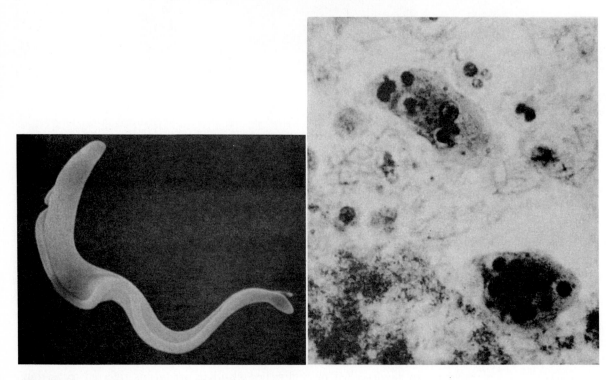

FIGURE 2-5 Protozoa.

tropical climates. Like bacteria, protozoa release toxins and enzymes that destroy cells or interfere with their functions. Examples of protozoa are shown in Figure 2-5. Malaria, amebic dysentery, and African sleeping sickness are all caused by protozoa.

METAZOA

Metazoa are multicellular parasitic animals (worms) that can be divided into three categories: roundworms, tapeworms, and flukes (Figure 2-6). They can infest any

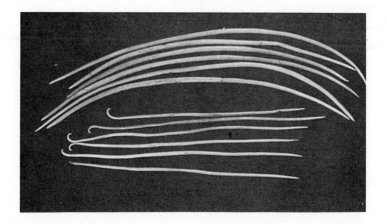

FIGURE 2-6 Worms.

compartment in the body and can travel across various tissue barriers from organ to bloodstream and to another organ. They will lodge in various parts of the body and may block the digestive tract, blood, and lymph vessels as they compete for the body's food. Three diseases caused by metazoa are pinworm, trichinosis, and tapeworm.

DISEASE AGENTS FOR NONINFECTIOUS DISEASE

The disease agents for noninfectious disease can be placed in the following categories.

NUTRIENTS—DEFICIENCY AND EXCESS

When we think of diseases related to nutrition, we usually think of deficiency diseases. However, some of the factors that have been identified as risks for non-infectious disease are due to an excess of nutrients. Table 2-1 on the following pages summarizes the importance and the results of deficiency and excess for the major nutrients. For instance, scurvy is a vitamin-deficiency disease due to insufficient vitamin C and a deficiency of protein and has been identified as the cause of kwash-iorkor, a disease prevalent in children in third world nations. On the other hand, too much sodium may be an agent of high blood pressure for some, whereas high fat intake has been implicated in heart disease and some cancer. Malnutrition also lowers resistance to infectious disease. Examination of Table 2-1 will help you to understand the significance of ingesting either too much or too little of any one nutrient.

OTHER CHEMICAL SUBSTANCES

The nutrients are all made of chemicals, but they are chemicals that the body needs for survival. Alcohol, the chemicals in cigarette smoke, and illicit drugs are not necessary for survival. They alter body processes in unnatural ways and in doing so produce conditions that may lead to disease and disorders. Alcoholism not only

TABLE 2-1 Diseases and symptoms of nutrient deficiency or excess

| Nutrient | Importance | Disease and/or Symptoms Caused by | |
		Deficiency	Excess
Carbohydrates			
Sugar and starch	Quick energy source.	None.	Obesity, dental caries.
Fiber	Protects against appendicitis, hemorrhoids, diverticulosis, colon cancer. Control of blood lipids, diabetes II, weight.	May be a factor in the development of appendicitis, hemorrhoids, diverticulosis, colon cancer.	Limits absorption of minerals and may limit absorption of vitamins.
Fat	Energy supply; protection of body organs; helps maintain structure and health of cells.	Eczema Skin disorders Retarded growth	Contributes to obesity, diabetes, cancer, hypertension, atherosclerosis.
Protein	Growth and development; formation of hormones; enzymes; antibodies; maintains acid-alkali balance; source of heat and energy.	Kwashiorkor Marasmas Fatigue; loss of appetite; diarrhea; vomiting; stunted growth; edema.	Difficulty in maintaining ideal weight; possible hypertrophy of liver and kidneys; contributes to obesity.
Water-Soluble Vitamins			
Thiamine (B$_1$)	Aids in energy metabolism; supports normal appetite and nervous system function.	Beriberi Symptoms include edema; abnormal heart rhythms; painful calf muscles; mental confusion.	Rapid pulse; weakness; headaches; insomnia; irritability.
Riboflavin (B$_2$)	Energy metabolism; supports normal vision and normal skin.	Ariboflavinosis symptoms: cracks at corners of mouth; magenta tongue.	Interferes with anticancer medication.
Niacin (B$_3$)	Energy metabolism; supports health of skin, nervous system, and digestive system.	Pellagra Symptoms include diarrhea, irritability, loss of appetite, weakness, mental confusion progressing to psychosis; dermatitis	Symptoms include diarrhea, nausea, vomiting; skin flush and rash; abnormal liver function; low blood pressure.
B$_6$	Aid in amino acid and fatty acid metabolism; helps convert tryptophan to niacin; helps to make red blood cells.	Symptoms include anemia, cracked corners of mouth, irritability, muscle twitching, dermatitis, kidney stones.	Symptoms include bloating, headaches, fatigue, depression; damage to nerves leading to loss of reflexes and sensation; difficulty walking.

TABLE 2-1 Diseases and symptoms of nutrient deficiency or excess—cont'd

Nutrient	Importance	Disease and/or Symptoms Caused by	
		Deficiency	**Excess**
Water-Soluble Vitamins—cont'd			
Folic acid	Used in new cell synthesis.	Symptoms include anemia, heartburn, diarrhea, constipation, suppression of immune system, frequent infections, mental confusion, faint, fatigue, smooth, red tongue.	Symptoms include diarrhea, insomnia, irritability, masking of vitamin B_6 deficiency symptoms.
B_{12}	Used in new cell synthesis; helps maintain nerve cells.	Pernicious anemia Symptoms include smooth tongue, fatigue, degeneration of peripheral nerves, progressing to paralysis; hypersensitivity of the skin.	None known.
Biotin	Energy metabolism, fat synthesis, amino acid metabolism, and glycogen synthesis.	Abnormal heart action, loss of appetite, nausea, depression, muscle pain, weakness, fatigue; drying, scaly dermatitis.	None known.
Pantothenic acid	Energy metabolism	Vomiting, intestinal distress, insomnia, fatigue.	Occasional diarrhea, possible water retention.
C	Collagen synthesis, antioxidant, thyroxin synthesis, amino acid metabolism; strengthens resistance to infection; helps in absorption of iron.	Scurvy Symptoms include anemia, atherosclerotic plaques, pinpoint hemorrhages, depression, frequent infections, bleeding gums, loosened teeth, muscle and joint pain, failure of wounds to heal.	Symptoms include nausea, abdominal cramps, diarrhea, headache, insomnia, fatigue, hot flashes, rashes, kidney stones.
Fat-Soluble Vitamins			
A	Vision; epithelial cells, mucous membranes, skin; bone and tooth growth; reproduction; hormone synthesis and regulation; cancer protection.	Hypovitaminosis A Deficiency of vitamin A causes disorders in almost every organ system in the body. A few of them are night blindness; rough, dry scaly skin; increased susceptibility to infections; frequent fatigue; loss of smell and appetite; anemia; vomiting; abdominal pain; jaundice; and enlargement of liver and spleen.	Hypervitaminosis A An excess of vitamin A produces symptoms in all the body systems that are affected by a deficiency. If excessive amounts continue to be ingested, death can occur.
D	Improves absorption and utilization of calcium and phosphorus required for bone formation.	Rickets Osteomalacia Symptoms include misshapen bones and teeth, retarded growth.	Hypervitaminosis D Symptoms include loss of appetite, headache, weakness, fatigue, irritability, kidney stones, irreversible renal damage. Death can occur.

Continued.

TABLE 2-1 Diseases and symptoms of nutrient deficiency or excess—cont'd

Nutrient	Importance	Disease and/or Symptoms Caused by	
		Deficiency	**Excess**
Fat-Soluble Vitamins—cont'd			
E	Antioxidant, stabilization of cell membranes, regulation of oxidation reactions.	Anemia, weakness, difficulty in walking, severe muscular wasting, fibrocystic breast disease.	Headache, dizziness, fatigue, visual problems, digestive discomfort.
K	Synthesis of blood-clotting proteins and a blood protein that regulates blood calcium.	Hemorrhaging.	Possible jaundice.
Major Minerals			
Sodium	Maintains normal extracellular fluid balance and acid-base balance; aids in nerve impulse transmission.	Muscle cramps, mental apathy, loss of appetite.	Hypertension.
Chloride	Maintains fluid and acid-base balance; aids in digestion.	Muscle cramps, mental apathy, loss of appetite, lack of growth in children.	Vomiting.
Potassium	Assists in many reactions, including the making of protein; cell integrity; transmission of nerve impulses; contraction of muscles, including heart.	Muscular weakness, paralysis, confusion.	Vomiting, muscular weakness.
Calcium	Principal mineral of bones and teeth; normal muscle contraction and relaxation, including heart muscle; nerve function; blood clotting; blood pressure; immune defenses.	Osteoporosis; stunted growth in children.	None (Excess calcium is excreted.)
Phosphorus	Part of bones, teeth, and cells; necessary in genetic material, energy transfer, and maintenance of acid-base balance.	Unknown.	May draw calcium out of body.
Magnesium	Necessary for bones, building of protein, enzyme action, muscular contraction, transmission of nerve impulses, and teeth.	Symptoms include depressed hormone secretion from pancreas; weakness, confusion.	Unknown.
Sulfur	Necessary for protein structure, part of biotin, thiamine, and insulin; aids in body's detoxification process.	Unknown.	Depressed growth.

predisposes the body to noninfectious diseases such as cirrhosis of the liver but also lowers resistance to infectious disease. Other *exogenous* chemicals can also produce disease. And there are *endogenous* chemicals, chemicals within our own bodies, that cause noninfectious disease.

The agents for alcoholism, tobacco addiction, or addiction to marijuana, cocaine, and other illicit drugs are easily identified. It is not always easy to track down the agent for illness that is produced by something in the environment. A number of substances are known to be disease agents. A few of the most common are lead, particularly in old paint, radon gas in our homes, asbestos in schools and other buildings, and sulfur dioxide in the air. We are just beginning to recognize how dangerous many of the chemicals in our environment are and to take measures to eliminate the danger.

Just as with nutritional deficiencies or excesses, a deficiency or excess of a normal body product can lead to disease. Everyone is familiar with the difference that steroids can make in the structure of the human body from the use of them by athletes. When the body secretes too much growth hormone, disorders such as *giantism* in children and *acromegaly* (parts of the body resume growth and become greatly enlarged) in adults appear. Too little of the same hormone in childhood leads to *dwarfism* (Figure 2-7).

A form of arthritis, *gout,* is caused by excess secretion of uric acid. In fact the most prevalent theory concerning rheumatoid arthritis is an unnecessary secretion

FIGURE 2-7 This photograph shows the effects of an excess of growth hormone (left) and a deficiency in growth hormone (right) compared with individuals of average stature.

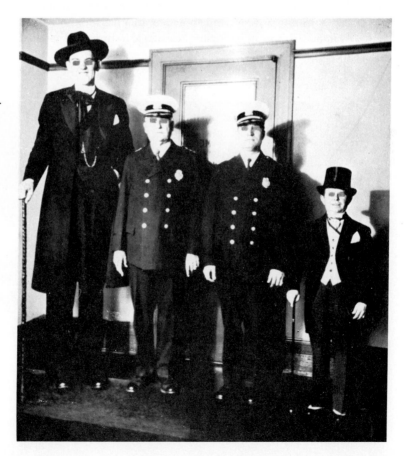

(excess) of body chemicals that attack the joint. Many other chronic diseases and disorders can be traced to endogenous factors such as these.

HEREDITY

As has been stated before, scientific research is identifying more and more disease states that are "in the genes." Genetic research is proceeding at an accelerated pace, with new findings published almost weekly. A gene or combination of genes is known to be responsible for some diseases such as cystic fibrosis or sickle cell anemia, whereas the absence or addition of a chromosome is the agent for others, such as Down syndrome. Heredity also affects the host's resistance to disease and will be discussed later in the chapter.

PSYCHOSOMATIC FACTORS

To many people, even some doctors, the term *psychosomatic* means an imaginary illness. This is a false impression, since by definition, *psychosomatic* means a disease or disorder influenced or caused by a person's mind. People who have imaginary illnesses are correctly referred to as *hypochondriacs*. Individuals who have a psychosomatic illness have an actual physiological disease or disorder that can be diagnosed by tests, and their mind has played a critical role in the occurrence of the disease.

Studies have demonstrated the fact that mental and emotional *stress* can depress the immune system. And some research has indicated that learning to manage stress can be effective in increasing resistance to disease. Evidence continues to accumulate

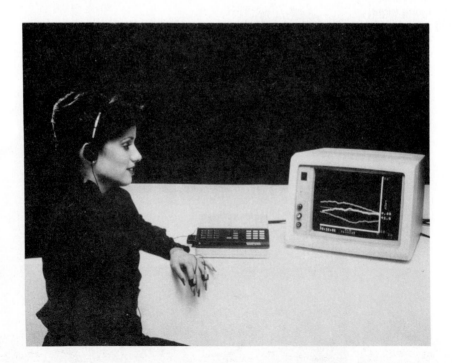

FIGURE 2-8
Biofeedback.

from research and clinical observations of the ability of the mind not only to cause disease but even to assist in, or actually bring about, a cure.

It has long been known that some individuals can learn to control their blood pressure and heartbeat through a technique called *biofeedback,* which trains them to control *autonomic* processes (Figure 2-8). There are even indications that by certain thought processes we can enhance our immune response. Evidence of success in this area has increased to the degree that a new field of specialization, ***psychoneuroimmunology,*** has emerged. All doctors have witnessed the difference that attitude and outlook can have on a patient's response to treatment. And most would agree that learning to manage stress, physical as well as mental, and a positive attitude, can increase the chances of prevention of, and recovery from, many diseases.

PHYSICAL FORCES

Some of the most common physical forces that act as agents of disease or disorder are mechanical forces, high or low temperatures, and radiation. The best example of a disease caused by mechanical force is *osteomyelitis,* an acute inflammation of bone and bone marrow resulting from pathogenic organisms but occurring at the site of traumatic injury. Most of us have experienced the effects of high temperature by burning ourselves. Burns may be minor or life threatening, depending on their degree of severity. Low temperatures can lead to frostbite and possible loss of fingers or toes. *Hypothermia* (significant loss of body heat) has been the cause of death for older individuals who cannot afford to heat their homes in winter or for those who have no homes.

A physical force that has been the cause of great concern in the years since the development of atomic power is *radiation.* We know that the ultraviolet rays of the sun can be carcinogenic as can X rays used in diagnosis of illness. The ability to control radiation has led to the ability to diagnose and, in the case of cancer, treat disease, while at the same time causing disease. Individuals who receive therapeutic doses of radiation may develop radiation sickness, and those exposed to radiation fallout develop acute radiation syndrome, which can lead to death, depending on the degree of exposure. The accident at the nuclear power plant at Chernobyl in the former Soviet Union is the fulfillment of our worst nightmares, and it will be years before the full toll on life and the environment is known.

HOST RESISTANCE TO INFECTIOUS DISEASE

The host defenses against infectious disease will be discussed in Chapter 3. It has been known for some time that the ability to resist any particular infectious disease varies with the individual. That is, each person is born with resistance to disease that is more or less effective than that which other individuals have. This is why some people never get colds; why some people who have inhaled the tuberculosis bacillus never get the disease; why some people do not become sick in the midst of an epidemic; why some people who smoke get lung cancer and others don't. The list could go on and on. Scientists are still trying to determine the exact cause for this difference in resistance to disease. Some of it seems to be present from birth, and it remains to be determined how much of our resistance to disease is inherited and how much is determined by environmental factors. It is known that the immune response can be slow or ineffective in the elderly, malnourished, seriously ill, debilitated, cancer afflicted, and AIDS afflicted.

HOST RESISTANCE TO NONINFECTIOUS DISEASE

As has already been stated, noninfectious diseases cannot be identified by a pathogenic organism. The *etiology* of noninfectious diseases lies in many different factors that are related to heredity and/or lifestyle. These are referred to as risk factors or predisposing factors, and for most noninfectious diseases, one or more of these factors has been identified. Unlike the risk factors in Table 2-2, there are risk factors that cannot be changed, such as race, heredity, sex, and age. Prevention and control for noninfectious diseases is aimed at reduction and/or elimination of as many of the risk factors as possible.

Through research and study of the causes of noninfectious disease, it has become apparent that the lifestyles of individuals play a major part in determining whether or not they will have certain noninfectious diseases. We suspect a relationship between the way we live and many diseases and disorders. We are *certain* there is a relationship between the way we live and our susceptibility to cardiovascular disease and some forms of cancer.

NUTRITION, WEIGHT, AND HEALTH

Nutrition plays an important part in everyone's health. We have only begun to discover many of the adverse effects of poor diets. Americans have become used to too much fat, too much salt, too much sugar, and too little of the whole grain foods and fruits and vegetables. And one of the worst problems is overnutrition, which leads to obesity. In a survey of some of the growing number of citizens reaching 100 and more years of age, it was found that one of the things they had in common was that none of them had ever been extremely obese.

Recent research has shown that many individuals inherit traits that give them a higher potential for gaining weight, and, for them, losing weight is much more difficult. Americans have typically admired the "chubby" baby as being well fed, but we now know that fat cells added by overfeeding babies and young children do not go away.

Mothers need to help their children learn wise ways to eat. Trying to lose weight by cutting calories has a very low rate of success. Over 90% of those who are able to lose weight on a diet regain what they have lost in a short time. It is now known that the best way to lose weight and keep it off is through a lifetime commitment to changed eating habits and regular exercise.

SLEEP

Getting adequate amounts of *sleep* is another factor in being able to resist disease. Individuals who get too much or too little sleep on a regular basis are more susceptible to disease. The amount of sleep necessary for good health varies among individuals, but 7 to 8 hours a night seems to be what is required for most people. Many studies have shown that more people report coming down with colds and

TABLE 2-2 Risk factors associated with five leading causes of death (United States)

Risk Factor	Cause of Death
Tobacco use	Cardiovascular disease
Elevated serum cholesterol	
Hypertension	
Obesity	
Diabetes	
Sedentary lifestyle	
Tobacco use	Cancer
Improper diet	
Alcohol	
Occupational or environmental exposures	
Hypertension	Cerebrovascular disease
Tobacco use	
Elevated serum cholesterol	
Nonuse of seat belts	Accidental injury
Alcohol or substance abuse	
Reckless driving	
Occupational hazards	
Stress/fatigue	
Tobacco use	Chronic lung disease
Occupational/environmental exposures	

missing work on Monday than any other day of the week, and this has been associated with lack of sleep and a break in regular routines over the weekend.

EXERCISE AND HEALTH

Our society is in the midst of a fitness revolution, and basic to this is the emphasis on getting enough *exercise* and the right kind for cardiovascular and respiratory effects to occur. Many studies in the United States and other countries have proved the benefits of adequate exercise as far as disease prevention and longevity are concerned. One long-term study done more than 25 years ago traced 50 pairs of identical twin brothers born in Ireland. In each pair, one brother stayed in Ireland and the other moved to the United States. The incidence of heart disease in the American brothers was significantly higher than in the Irish brothers. When their lifestyles were studied, only two differences were found consistently: the Irish brothers ate more potatoes and less meat and walked everywhere, while the American brothers ate fewer potatoes, more meat, and rode everywhere.

Even though most Americans know how important exercise is, many of those who have taken up walking or jogging (the percentage is very small) still try to get the closest parking place available, take elevators or escalators instead of stairs, and ride when they could walk. The rest make no effort at all to increase their activity level. If exercise is going to improve the chances of resisting disease, then each individual needs to get the optimum amount. The majority of Americans fall far short of this goal.

SMOKING AND ALCOHOL

The elimination of *smoking,* which has been proved to cause lung cancer and other diseases of the lung, as well as have an adverse effect on the heart, and moderation in *drinking* or no drinking at all, are two behaviors that would lead to the prevention of untold physical and mental suffering and disease. Smoking and drinking (to excess), cause disease and suffering not only in the individual who uses these substances but in anyone else who is involved. Some laws have been enacted to protect innocent bystanders from passive smoke, but we have a long way to go before these two factors, which so obviously lower the resistance of the host, are eliminated or controlled.

STRESS MANAGEMENT

The benefits of *stress management* have been discussed. It is not possible to live a life free of stressors. Mental and physical stressors that cannot be eliminated are present in everyone's life. Learning to manage stress can be one of the most effective single steps in preventing disease.

The optimum level of resistance to disease will occur in individuals as they strive to achieve a lifestyle that includes wise eating habits, adequate sleep, regular exercise, elimination of unnecessary drugs, and effective stress management.

ENVIRONMENT AND DISEASE

Environmental factors can be thought of in three categories, biologic, physical and social. In developed nations, the control of *biologic* environmental factors by sanitary measures to ensure clean water, air, food, adequate disposal of waste products, and pest control has erased the threat of many infectious diseases. During times of disaster when sanitation measures are overwhelmed or in third world countries where they are still inadequate, the flourishing of infectious diseases that were once rare reminds us of our vulnerability and the need for continual vigilance in maintaining a safe environment.

Physical factors such as climate and geography can also have an effect on disease. Some diseases flourish in warm, tropical climates, and others occur mainly in temperate climates. Geographical features such as low, swampy lands that provide ideal breeding grounds for insect vectors are conducive to disease.

The institutions, cultural norms, and economic features of a *society* can include patterns of hygiene, sanitation, and personal relations that produce an environment that is more favorable to disease. The Japanese practice of eating raw fish (which may be contaminated), the use of "earth" toilet facilities in undeveloped nations, rubbing noses among the Eskimos, and many other societal customs and conditions provide environmental factors that can unbalance the equilibrium between disease agent, host, and environment, providing the conditions for disease to take place.

CHAIN OF INFECTION

As part of the foundation for studying the individual infectious diseases, it is important to look at the chain of infection by which pathogenic organisms are able to continue to exist in the environment.

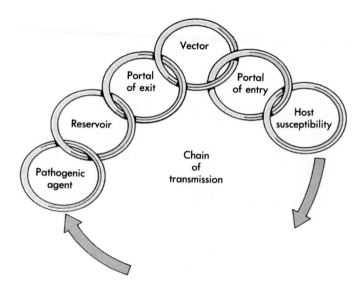

FIGURE 2-9 Chain of infection.

Pathogenic organisms or agents are all "hitchhikers." They have to find a way to get from one host to another, from one place to another, from their *reservoir* (humans, plants, animals, or organic matter upon which they exist or are stored) to a susceptible host. Their transportation is referred to as a *mode of conveyance* or *vector*. They also need to find a way to get into their new host, a *portal of entry,* and a way to leave, a *portal of exit* or *avenue of escape* if they are not destroyed.

The "chain of transmission" is shown in Figure 2-9. Our success in preventing and controlling infectious diseases has come through being able to break one or more of the "links" in the chain.

Transmission may be by *direct* or *indirect contact*. Direct contact would be by skin or mucous membrane: by kissing or sexual intercourse; through droplet infection in the spray of a sneeze or a cough; or through blood transfusion. Indirect contact can be made by using, touching, or ingesting any object or food that has been contaminated with the pathogenic organisms. Pathogens may be carried in the air in evaporated residue of human discharges and in dust arising from contaminated bedding or soil. Insects, sometimes borne by animals and sometimes flying or crawling, may harbor a pathogen and transmit it through a bite or by depositing it on some animal, human, or object.

STAGES OF DISEASE

A knowledge of the progression of an infection once a pathogenic agent enters the body will also help you to understand infectious diseases. The stages of a disease are divided as shown in Figure 2-10. Although the divisions between these stages are not always apparent, most individuals follow the general pattern.

1. Incubation—Occurs between the time when the agent enters the body and the first symptoms.
2. Prodrome—General symptoms occur: headache, fever, nausea, irritability, and runny nose. The disease is already highly communicable.

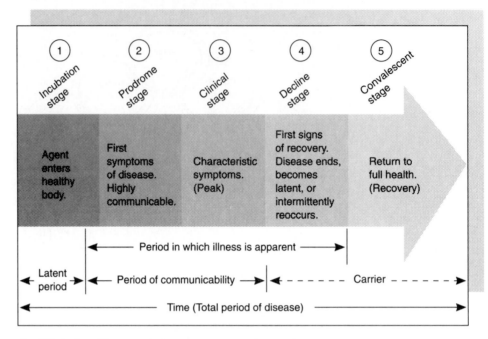

FIGURE 2-10 Stages of disease.

3. Clinical—Characteristic symptoms appear. This is the peak or most intense stage of the disease. Communicability of disease organisms is most probable at this time.
4. Decline—Symptoms begin to fade and recovery begins. Relapses may occur if too much is attempted too soon.
5. Convalescent—Rebuilding of the body occurs. The host is immune to the disease, but the agent may still be transmitted if a carrier state exists.

SUMMARY

Ancient peoples attributed disease to gods or to evil spirits. The theory of contagion did not develop until biblical times, when isolation of lepers led to a decrease in leprosy. In the nineteenth century, the discovery of micoorganisms and their relation to infection led to the germ theory of disease. Finally, the modern theory of multiple causation evolved. The classic epidemiologic model of disease is based on the need for a balance between the virulence of the disease agent, the resistance of the host, and factors in the biologic, physical, and social environment. Pathogenic organisms can be identified for most infectious diseases, but there are many different causes for noninfectious diseases. These are malnutrition or overnutrition, chemical substances, inherited susceptibility, psychosomatic factors, and physical forces. Some causes of noninfectious disease also play a role in infectious disease as they lower the resistance of the host. The lifestyles of individuals determine their ability to resist infection and also play a major part in determining whether or not they contract some noninfectious diseases. The important lifestyle factors are nutrition, sleep, exercise, drug use, and stress management. Biologic, physical, and social factors in the environment also affect the occurrence of disease. The chain of infection, methods of disease transmission, and stages of infectious disease are also important concepts in disease occurrence.

QUESTIONS FOR REVIEW

1. What theories of disease causation have human beings believed in through the ages (in chronological order)?
2. What was learned from the isolation of lepers in biblical times?
3. Why was it necessary to develop the theory of multiple causation?
4. What is meant by prevalence rate and incidence rate?
5. What are the differences among the primary, secondary, and tertiary levels of disease prevention?
6. How does the classic epidemiologic theory of disease apply to infectious and noninfectious disease?
7. What are six broad categories for classifying pathogenic agents?
8. How does a virus cause disease?
9. What is the difference between viral infection and viral disease?
10. How is it possible to get a bacterial disease without being exposed to someone who carries the disease agent?
11. How are rickettsiae like or different from bacteria?
12. What are some examples of fungi that are pathogenic and some that are not pathogenic?
13. How do protozoa cause disease?
14. How do metazoa cause disease?
15. What are the "disease agents" for noninfectious disease?
16. What are the roles of exogenous and endogenous chemicals in causing disease?
17. In what way does heredity determine whether or not an individual gets a disease?
18. How do psychosomatic factors influence an individual's susceptibility to disease?
19. What is the difference between having a psychosomatic disease and being a hypochondriac?
20. What physical forces play a part in disease occurrence?
21. What factors affect the resistance of the host to infectious and noninfectious disease?
22. What are the biologic, physical, and social factors in the environment that play a part in disease occurrence?
23. What is the chain of infection, and why is it important?
24. What are the stages of disease, and what occurs to the victim during each stage?

FURTHER READING

Anspaugh, Lynn R., Robert J. Catlin, and Marvin Goldman. "The Global Impact of the Chernobyl Reactor Accident." *Science,* Dec. 16, '88, 242:1513-1519.

Benevich, Teri. "New Sources Add to Lead Poisoning Concerns." *Journal of the American Medical Association,* Feb. 9, '90, 263:790-791.

Benzaia, Diana. "New Ways to Fight Allergies." *Consumers Digest,* May-June '89, 28:56-59.

Blumenthal, Dale. "The Health-Diet Link: Charting a Rising Awareness." *FDA Consumer,* Oct. '89, 23:22-27.

Boyd, Robert F. *General Microbiology.* St. Louis: Mosby, 1988.

Braus, Pat. "The Who and Where of Heart Disease." *American Demographics,* Nov. '90, 12: 32-37.

Control of Communicable Disease in Man. Abram S. Benenson, ed. Fifteenth Edition, Washington, D.C.: American Public Health Association, 1990.

Cook-Mozaffari, Paula, et al. "Cancer near Potential Sites of Nuclear Installations." *The Lancet,* Nov. 11, '89, 2:1145-1147.

"Coronary Heart Disease Attributable to Sedentary Lifestyle." *Journal of the American Medical Association,* Sept. 19, '90, 264:1390-1391.

Dunnette, David A. "Assessing Risks and Preventing Disease from Environmental Chemicals." *Journal of Community Health,* Fall '89, 14:169-186.

Farley, John. "Parasites and the Germ Theory of Disease." *The Milbank Quarterly,* Spring '89, 67:50-68.

Gerhardt, Ann L. "Vitamin megadoses: Use, abuse, and toxicity." *Consultant,* May '88, 28:151-155.

Jaret, Peter. "The Disease Detectives." *National Geographic,* Jan., 1991, 179:114-140.

Leaf, Alexander. "Potential Health Effects of Global Climatic and Environmental Changes." *New England Journal of Medicine,* Dec. 7, '89, 321:1577-1583.

Lewin, Roger. "Stress Proteins: Are Links in Disease." *Science,* June 24, '88, 240:1732-1733.

Lieber, Charles S. "The Influence of Alcohol on Nutritional Status." *Nutrition Reviews,* July '88, 46:241-254.

Manton, Kenneth G. "Life-style Risk Factors," *Annals of the American Academy of Political and Social Science,* May '89, 503:72-88.

Marantz, Paul R. "Blaming the Victim: The Negative Consequence of Preventive Medicine." *American Journal of Public Health,* Oct. '90, 80:1186-1187.

McCance, Kathryn L. and Sue E. Huether. *Pathophysiology: The Biologic Basis for Disease in Adults and Children.* St. Louis: Mosby, 1990.

McClelland, David C. "Motivational Factors in Health and Disease." *American Psychologist,* April '89, 44:675-683.

Mee, Charles L. "How a Mysterious Disease Laid Low Europe's Masses." (bubonic plague in the 1300s), *Smithsonian,* Feb. '90, 20:66-74.

Murray, et al. *Medical Microbiology.* St. Louis: Mosby, 1990.

O'Reilly, Brian. "New Truths about Staying Healthy." *Fortune,* Sept. 25, '89, 120:57-62.

Ornish, Dean, et al. "Can Lifestyle Changes Reverse Coronary Heart Disease?" *Lancet,* July 21, '90, 336:129-133.

Pacelli, Lauren C. "Life-style Can Reverse Atherosclerosis." *Physician and Sports Medicine,* Dec. '90, 18:19-21.

Pichoushkov, Anatolij Vasilievich. "A Disease Consigned to the History Books." (polio), *World Health,* Dec., '89, p. 10-12.

Rose, Geoffrey and Martin Shipley. "Effects of Coronary Risk Reduction on the Pattern of Mortality." *Lancet,* Feb. 3, '90, 335:275-277.

Stamford and Porter Shimer, "Runs in the Family?" *Reader's Digest,* Oct. '90, 137:15-16.

Stehr-Green, Paul A. "Exposure to Toxic Waste Sites: An Investigative Approach." *Public Health Reports,* Jan-Feb. '89, 104:71-74.

Sullivan, Louis W. "Healthy People 2000." *New England Journal of Medicine,* Oct. 11, '90, 323:1065-1067.

Sytkowski, Pamela A., et al. "Changes in Risk Factors and the Decline in Mortality from Cardiovascular Disease." *New England Journal of Medicine,* June 7, '90, 322:1635-1641.

Thompson, Keith. "Preventing Hypertension through Life-style Changes." *Physician and Sports Medicine,* Feb. '90, 18:19-20.

Vollhardt, Lawrence T. "Psychoneuroimmunology: A Literature Review." *American Journal of Orthopsychiatry,* Jan. '91, 61:35-47.

Weiss, Rick. "The Viral Advantage: A Crowded World Ensures Prosperous Futures for Disease-Causing Viruses." *Science News,* Sept. 23, '89, 136:200-203.

Williams, Roger R. "Nature, Nurture, and Family Predisposition." *New England Journal of Medicine,* Mar. 24, '88, 318:769-771.

Chapter 3

The Body's Defenses: Immunity and Immune Disorders

OBJECTIVES

1 Describe the role that the external barriers play in protecting us from disease.

2 Differentiate between nonspecific and specific natural immunity.

3 Relate what happens in the combined immune response.

4 Explain the four types of acquired immunity.

5 Explain the processes that occur in the acute inflammatory response.

6 Explain the cause of the signs of the inflammatory response.

7 Distinguish between resolution, regeneration, and repair.

8 Discuss the factors that may hasten or delay healing.

9 Explain the terms *autoimmune* and *hypersensitivity*.

10 Describe and state the cause(s), symptoms, prevention, and treatment for the following:

Allergic rhinitis
Urticaria and angioedema
Asthma
Rheumatoid arthritis
Lupus erythematosus

NATURAL NONSPECIFIC IMMUNITY

EXTERNAL BARRIERS

External barriers are the body's first line of defense against invaders (Figure 3-1). The *skin* provides a natural barrier to most pathogenic (disease-causing) agents. In addition to being a mechanical barrier, the skin also keeps most bacteria from surviving because of the lactic acid and fatty acids in *sweat* and the low pH generated by *sebaceous secretions*.

Another effective defense mechanism is the *mucus* secreted by the membranes lining the inner surfaces of the body. The mucus serves to keep bacteria from attaching to the surfaces, and pathogens and other foreign particles are trapped in the mucus and removed from the body by mechanical means such as the action of the *cilia, sneezing,* and *coughing.*

Body fluid secretions also protect epithelial surfaces by mechanical and chemical means. The washing action of *tears, saliva,* and *urine* removes bacteria and foreign particles from the body, while body fluids such as *tears, gastric juice, semen, nasal secretions,* and *saliva* contain bacteriocidal components that destroy pathogens before they can infect the body.

A very different protective function is fulfilled by *"friendly" bacteria,* which naturally inhabit various parts of the body and suppress the growth of pathogenic organisms. For instance, there are bacteria in the vagina that produce lactic acid and metabolize glycogen secreted by the vaginal epithelium. When enough of these nonpathogenic bacteria are destroyed by antibiotic use, the resulting increase in glycogen allows the yeast *Candida albicans* to grow, which can result in candidiasis, a yeast infection.

INFLAMMATION

When pathogenic agents penetrate external barriers, the first reaction of the body is the inflammatory response. Infection is just one cause of inflammation, which

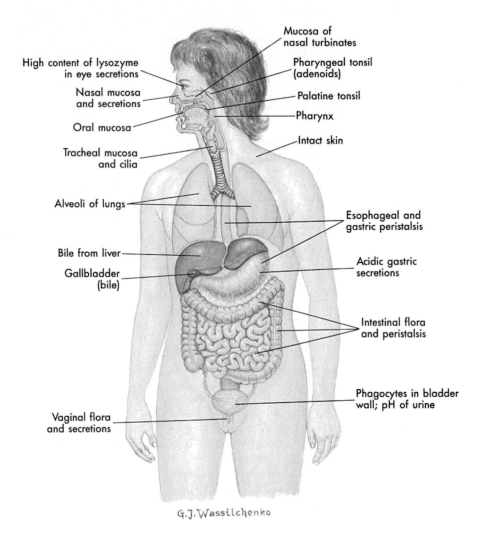

High content of lysozyme in eye secretions

Nasal mucosa and secretions

Oral mucosa

Tracheal mucosa and cilia

Alveoli of lungs

Bile from liver

Gallbladder (bile)

Vaginal flora and secretions

Mucosa of nasal turbinates

Pharyngeal tonsil (adenoids)

Palatine tonsil

Pharynx

Intact skin

Esophageal and gastric peristalsis

Acidic gastric secretions

Intestinal flora and peristalsis

Phagocytes in bladder wall; pH of urine

G.J. Wassilchenko

FIGURE 3-1   First line of defense.

can also occur as the result of a simple blow, exposure to the sun, contact with certain chemicals, and in many other ways. Any time the cells or tissues of the body are injured, internally or on the surface, by whatever agent, the inflammatory response occurs. An inflammatory response (produced by bacterial penetration) is diagrammed in Figure 3-2.

Although inflammation may not seem like a desirable thing to have at the time you are injured, it is actually the necessary response of the body for the healing process to begin. Everyone experiences inflammation from time to time. The signs are redness, warmth, pain, swelling, and loss of function. Sometimes inflammation is a mild reaction to a slight injury, but at other times it may be a strong reaction to a severe injury, and at some point can become chronic. A comprehension of the inflammatory process is basic to the understanding of disease.

ACUTE INFLAMMATORY RESPONSE

The acute or immediate inflammatory response occurs in the blood vessels in the area of the injury. At first there is a brief period when the blood vessels constrict;

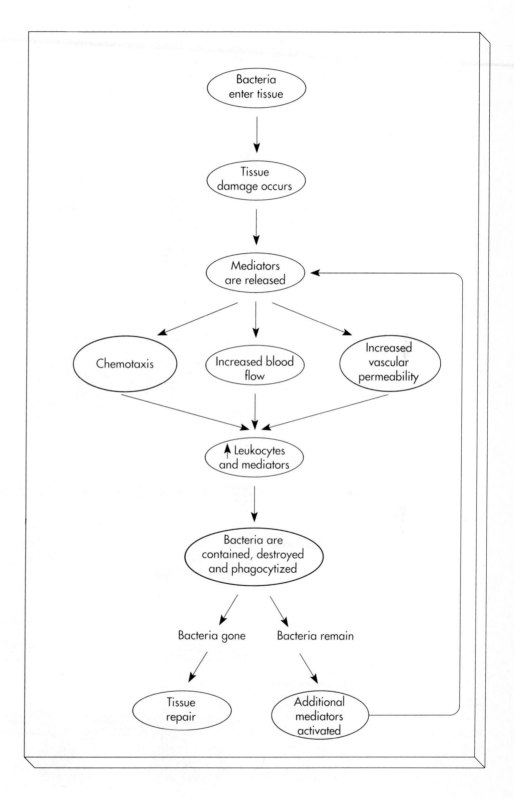

FIGURE 3-2 The inflammatory response.

then they dilate, resulting in an increased flow of blood to the area and an increased amount of fluid leaving the vessels for tissue spaces. At the same time, the permeability (ease of penetration) of the blood vessels increases, allowing the passage of plasma proteins, as well as fluid, into the tissue spaces. The blood remaining in the venules becomes thicker and slows down, thus permitting a process called **pavementing** (Figure 3-3), in which the leukocytes (white blood cells), which are

FIGURE 3-3   Pavementing.

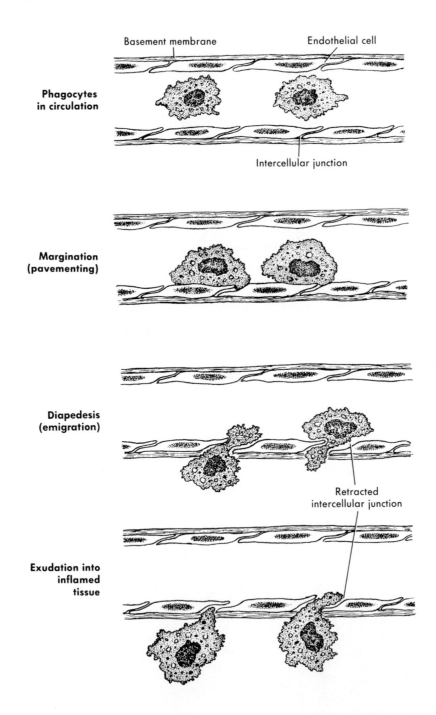

Basement membrane

Endothelial cell

Phagocytes in circulation

Intercellular junction

Margination (pavementing)

Diapedesis (emigration)

Retracted intercellular junction

Exudation into inflamed tissue

normally traveling in the mainstream of the blood, form a layer covering the endothelium (lining) of the venules.

The leukocytes then move along the endothelium in an amoeba-like fashion, to a point where they can leave the blood vessel. This process is called diapedesis or **emigration**.

Once the leukocytes have left the blood vessel, they travel toward the sight of injury through another process, **chemotaxis.** Chemotaxis is the movement of an organism or cells in response to a chemical attractant. In the inflammatory response, chemicals called **mediators** lure the leukocytes to the inflammatory site, where they release enzymes (proteins that act as catalysts) and begin the process of phagocytosis (engulfing and destroying foreign particles or organisms).

CHEMICAL MEDIATORS OF INFLAMMATION

Histamine was the first chemical identified as a mediator of the inflammatory response. As scientists realized that more than one chemical must be involved, the search for others got under way. Now there are many chemicals that are thought to take part in the inflammatory response. These mediators come from the plasma, cells, or possibly from damaged tissue. Histamine, bradykinin, complement, prostaglandins, leukotrienes, lysosomal enzymes, oxygen metabolites, platelet activating factor (PAF), interleukin-1 (IL-1), and tumor necrosis factor (TNF) are considered the principal mediators. Table 3-1 summarizes some of their actions.

When the leucocytes reach the site of injury, some of them, the neutrophils and the monocytes (which become macrophages), perform phagocytic action, while the others, basophils, mast cells, and eosinophils, release chemicals. If the cell injury is due to viral infection, *interferon,* a protein that protects the body against viral infection and possibly some forms of cancer, is released. It is nonspecific in that it protects against many different viruses, and infection by one virus can produce protection against other kinds of viruses. Viruses stimulate cells to produce interferon, and interferon in turn produces antiviral proteins that disrupt viral reproduction.

When interferon was discovered in 1957, great hopes existed for its use in bolstering the immune system and treating cancer. Although these hopes have not been fulfilled to date, it has been effective in a few cases. One of these is its ability to treat a rare form of leukemia.

TABLE 3-1 Chemical mediators

Mediators	Actions
Histamine	Increased vascular permeability
Bradykinin	Increased vascular permeability, pain
Complement	Increased vascular permeability, chemotaxis, facilitates phagocytosis
Prostaglandins	Vasodilation, fever, pain, potentiate other mediators in vascular permeability
Leukotrienes	Increased vascular permeability, chemotaxis
Lysosomal enzymes	Increased vascular permeability, chemotaxis
Oxygen metabolites	Increased vascular permeability
Platelet activating factor (PAF)	Increased vascular permeability, chemotaxis
Interleukin-1 (IL-1) and tumor necrosis factor (TNF)	Fever, chemotaxis

Another nonspecific defense of the body is found in complement, a complex of interrelated and interacting proteins manufactured in the liver. Complement is active in inflammation and phagocytosis and also assists the action of antibodies in the specific response if the infecting agent is not destroyed by the nonspecific defenses.

Inflammatory Exudates.   The increased permeability of the blood vessels allows certain fluids to escape along with the leukocytes and cellular debris. The *exudate* has various functions. The role of the leukocytes has already been mentioned. The fluid of the exudate also dilutes poisonous substances that may be present at the site of injury. The plasma fluid contains antibodies to microbial invasion, and fibrinogen (blood clotting factor), which can form a barrier to invaders. Fibrinogen also aids in phagocytosis by trapping microorganisms for the leukocytes.

The nature of the exudate changes according to the severity of the injury. Mild damage produces a watery exudate, which is called **serous.** More severe injury may lead to the release of more fibrin, and the exudate is then described as **fibrinous.** **Purulent** exudate, or pus, also occurs in a more severe injury, and if the lesion is deep enough to penetrate blood vessels and allow red blood cells to escape, then the exudate is called **hemorrhagic.**

HEALING

When an injury is mild, resolution occurs, with the site returning to normal. However, if there has been extensive damage, the inflammatory response does not resolve; a chronic abscess may form, pus is produced continuously, and fibrous tissue is laid down around the abscess, walling it off. If the inflammatory agent is destroyed or neutralized, healing may still occur. But if the body is unable to remove or destroy the inflammatory agent, then the result is chronic inflammation. Chronic inflammation may also occur without an acute phase as the result of certain disease processes, such as tuberculosis, syphilis, autoimmune diseases, and hypersensitivity, all of which will be discussed in later chapters.

When significant amounts of tissue have been destroyed, resolution cannot occur. Whether loss of tissue occurs from an accidental or surgical incision, physical or chemical agents, ischemia, or severe inflammation leading to necrosis (cell death), it is replaced by **regeneration** and **repair.** The replacing of lost tissue by tissue of the same type is regeneration. This type of healing is referred to as primary healing and occurs most often when a surgical incision has been made as shown in Figure 3-4. The replacing of lost tissue by granulation tissue, which becomes a fibrous connective-tissue scar, is repair and referred to as secondary healing (Figure 3-5). Most cells in the body have some capacity to regenerate, with the exception of central nervous system (CNS) nerve cells, skeletal cells, and cardiac muscle cells.

If neurons are destroyed in the CNS, they are permanently lost. In the peripheral nervous system (PNS), regeneration may occur if the cell body is not destroyed. Healing in any part of the body follows the same pattern, beginning with the inflammatory reaction and ending with resolution or regeneration and repair. There are local variations, depending on the type of tissue involved.

FACTORS AFFECTING INFLAMMATION AND HEALING

For some individuals, in some cases, the inflammatory response and healing may be impaired. Many factors can lead to slow healing or no healing (Figure 3-6). One of the most crucial factors in an effective inflammatory response is an

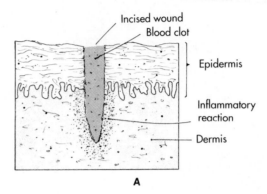

A

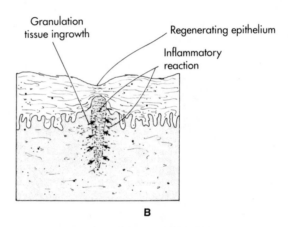

B

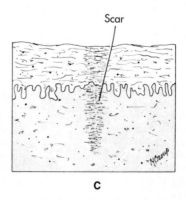

C

FIGURE 3-4   Regeneration or primary healing. The edges of an incised wound are held together by a blood clot or sutures **(A)**; there is an ingrowth of granulation tissue, **(B)**; a scar forms **(C)**.

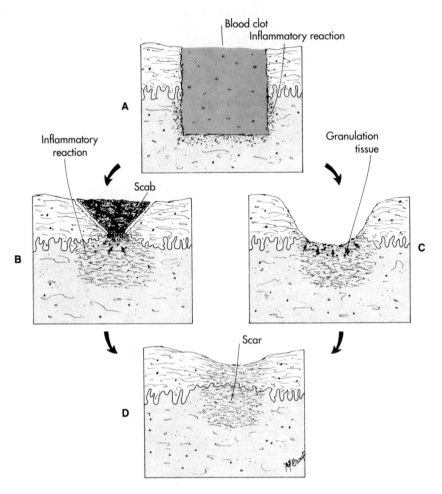

FIGURE 3-5 Repair or secondary healing is much like regeneration but involves more extensive regeneration and a more abundant scar. **(A)**, wound; **(B)**, healing under a scab; **(C)**, an open wound with visible granulation tissue. Secondary healing results in a large scar; often an area remains hairless, **(D)**.

FIGURE 3-6 Factors that affect healing.

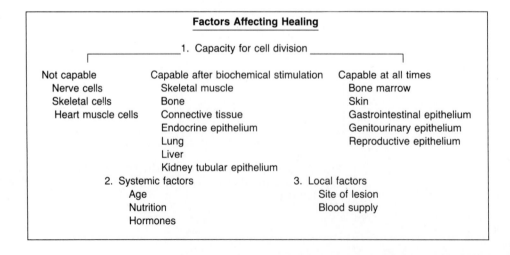

Factors Affecting Healing

1. Capacity for cell division

Not capable	Capable after biochemical stimulation	Capable at all times
Nerve cells	Skeletal muscle	Bone marrow
Skeletal cells	Bone	Skin
Heart muscle cells	Connective tissue	Gastrointestinal epithelium
	Endocrine epithelium	Genitourinary epithelium
	Lung	Reproductive epithelium
	Liver	
	Kidney tubular epithelium	

2. Systemic factors
   Age
   Nutrition
   Hormones

3. Local factors
   Site of lesion
   Blood supply

adequate blood supply. If the blood supply to the area of injury is impaired for any reason, the inflammatory response will be slow and healing prolonged. Nutrition is another important factor. Lack of sufficient protein, vitamin C, and zinc have been shown to delay healing, and adequate calcium and vitamin D are crucial in the healing of bones.

Although age has been thought by some to be a factor in slow healing, there is little to support this idea, and if healing in the elderly does occur more slowly, it is probably due to malnutrition or inadequate circulation. Antiinflammatory drugs such as the glucocorticoids inhibit inflammation and wound healing if they are present in large amounts. The presence of infection or foreign bodies will also impede healing. Diabetics have an increased susceptibility to infection, and this along with other deficiencies caused by the disease lead to inadequate healing.

NATURAL SPECIFIC IMMUNITY

There are two kinds of specific immunity to disease: (1) **humoral,** or **antibody-mediated immunity,** and (2) **cell-mediated immunity.** Both kinds are provided by the action of lymphocytes. In humoral immunity, *B lymphocytes,* or *B cells,* produce antibodies that protect against extracellular antigens such as bacteria, toxins, parasites, and viruses outside of cells. In cell-mediated immunity, *T lymphocytes (T cells)* produce **lymphokines,** which provide protection against intracellular antigens such as viruses, intracellular bacteria and fungi, and tumors and regulate humoral and cell-mediated immune responses. Three types of T cells have been identified. Helper T cells are needed for antibody production by B cells. Killer T cells are active in destroying foreign cells and in the rejection of tissue transplants. Suppressor T cells act to suppress the production of antibodies (see Figure 3-7). They keep the immune response from getting out of control.

THE COMBINED IMMUNE RESPONSE

When a microbial invader **(antigen)** enters the body, chemical messages are sent out from the point of entry, and phagocytes, B cells, and T cells all arrive at the scene. As the phagocytes begin to attack, antigens reach the B and T cells, which begin clonal expansion. B cells form immunoglobulin (antibodies), which partici-

DID YOU KNOW?

T Cells and Autoimmune Disorders

Nearly everyone has errant T cells that could at any time attack a healthy organ if an environmental trigger occurs. These triggers are thought to be bacteria or viruses, and it is also believed that a genetic susceptibility plays a part. Scientists seem to be close to unraveling the puzzle, spurred on by the diagnosis of Grave's disease for former President George Bush and his wife within 3 years of each other, as well as by the AIDS epidemic (HIV affects the immune system also). Fortunately, Grave's disease is easily treated, but for many autoimmune disorders there is no treatment, only a downhill slide to disability and, sometimes, death.

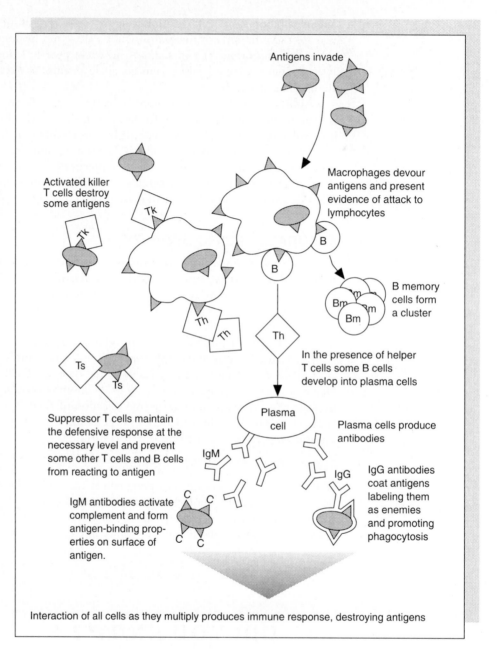

FIGURE 3-7 The immune response is a coordinated effort to destroy foreign invaders (antigens). It involves four varieties of lymphocyte: macrophages, neutrophils, B cells and T cells. Macrophages engulf invading antigens such as bacteria and at the same time, inform other lymphocytes of the attack. B cells and helper and killer T cells swarm around the macrophages and begin to multiply. Suppressor T cells take their cue from the number of antigens as to when to suppress the response. All four varieties of lymphocytes produce active cells and memory cells. Memory cells stay in the bloodstream and are prepared in case the same antigen attacks again. The interaction and multiplication of these cells provides a strong defense against invaders.

Within the figure:

Antigens invade

Activated killer T cells destroy some antigens

Macrophages devour antigens and present evidence of attack to lymphocytes

B memory cells form a cluster

In the presence of helper T cells some B cells develop into plasma cells

Plasma cell

Plasma cells produce antibodies

Suppressor T cells maintain the defensive response at the necessary level and prevent some other T cells and B cells from reacting to antigen

IgM antibodies activate complement and form antigen-binding properties on surface of antigen.

IgG antibodies coat antigens labeling them as enemies and promoting phagocytosis

Interaction of all cells as they multiply produces immune response, destroying antigens

pates in the inflammatory response. Antibodies attach to antigen on the surface of the microbes, causing clumping and immobilization. Complement is activated in response to this action and enhances the phagocytosis of the invaders by causing destruction of the invader's cell membrane (Figure 3–7). In the meantime, more T cells have been produced, T lymphocytes have combined with microbial antigens, and other chemicals are released. If the effort is successful, B and T lymphocytes withdraw, and **macrophages** perform the clean up.

ACQUIRED IMMUNITY

We have been discussing natural immunity to disease. Everyone is born with these defense mechanisms, but we also acquire immunity to disease. Acquired immunity can be acquired naturally or artificially, and it can be active or passive. Thus there are four kinds of acquired immunity: active natural, active artificial, passive natural, and passive artificial.

ACTIVE NATURAL IMMUNITY

Active natural immunity occurs when an individual is exposed to a disease-causing microorganism and the body learns to produce the antibodies necessary to destroy the organism. Normally the symptoms and the disease will be present with the first infection (in some cases the person may be asymptomatic yet still produce the antibodies). On subsequent exposure, the body is prepared with the specific antibodies, and the individual is immune to the disease. Most people over age 40 years were infected with the mumps virus as children. When exposed to mumps as an adult, they do not become ill. (Mumps is one childhood disease that does not always produce apparent symptoms.)

ACTIVE ARTIFICIAL IMMUNITY

Active artificial immunity occurs through vaccination with a form of the microorganism. It may be dead, attenuated (weakened), or altered so that it will not produce the disease but will cause the body to produce antibodies. Since the body has learned to make the antibodies, this type of vaccination is long lasting and preferable. Most people under age 20 years have received the measles, mumps, and rubella (MMR) vaccine and will not become sick with these diseases. Recommendations for vaccinations for children and adults are shown in Tables 3-2, 3-3, and 3-4.

PASSIVE NATURAL IMMUNITY

Passive natural immunity results from the transfer of antibodies from a mother to her baby through the placenta. The mother has been exposed to a number of pathogenic organisms during her life, and this protection is passed on to the baby in the form of antibodies. If the mother nurses the baby, then more protection is gained by antibodies in the milk. However, in both cases, since the baby's body has not learned to make the antibodies, the protection lasts only for a few months until the antibodies are broken down.

PASSIVE ARTIFICIAL IMMUNITY

Passive artificial immunity is acquired through inoculation with antibodies. Since it gives protection only as long as the antibodies are not used or eliminated from the system, this type of therapy is generally reserved for those who have been exposed to a disease such as rabies or tetanus or are at high risk for an infection because of age or physical condition. Immune serum or serum-containing antibodies, which is given to counteract one or more specific **toxin**(s), is also referred to as **antisera** or **antitoxin**. Figure 3-8 is a model of the different types of immunity.

Text continued on p. 74.

TABLE 3-2 Recommended schedule of vaccinations for all children*

2 Months	4 Months	6 Months	12 Months	15 Months	4-6 Years (Before Beginning School)
DTP	DTP	DTP		DTP*	DTP
Polio	Polio			Polio*	Polio
				MMR†	MMR§
HbCV:					
Option 1‖	HbCV	HBCV		HbCV	
Option 2‖	HbCV		HbCV		

	At Birth (Before Hospital Discharge)	1-2 Months	4 Months	6-18 Months
HBv:				
Option 1	HBv	HBv**		HBv**
Option 2		HBv**	HBv**	HBv**

DTP, Diphtheria, tetanus, and pertussis vaccine.

Polio, Live oral polio vaccine (OPV) drops or inactivated (killed) polio vaccine (IPV) shots.

MMR, Measles, mumps, and rubella vaccine.

HbCV, *Haemophilus influenzae* type b conjugate vaccine.

HBv, Hepatitis B vaccine.

*Many experts recommend these vaccines at 18 months.

†In some areas this dose of MMR vaccine may be administered at 12 months.

§Many experts recommend this dose of MMR vaccine be administered at entry into middle school or junior high school.

‖HbCV vaccine is administered in either a four-dose schedule (1) or a three-dose schedule (2), depending on the type of vaccine used.

**HBv can be administered at the same time as DTP and/or HbCV.

Source: U.S. Center for Disease Control.

TABLE 3-3 Vaccines and toxoids recommended for adults, by age groups, United States*

Age Group (Years)	Vaccine/Toxoid					
	Td†	Measles	Mumps	Rubella	Influenza	Pneumococcal Polysaccharide
18-24	X	X	X	X		
25-64	X	X§	X§	X		
≥65	X				X	X

*Tables 3-2, 3-3 and 3-4 have been adapted from *MMWR* Nov. 15, 1991 Vol 40, N. RR-12, pp 56-69.

†Td = Tetanus and diphtheria toxoids, adsorbed (for adult use), which is a combined preparation containing <2 flocculation units of diphtheria toxoid.

§Indicated for persons born after 1956.

Source: U.S. Centers for Disease Control.

TABLE 3-4 Immunobiologics and schedules for adults (≥18 years of age)†, United States

Immunobio-logic Generic Name	Primary Schedule and Booster(s)	Indications	Major Precautions and Contraindica-tions‡	Special Considera-tions
Toxoids				
Tetanus/diphtheria toxoid, adsorbed (for adult use)(Td)	Two doses intramuscularly (IM) 4 weeks apart; third dose 6-12 months after second dose. Booster every 10 years.	All adults.	Except in the first trimester, pregnancy is not a contraindication; history of a neurologic reaction or immediate hypersensitivity reaction following a previous dose; history of severe local (Arthus-type) reaction following previous dose; such individuals should not be given further routine or emergency doses of Td for 10 years.	Tetanus prophylaxis in wound management.
Live Virus Vaccines				
Measles vaccine, live	One dose subcutaneously (SC); second dose at least 1 month later, at entry into college or post-high school education, beginning medical facility employment, or before traveling. Susceptible travelers should receive one dose.	All adults born after 1956 without documentation of live vaccine on or after first birthday, physician-diagnosed measles, or laboratory evidence of immunity; persons born before 1957 are generally considered immune.	Pregnancy; immunocompromised persons§; history of anaphylactic reactions following egg ingestion or receipt of neomycin.	MMR is the vaccine of choice if recipients are likely to be susceptible to rubella and/or mumps as well as to measles. Persons vaccinated between 1963 and 1967 with a killed measles vaccine alone, killed vaccine followed by live vaccine, or with a vaccine of unknown type should be revaccinated with live measles virus vaccine.
Mumps vaccine, live	One dose SC; no booster.	All adults believed to be susceptible can be vaccinated. Adults born before 1957 can be considered immune.	Pregnancy; immunocompromised persons§; history of anaphylactic reaction following egg ingestion.	MMR is the vaccine of choice if recipients are likely to be susceptible to measles and rubella as well as to mumps.

Source: U.S. Centers for Disease Control.

TABLE 3-4 Immunobiologics and schedules for adults (≥18 years of age)†, United States—cont'd

Immunobiologic Generic Name	Primary Schedule and Booster(s)	Indications	Major Precautions and Contraindications‡	Special Considerations
Live Virus Vaccines—cont'd				
Rubella vaccine, live	One dose SC; no booster.	Indicated for adults, both male and female, lacking documentation of live vaccine on or after first birthday or laboratory evidence of immunity, particularly young adults who work or congregate in places such as hospitals, colleges, and military, as well as susceptible travelers.	Pregnancy; immunocompromised persons§; history of anaphylactic reaction following receipt of neomycin.	Women pregnant when vaccinated or who become pregnant within 3 months of vaccination should be counseled on the theoretical risks to the fetus. The risk of rubella vaccine–associated malformations in these women is so small as to be negligible. MMR is the vaccine of choice if recipients are likely to be susceptible to measles or mumps as well as to rubella.
Smallpox vaccine (vaccinia virus)	THERE ARE NO INDICATIONS FOR THE USE OF SMALLPOX VACCINE IN THE GENERAL CIVILIAN POPULATION.			Laboratory workers working with orthopox viruses or health-care workers involved in clinical trials of vaccinia-recombinant vaccines.
Yellow fever attenuated virus, live (17D strain)	One dose SC 10 days to 10 years before travel; booster every 10 years.	Selected persons traveling or living in areas where yellow fever infection exists.	Although specific information is not available concerning adverse effects on the developing fetus, it is prudent on theoretical grounds to avoid vaccinating a pregnant woman unless she must travel where the risk of yellow fever is high. Immunocompromised persons§; history of hypersensitivity to egg ingestion.	Some countries require a valid International Certificate of Vaccination showing receipt of vaccine. If the only reason to vaccinate a pregnant woman is an international requirement, efforts should be made to obtain a waiver letter.

TABLE 3-4 Immunobiologics and schedules for adults (≥18 years of age)†, United States— cont'd

Immunobiologic Generic Name	Primary Schedule and Booster(s)	Indications	Major Precautions and Contraindications‡	Special Considerations
Live Virus and Inactivated Virus Vaccines				
Polio vaccines: Enhanced potency inactivated poliovirus vaccine (eIPV); Oral poliovirus vaccine, live (OPV)	eIPV preferred for primary vaccination; two doses SC 4 weeks apart; a third dose 6-12 months after second; for adults with a completed primary series and for whom a booster is indicated, either OPV or eIPV can be administered. If immediate protection is needed, OPV is recommended.	Persons traveling to areas where wild poliovirus is epidemic or endemic. Certain health-care personnel.	Although there is no convincing evidence documenting adverse effects of either OPV or eIPV on the pregnant woman or developing fetus, it is prudent on theoretical grounds to avoid vaccinating pregnant women. However, if immediate protection against poliomyelitis is needed, OPV is recommended. OPV should not be given to immunocompromised individuals or to persons with known or possibly immunocompromised family members.§ eIPV is recommended in such situations.	Although a protective immune response to eIPV in the immunocompromised person cannot be assured, the vaccine is safe, and some protection may result from its administration.
Inactivated Virus Vaccines				
Hepatitis B (HB) inactivated-virus vaccine	Two doses IM 4 weeks apart; third dose 5 months after second; booster doses not necessary within 7 years of primary series. Alternate schedule for one vaccine: three doses IM 4 weeks apart; fourth dose 10 months after the third.	Adults at increased risk of occupational, environmental, social, or family exposure.	Data are not available on the safety of the vaccine for the developing fetus. Because the vaccine contains only noninfectious HBsAg particles, the risk should be negligible. Pregnancy should *not* be considered a vaccine contraindication if the woman is otherwise eligible.	The vaccine produces neither therapeutic nor adverse effects on HBV-infected persons. Prevaccination serologic screening for susceptibility before vaccination may or may not be cost effective depending on costs of vaccination and testing and on the prevalence of immune persons in the group.

Continued.

TABLE 3-4 Immunobiologics and schedules for adults (≥18 years of age)†, United States—cont'd

Immunobio-logic Generic Name	Primary Schedule and Booster(s)	Indications	Major Precautions and Contraindica-tions‡	Special Considera-tions
Inactivated Virus Vaccines—cont'd				
Influenza vaccine (inactivated whole virus and split-virus vaccine)	Annual vaccination with current vaccine. Either whole or split virus vaccine may be used.	Adults with high-risk conditions, residents of nursing homes or other chronic-care facilities, medical-care personnel, or healthy persons ≥65 years.	History of anaphylactic hypersensitivity to egg ingestion.	No evidence exists of maternal or fetal risk when vaccine is administered in pregnancy because of an underlying high-risk condition in a pregnant woman. However, it is reasonable to wait until the second or third trimester, if possible, before vaccination.
Human diploid cell rabies vaccine (HDCV) (inactivated, whole virion); rabies vaccine, adsorbed (RVA)	Preexposure prophylaxis: two doses 1 week apart; third dose 3 weeks after second. If exposure continues, booster doses every 2 years, or an antibody titer determined and a booster dose administered if titer is inadequate (<5). Postexposure prophylaxis: all postexposure treatment should begin with soap and water. (1) Persons who have (a) previously received postexposure prophylaxis with HDCV, (b) received recommended IM preexposure series of HDCV, (c) received recommended ID preexposure series of HDCV in the United States, or	Veterinarians, animal handlers, certain laboratory workers, and persons living in or visiting countries for >1 month where rabies is a constant threat.	If there is substantial risk of exposure to rabies, preexposure vaccination may be indicated during pregnancy. Corticosteroids and immunosuppressive agents can interfere with the development of active immunity; history of anaphylactic or Type III hypersensitivity reaction to previous dose of HDCV.	Complete preexposure prophylaxis does not eliminate the need for additional therapy with rabies vaccine after a rabies exposure. The decision for postexposure use of HDCV depends on the species of biting animal, the circumstances of biting incident, and the type of exposure (e.g., bite, saliva contamination of wound). The type of and schedule for postexposure prophylaxis depends upon the person's previous rabies vaccination status, or the result of a previous or current serologic test for rabies antibody. For postexposure prophylaxis, HDCV should always be administered IM, *not* ID.

TABLE 3-4 Immunobiologics and schedules for adults (≥18 years of age)†, United States—cont'd

Immunobiologic Generic Name	Primary Schedule and Booster(s)	Indications	Major Precautions and Contraindications‡	Special Considerations
Inactivated Virus Vaccines—cont'd				
	(d) have a previously documented rabies antibody titer considered adequate: two doses of HDCV, 1.0 mL IM, one each on days 0 and 3. (2) Persons not previously immunized as above: HRIG 20 IU/kg body weight, half infiltrated at bite site if possible; remainder IM; and five doses of HDCV, 1.0 mL IM, one each on days 0, 3, 7, 14, 28.			
Inactivated Bacteria Vaccines				
Cholera vaccine	Two 0.5-mL doses SC or IM or two 0.2-mL doses ID 1 week to 1 month apart; booster doses (0.5 mL IM or 0.2 mL ID) every 6 months.	Travelers to countries requiring evidence of cholera vaccination for entry.	No specific information on vaccine safety during pregnancy. Use in pregnancy should reflect actual increased risk. Persons who have had severe local or systemic reactions to a previous dose.	One dose generally satisfies international health regulations. Some countries may require evidence of a complete primary series or a booster dose given within 6 months before arrival. Vaccination should not be considered an alternative to continued careful selection of foods and water.
Haemophilus influenzae type b conjugate vaccine (HbCV)	Dosage for adults has not been determined.	May be considered for adults at highest theoretical risk (e.g., those with anatomic or functional asplenia or HIV infection).	No specific information on vaccine safety during pregnancy.	No efficacy data available for adults; not indicated for adult contacts of children with invasive disease.

Continued.

TABLE 3-4　Immunobiologics and schedules for adults (≥18 years of age)†, United States—cont'd

Immunobiologic Generic Name	Primary Schedule and Booster(s)	Indications	Major Precautions and Contraindications‡	Special Considerations
Inactivated Bacteria Vaccines—cont'd				
Meningococcal polysaccharide vaccine (tetravalent A, C, W135, and Y)	One dose in volume and by route specified by manufacturer; need for boosters unknown.	Travelers visiting areas of a country that is recognized as having epidemic meningococcal disease.	Pregnancy unless there is substantial risk of infection.	
Plague vaccine	Three IM doses; first dose 1.0 mL; second dose 0.2 mL 1 month later; third dose 0.2 mL 5 months after second; booster doses (0.2 mL) at 1- to 2-year intervals if exposure continues.	Selected travelers to countries reporting cases, or in which avoidance of rodents and fleas is impossible; all laboratory and field personnel working with *Yersinia pestis* organisms possibly resistant to antimicrobials; those engaged in *Y. pestis* aerosol experiments or in field operations in areas with enzootic plague where regular exposure to potentially infected wild rodents, rabbits, or their fleas cannot be prevented.	Pregnancy, unless there is substantial and unavoidable risk of exposure; persons with known hypersensitivity to any of the vaccine constituents (see manufacturer's label); patients who have had severe local or systemic reactions to a previous dose.	Prophylactic antibiotics may be recommended for definite exposure whether or not the exposed person has been vaccinated.
Pneumococcal polysaccharide vaccine (23 valent)	One dose; revaccination recommended for those at highest risk ≥6 years after the first dose.	Adults who are at increased risk of pneumococcal disease and its complications because of underlying health conditions; older adults, especially those ≥65 years of age who are healthy.	The safety of vaccine for pregnant women has not been evaluated; it should not be given during pregnancy unless the risk of infection is high. Previous recipients of any type of pneumococcal polysaccharide vaccine who are at highest risk of fatal infection or antibody loss may be revaccinated >6 years after the first dose.	

TABLE 3-4 Immunobiologics and schedules for adults (≥18 years of age)†, United States—cont'd

Immunobiologic Generic Name	Primary Schedule and Booster(s)	Indications	Major Precautions and Contraindications‡	Special Considerations
Inactivated Bacteria and Live-Bacteria Vaccines				
Typhoid vaccine, SC and oral	Two 0.5-mL doses SC 4 or more weeks apart, booster 0.5 mL SC or 0.1 mL ID every 3 years if exposure continues. Four oral doses on alternate days. The manufacturer recommends revaccination with the entire four-dose series every 5 years.	Travelers to areas where there is a recognized risk of exposure to typhoid.	Severe local or systemic reaction to a previous dose. Acetone-killed and -dried vaccines should not be administered ID.	Vaccination should not be considered an alternative to continued careful selection of foods and water.
Live Bacteria Vaccine				
Bacille Calmette-Guérin vaccine (BCG)	One dose ID or percutaneously. (See package label.)	For children only, who have prolonged close contact with untreated or ineffectively treated active tuberculosis patients; groups with excessive rates of new infection in which other control measures have not been successful.	Pregnancy, unless there is unavoidable exposure to infective tuberculosis; immunocompromised patients.§	In the United States, tuberculosis control efforts are directed towards early identification and treatment of cases, and preventive therapy with isoniazid.
Immune Globulins				
Cytomegalovirus immune globulin (IV)	Bone marrow transplant recipients: 1.0 g/kg weekly; kidney transplant recipients: 150 mg/kg initially, then 50-100 mg/kg every 2 weeks.	As prophylaxis for bone marrow and kidney transplant recipients.		Prophylaxis must be continued for 3-4 months to be effective.
Immune globulin (IG)	Hepatitis A prophylaxis: *Preexposure:* one IM dose of 0.02 mL/kg for anticipated risk of 2-3 months; IM dose of 0.06 mL/kg for anticipated risk of 5 months; repeat appropriate dose at above intervals if exposure continues.	Nonimmune persons traveling to developing countries.		For travelers, IG is not an alternative to continued careful selection of foods and water. Frequent travelers should be tested for hepatitis A antibody. IG is not indicated for persons with antibody to hepatitis A.

Continued.

TABLE 3-4 Immunobiologics and schedules for adults (≥18 years of age)†, United States—cont'd

Immunobiologic Generic Name	Primary Schedule and Booster(s)	Indications	Major Precautions and Contraindications‡	Special Considerations
Immune Globulins—cont'd				
	Postexposure: one IM dose of 0.02 mL/ kg administered within 2 weeks of exposure.	Household and sexual contacts of persons with hepatitis A; staff, attendees, and parents of diapered attendees in day care center outbreaks.		
	Measles prophylaxis: 0.25 mL/kg IM (maximum 15 mL) administered within 6 days after exposure.	Exposed susceptible contacts of measles cases.	IG should *not* be used to control measles.	IG administered within 6 days after exposure can prevent or modify measles. Recipients of IG for measles prophylaxis should receive live measles vaccine 3 months later.
Hepatitis B immune globulin (HBIG)	0.06 mL/kg IM as soon as possible after exposure (with HB vaccine started at a different site); a second dose of HBIG should be administered 1 month later (percutaneous/mucous membrane exposure) or 3 months later (sexual exposure) if the HB vaccine series has not been started.	Following percutaneous or mucous membrane exposure to blood known to be HBsAg positive (within 7 days); following sexual exposure to a person with acute HBV or an HBV carrier (within 14 days).		
Tetanus immune globulin (TIG)	250 U IM.	Part of management of nonclean, non-minor wound in a person with unknown tetanus toxoid status, with less than two previous doses or with two previous doses and a wound more than 24 hours old.		

TABLE 3-4 Immunobiologics and schedules for adults (≥18 years of age)†, United States—cont'd

Immunobiologic Generic Name	Primary Schedule and Booster(s)	Indications	Major Precautions and Contraindications‡	Special Considerations
Immune Globulins—cont'd				
Rabies immune globulin, human (HRIG)	20 IU/kg, up to half infiltrated around wound; remainder IM.	Part of management of rabies exposure in persons lacking a history of recommended preexposure or postexposure prophylaxis with HDCV.		Although preferable to administer with the first dose of vaccine, can be administered up to the eighth day after the first dose of vaccine.
Vaccinia immune globulin	0.6 mL/kg in divided doses over 24-36 hours; may be repeated every 2-3 days until no new lesions appear.	Treatment of eczema vaccinatum, vaccinia necrosum, and ocular vaccinia.		Of no benefit for postvaccination encephalitis.
Varicella-zoster immune globulin (VZIG)	Persons >50 kg: 125 U/10 kg IM; persons >50 kg: 625 U.	Immunocompromised patients known or likely to be susceptible with close and prolonged exposure to a household contact case or to an infectious hospital staff member or hospital roommate.		

†Several vaccines and toxoids are in "Investigational New Drug" (IND) status and available only through the U.S. Army Research Institute for Infectious Diseases (telephone 301-663-2403). These are: (a) eastern equine encephalitis vaccine (EEE), (b) western equine encephalitis vaccine (WEE), (c) Venezuelan equine encephalitis vaccine (VEE), and (d) tularemia vaccine. Pentavalent (ABCDE) botulinum toxoid is available only through CDC's Drug Service.

‡When any vaccine or toxoid is indicated during pregnancy, waiting until the second or the third trimester, when possible, is a reasonable precaution that minimizes concern about teratogenicity.

§Persons immunocompromised because of immune deficiency diseases, HIV infection (who should primarily not receive OPV and yellow fever vaccines) (see text), leukemia, lymphoma, or generalized malignancy or immunosuppressed as a result of therapy with corticosteroids, alkylating drugs, antimetabolites, or radiation.

¶Some persons have recommended 125 U/10 kg regardless of total body weight.

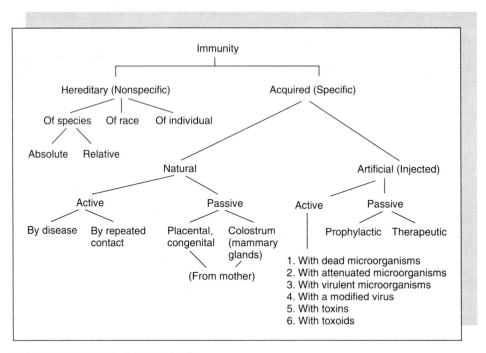

FIGURE 3-8 Diagram of types of immunity.

IMMUNE DISORDERS

Because the body's response to foreign invaders is so complex, there are times when it may malfunction. Instead of protecting us from disease and discomfort as it does most of the time, the immune response may become overactive or mis-directed. The conditions that then occur are referred to as hypersensitivity (allergies) and autoimmune disorders.

HYPERSENSITIVITY (ALLERGIES)

Allergies occur because of an inappropriate reaction of the immune system. As has been discussed previously in this chapter, the function of the immune system is to recognize foreign invaders (antigens), such as bacteria and viruses, and to form antibodies and sensitized lymphocytes that will interact with these disease agents when next encountered and destroy them. In allergies, for some unknown reason, the immune system forms antibodies against harmless substances because they are identified as potentially harmful antigens.

One out of seven people in the United States today has an allergy. The substance that causes an allergic reaction is called an allergen, and these allergens can be introduced into the body by different routes. These routes are inhalation, ingestion, injection, and direct contact. The list of possible allergens is endless, and in many cases there is an inherited tendency to develop an allergy. Some of the most common allergens are pollen, animal dander, and other particulates in the air; milk, straw-berries, and almost any other food; penicillin and many other drugs; poison ivy and other plant life; synthetic materials, chemicals, and insect venom.

The symptoms are also diverse, ranging from a mild rash to life-threatening anaphylactic shock (Figure 3-9). Most allergic reactions are acute and not recurrent, since the allergen is readily identified and can be avoided. However, the most common allergic reaction, allergic rhinitis, is often a chronic condition.

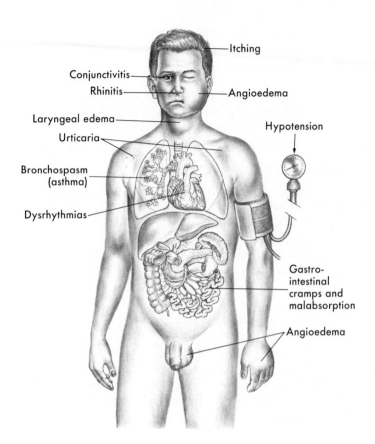

FIGURE 3-9 Hypersensitivity reactions may affect various body systems.

ALLERGIC RHINITIS

Allergic rhinitis, generally called hay fever, is a reaction to an airborne allergen. For some individuals it may be a seasonal problem, caused by certain pollens, while for others it is year-round and caused by many different allergens.

Cause   A predisposition to allergic rhinitis is inherited. The major allergens that induce the reaction are pollen, mold spores, house dust, animal dander, cigarette smoke, and upholstery.

Symptoms   Histamine and other chemicals released by the body in response to an allergen are responsible for the allergic reaction. For some individuals, the symptoms may be mild, with runny nose, watery, itchy eyes, and sneezing. For others, however, these may be accompanied by malaise, fever, headache, and sinus pain. In perennial allergic rhinitis, chronic nasal obstruction is common and often results in eustachian tube obstruction and if untreated may lead to asthma, otitis media (middle ear infection) with hearing loss, and other respiratory problems.

Prevention   The best method of prevention is desensitization and avoidance of allergens.

Treatment   Antihistamines will reduce symptoms. Nasal sprays may be used, but continued use can cause a **rebound effect** when the drug is suddenly discontinued, leading to a return of the allergic symptoms. Decongestants are of little value. A process called desensitization is considered to be the most effective treatment. In order for a person to undergo desensitization, specific allergens must be identified. The specialist will then administer repeated small doses of the allergen until the person no longer has an allergic reaction. Sometimes a change of residence is recommended to provide an environment as free of the allergen as possible.

URTICARIA AND ANGIOEDEMA

Urticaria is a skin condition that is more commonly called hives. It is characterized by the development of itchy wheals (raised white lumps surrounded by an area of red inflammation) (Figure 3-10).

Sometimes a more severe condition called angioedema (swelling in areas of skin, mucous membranes, or internal organs) occurs with urticaria, or it may occur by itself. These reactions may occur in 20% of the population at one time or another.

Cause   It is sometimes difficult to identify the cause, but urticaria and angioedema are often due to a reaction to a particular food, food additive, insect sting, or drug. In any case, the reaction is thought to be related to the release of histamine. In some individuals, exposure to cold, heat, water, or sunlight may also cause urticaria and angioedema. There are also a number of other disorders that can cause these reactions, including Hodgkin's disease, systemic lupus erythematosus, and psychogenic disease.

Symptoms   The main symptom of urticaria is a rash. Itchy, raised white lumps surrounded by an area of red inflammation appear. These lesions vary in size, and large ones may merge into large patches. Angioedema produces sudden swellings in the skin, throat, and other areas.

Prevention   Avoidance of allergens, if possible, is the best means of prevention.

FIGURE 3-10 Urticaria.

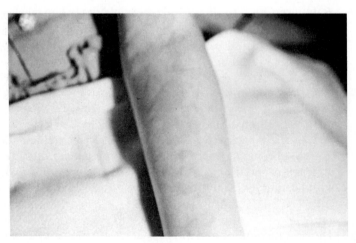

Treatment Antihistamines can ease the itching and swelling for every kind of urticaria. Medicated lotions can also reduce the discomfort from itching.

ASTHMA

Asthma attacks can be very terrifying experiences for everyone involved because of the difficulty the victim has in breathing. Spasms of the bronchial tubes, increased mucus secretion, and swelling of the mucous membranes are responsible for the airway obstruction.

Extrinsic asthma begins in childhood and is usually accompanied by other allergies, such as allergic rhinitis. In *intrinsic* asthma, which is more common in adults, no extrinsic allergen can be identified. Most of these cases are preceded by a severe respiratory infection. About one in 10 children experiences asthma as does one in 20 of the general population. It can strike at any age, but half of all cases occur in children under age 10 years, and it affects twice as many boys as girls in this age group. When it occurs in the 10- to 30-year age group, the incidence is equal among the sexes.

Cause A predisposition for asthma seems to be inherited, since three fourths of children with two asthmatic parents have the disorder, and about one third of asthmatic children share the disease with at least one other member of the family. Extrinsic asthma attacks are brought on by exposure to allergens, whereas attacks of intrinsic asthma can be due to a number of factors, including emotional stress, fatigue, endocrine changes, temperature and humidity changes, and exposure to noxious fumes. Many asthmatics have both intrinsic and extrinsic asthma.

Symptoms Asthma attacks may begin abruptly or insidiously. An acute attack leads to sudden difficulties in breathing, wheezing, tightness in the chest, and a cough with thick, clear or yellow sputum. The victims may be unable to speak and feel as if they are suffocating. If the attack comes on gradually, these symptoms are mild at first but may progress to become as severe as the acute attack. Without treatment, the disease can lead to respiratory failure and death.

Prevention In extrinsic asthma, avoidance of known allergens is the best prevention. For intrinsic asthma, predisposing factors need to be avoided or removed as much as possible.

DID YOU KNOW?

Relief Is a Spray Away

Doctors have been prescribing a corticosteroid nasal spray for hay fever, and sufferers are finding it to be effective in reducing their symptoms. It takes a week or so before the effects are evident, but this spray does not have the rebound effect of over-the-counter sprays. Corticosteroid sprays do not have the steroid side effects, since they act only on the nasal tissue and mucus production.

Treatment   Acute attacks may be relieved by a number of drugs. For persistent asthma, adrenocortical hormones may be required. These hormones provide dramatic relief but cannot be used on a long-term basis because of dangerous side effects. Sedatives and expectorants are sometimes used. Controlling the predisposing factors and removing allergens is considered to be the best treatment.

AUTOIMMUNITY

RHEUMATOID ARTHRITIS

Rheumatoid arthritis is a chronic systemic inflammatory disease that primarily attacks peripheral joints and surrounding muscles, tendons, ligaments, and blood vessels. The disease generally progresses slowly but is potentially crippling, and 10% of its victims suffer total disability.

One of the distinguishing characteristics of the disease is the tendency for the pain that occurs as a result of the inflammation to fluctuate in severity, at times even disappearing altogether for a time (spontaneous remission). This characteristic has resulted in many claims of miraculous cures by different methods when in fact the "cure" received credit for what was a natural decrease in pain or natural remission at an opportune time. Many unscrupulous quacks have taken advantage of this phenomenon to promote their worthless products.

The disease occurs worldwide but is found three times as often in women as in men. Although rheumatoid arthritis can occur at any age, it generally appears in women between the ages of 30 and 60. More than 6.5 million people are affected in the United States.

Cause   The cause is unknown. However, the most widely held theory is that it is an autoimmune disease. The belief is that the changes in the joints are related to an antigen-antibody reaction that is poorly understood. Individuals who get rheumatoid arthritis are believed to have a genetic susceptibility.

Symptoms   Rheumatoid arthritis develops insidiously with nonspecific symptoms. These include fatigue, malaise, anorexia, persistent low-grade fever, weight loss, lymphadenopathy, and vague joint pain. Later, more specific symptoms appear in affected joints. They may stiffen after use and become tender and painful. At first the pain occurs only upon moving the joint, but eventually it is present even at rest. As the disease progresses, joint function diminishes. Deformities are common: joints may swell and wrists and fingers assume unnatural positions (Figure 3-11). The most common overt sign is the gradual appearance of rheumatoid nodules, usually in pressure areas. Inflammation of the blood vessels can lead to skin lesions and leg ulcers. Other complications of rheumatoid arthritis include osteoporosis, myositis, cardiopulmonary lesions, lymphadenopathy, and peripheral neuritis.

Prevention   None known at present.

Treatment   No modern drug has proved as effective for relieving the pain and inflammation of rheumatoid arthritis as aspirin. Unfortunately, many individuals cannot tolerate

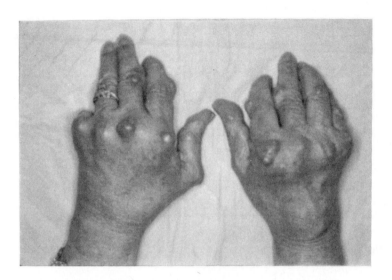

FIGURE 3-11   Rheumatoid arthritis.

aspirin and develop stomach problems. Nonsteroidal anti-inflammatory drugs (NSAIDS) have been effective but may also cause stomach problems. Corticosteroids are very effective but have prohibitive side effects. Gold salts and immunosuppressives are used when other therapies are not effective. Methotrexate, a drug originally used in cancer chemotherapy, has been found to be effective, in much smaller doses, for rheumatoid arthritis but is generally a second-line choice. Rest is of great importance during the acute phase, with 8 to 10 hours of sleep every night and frequent rest periods between daily activities. Physiotherapy helps to restore function and prevent crippling deformities. In advanced disease, surgical repair may be necessary.

LUPUS ERYTHEMATOSUS

This chronic inflammatory disorder of the connective tissues appears in two forms, cutaneous and systemic. Cutaneous lupus erythematosus is a mild form that affects only the skin, while the systemic kind affects the skin and a number of organ systems and can be fatal. Systemic lupus erythematosus (SLE) resembles rheumatoid arthritis in that there are times of complete remission and at different times the symptoms may be mild or severe.

The disease occurs eight times more frequently in women than in men, and this increases to 15 times more often for women during childbearing years. The disease is found worldwide but is more prevalent among Asians and blacks.

Cause   Physical or mental stress, streptococcal or viral infections, exposure to sunlight or ultraviolet light, immunization, pregnancy, and abnormal estrogen metabolism may make a person more susceptible to SLE. Individuals who develop cutaneous lupus erythematosus go on to SLE in about 5% of the cases. The exact cause of these diseases is unknown, but evidence suggests an autoimmune defect.

Symptoms   There are a variety of symptoms that may occur in individuals with SLE. They may appear suddenly or slowly and, in 90% of patients, are similar to arthritis symptoms. Other symptoms include fever, weight loss, malaise, fatigue, and skin rashes. A butterfly rash over the nose and cheeks occurs in less than 50% of the patients (Figure 3-12). Skin lesions generally appear in areas exposed to light. Individuals who have the more serious form of the disease can develop myocarditis, renal involvement leading to kidney failure, convulsive disorders, and other complications that can lead to death. In cutaneous lupus erythematosus, there are raised, red, scaling plaques that, if not treated, can lead to scarring and permanent disfigurement. These lesions can appear anywhere on the body, but they usually erupt on the face, scalp, ears, neck, and arms.

Prevention   None known at present.

Treatment   If the disease is mild, little or no treatment is required. For the systemic form, corticosteroids are the treatment of choice. Some individuals who are particularly sensitive to light need to wear protective clothing and use a screening agent when out in the sun.

FIGURE 3-12 Lupus erythematosus.

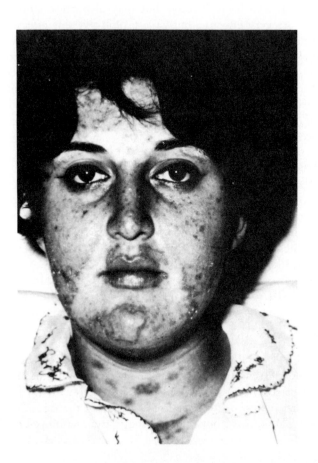

SUMMARY

The human body is protected by *natural immunity* and *acquired immunity*. In natural immunity there are nonspecific and specific defense mechanisms. Nonspecific mechanisms are the external barriers to injury and infection, such as the skin and mucus and the inflammatory response. The body is also able to repair damage to tissue, but there are factors that influence the speed and extent of repair possible. Specific defense mechanisms are composed of antibody-mediated and cell-mediated responses. B cells, T cells, and complement are all active in the immune response to infection.

There are four kinds of acquired immunity. Acquired active natural immunity is present after an individual has been exposed to a disease and the body has learned to produce antibodies. Acquired active artificial immunity occurs when an individual has been vaccinated with a disease agent. Acquired passive natural immunity results from the passage of antibodies from the mother to the fetus or baby. Finally, acquired passive artificial immunity is a result of inoculation with antibodies.

The immune system sometimes malfunctions, and this leads to conditions referred to as hypersensitivity and autoimmune disorders. The most common hypersensitivity disorders are allergic rhinitis, urticaria and angioedema, and asthma. Two of the most common autoimmune disorders are rheumatoid arthritis and lupus erythematosus.

QUESTIONS FOR REVIEW

1. What are the external barriers to infection in natural, nonspecific immunity?
2. How do the external barriers protect us from disease?
3. What do the "friendly" bacteria do to protect us from disease?
4. What produces the inflammatory response?
5. What are the signs of inflammation?
6. Explain what occurs during the inflammatory response.
7. What is chemotaxis?
8. What are the principal chemical mediators of the inflammatory response?
9. How does interferon work to assist the body in the inflammatory response?
10. What is complement?
11. What are inflammatory exudates, and how do they perform in the inflammatory response?
12. When does resolution occur, and when do regeneration and repair occur in the inflammatory response?
13. What factors cause a difference in the time required for healing?
14. How are humoral and cell-mediated immunity different?
15. What occurs during the combined immune response?
16. What is the difference between acquired active natural immunity and acquired active artificial immunity?
17. What is the difference between acquired passive natural immunity and acquired passive artificial immunity?
18. How are *autoimmune* and *hypersensitivity* defined?
19. What are the characteristics of allergic rhinitis, urticaria, angioedema, and asthma?
20. What are common allergens or risk factors, symptoms, prevention, and treatment for

Allergic rhinitis?

Urticaria and angioedema?

Asthma?

21. What are the characteristics of rheumatoid arthritis and lupus erythematosus?
22. What are the risk factors, symptoms, prevention, and treatment for
    Rheumatoid arthritis?
    Lupus erythematosus?

FURTHER READING

Allison, Malorye. "The Down Side of NSAIDS." *Harvard Health Letter,* Nov. '90, 3-5.

Ben-Chetrit, E. "Lucky Lady". *New England Journal of Medicine,* Mar., '93, 328 9:636-639.

Benzaia, Diana. "New Ways to Fight Allergies." *Consumers Digest,* May-June '89, 18: 56-59.

Bernstein, JA. "Allergic Rhinitis. Helping Patients Lead an Unrestricted Life. *Postgraduate Medicine,* May 1, '93, 93(6):124-8, 131-2.

Boyd, Robert F. *General Microbiology.* St. Louis: Mosby, 1988.

Brewerton, Derrick A. "Causes of Arthritis," *Lancet,* Nov. 5, '88, 1063-1066.

"Bronchial Inflammation and Asthma Treatment." *Lancet,* Jan. 12, '91, 337:82-83.

Brown, Gregory K., Perry M. Nicassio and Kenneth A. Wallston. "Pain Coping Strategies and Depression in Rheumatoid Arthritis." *Journal of Consulting and Clinical Psychology,* Oct. '89, 57:652-657.

Cervera, R, et al. "Systemic Lupus Erythematosus: Clinical and Immunologic Patterns of Disease Expression in a Cohort of 1,000 Patients." The European Working Party on Systemic Lupus Erythematosus. *Medicine,* (Baltimore) (MNY), Mar. '93, 72(2):113-124.

Cohn, Irun R. "The Self, the World and Autoimmunity." *Scientific American,* Apr. '88, 52-60.

Condemi, John J. "The Autoimmune Diseases." *Journal of the American Medical Association,* Nov 27, '87, 258:2920-2929.

Control of Communicable Disease in Man. Abram S. Benenson, ed. Fifteenth Edition, Washington, D. C.: American Public Health Association, 1990.

Collier, David H. "Gout and Arthritis: Are They Really Affected by Diet?" *Consultant,* May '89, 29:63-69.

Ding, John E. Young and Zanvil A. Cohn. "How Killer Cells Kill." *Scientific American,* Jan. '88, 38-46.

Ershler, WB. "The influence of an Aging Immune System on Cancer Incidence and Progression." *Journal of Gerontology,* Jan. '93, 48(1):B3-7.

"Fighting Hay Fever." *Consumers' Research Magazine,* May '89, 72:30-33.

Gamlin, Linda. "The Human Immune System." *New Scientist,* Mar. 10, '88, 117:151-154.

Gantz, Nelson M., et al. "Questions and Answers on Sinusitis." *Patient Care,* Aug. 14, '88, 22:53-65.

"Gout." *Harvard Medical School Health Letter,* Apr. '89, 14:1-3.

Harris, Edward D., Jr. "Rheumatoid Arthritis: Pathophysiology and Implications for Therapy." *New England Journal of Medicine,* May 3, '90, 322:1277-1289.

Jacobs, Robert L., Eli O. Meltzer, John C. Selner and Raymond G. Slavin. "Rhinitis: Not Just Hay Fever." *Patient Care,* Mar. 30, '89, 23:168-178.

Kaliner, Michael, et al. "Rhinitis and Asthma." *Journal of the American Medical Association,* Nov. 27, '87, 258:2851-2873.

Lockshin, Michael D. "Therapy for Systemic Lupus Erythematosus." *New England Journal of Medicine,* Jan. 17, '91, 324:189-191.

McCarthy, Paul. "Wheezing or Breezing through Exercise-Induced Asthma." *Physician and Sports Medicine,* July '89, 17:125-130.

Marcos, A., et al. "Evaluation of Immunocompetence and Nutritional Status in Patients with Bulimia Nervosa." Jan. '93, 57(1):65-69.

Marwick, Charles. "As Immune System Yields Its Secrets, New Strategies against Disease Emerge." *Journal of the American Medical Association,* Nov. 24, '89, 262:2786-2787.

Marx, Jean L. "What T Cells See and How They See It." *Science,* Nov. 11, '88, 242: 863-865.

Mazow, Jack B. "Allergic Rhinitis: Formulating the Best Treatment Plan." *Consultant,* Apr. '89, 29:143-147.

McCance, Kathryn L. and Sue E. Huether. *Pathophysiology: The Biologic Basis for Disease in Adults and Children.* St. Louis: Mosby, 1990.

Meenan, Robert F., et al. "The Stability of Health Status in Rheumatoid Arthritis: A Five-Year Study of Patients with Established Disease." *American Journal of Public Health,* Nov. '88, 78:1484-1487.

Molfino, Nestor A., Luis J. Nannini, Alberto N. Martelli and Arthur S. Slutsky. "Respiratory Arrest in Near-Fatal Asthma." *New England Journal of Medicine,* Jan. 31, '91, 324:285-288.

Murray, et al. *Medical Microbiology.* St. Louis: Mosby, 1990.

Norman, Philip S. "Allergic Rhinitis; Combined Therapy for More Satisfactory Control." *Consultant,* Feb. '88, 28:69-74.

Owens, Gregory R. "Exercise-Induced Asthma: Optimal Testing Methods and Preventive Measures." *Consultant,* Nov. '90, 30:30-35.

Rennie, John. "The Body against Itself; Trends in Immunology." *Scientific American,* Dec. '90, 263:106-115.

Robertson, Miranda. "The New Biology of Immune Recognition." *Nature,* Nov. 22, '90, 348:281-282.

Roitt, Ivan. *Essential Immunology.* Boston: Blackwell Scientific Publications, 1990.

"Sinusitis: When the Holes in Your Head Hurt." *Current Health 2,* Jan. '88, 14:16-18.

Spencer-Green, G. "Drug Treatment of Arthritis. Update on Conventional and Less Conventional Methods. *Post-graduate Medicine,* May 15, 1993. 93(7):129-140.

Stehlin, Dori. "How to Take Your Medicine; Nonsteroidal Anti-inflammatory Drugs." *FDA Consumer,* June '90, 24:32-35.

Stehlin Dori. "Living with Lupus," *FDA Consumer,* Dec.-Jan. '89, 23:8-12.

Sternberg, EM, GP Chrousos, RL Wilder and PW Gold. "The Stress Response and the Regulation of Inflammatory Disease." *Annals of Internal Medicine,* Nov. 15, '92, 117:(10), 854-856.

Stinson, Stephen. "Better Understanding of Arthritis Leading to New Drugs to Treat It." *Chemical & Engineering News,* Oct. 16, '89, 67:37-51.

Touger-Decker, Riva. "Nutritional Considerations in Rheumatoid Arthritis." *Journal of the American Dietetic Association,* Mar. '88, 88:327-331.

White MV and MA Kaliner. "Mediators of Allergic Rhinitis." *Journal of Allergy Clinical Immunology.* Oct. '92, 90 (4 pt 2):699-704.

Unit

2

Infectious Diseases

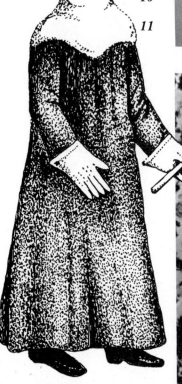

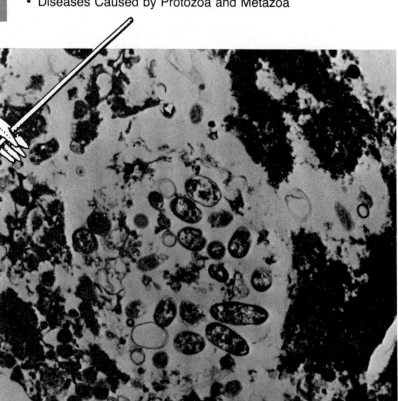

(above) Doctor's protective wear from 14th century plague epidemic.

(right) Electron micrograph of *Legionella pneumophila*

Since the relationship between disease and bacteria was discovered by Pasteur, Lister, and Koch in the nineteenth century, great strides have been made in the fight against infectious disease. Effective treatment and cures have been found for many diseases that at one time led to much suffering, scarring, crippling, and death.

More important than being able to treat and cure infectious disease, however, is the ability to prevent it from occurring. Jenner's discovery of the smallpox vaccination in the eighteenth century provided the means for preventing and eventually eradicating this disfiguring and potentially fatal disease, and today we are able to prevent infection with a number of diseases by vaccination or inoculation.

In the past three decades, doctors, scientists, and health educators have begun to focus their attention, not on what causes people to get sick, but what causes some people, exposed to the same diseases, to stay well. This change in focus has coincided with rapid development in the science of immunology. Increasing evidence of a mind-body link in the development of disease and disorders has led to a new disciplined psychoneuroimmunology, mentioned in Chapter 2.

All persons may be created equal in their right to life, liberty and the pursuit of happiness but they are not created or born equal in biochemical makeup. About 10% of the population never have a cold. In any disease epidemic some individuals escape the disease even though they have never had an apparent infection or been vaccinated against it. The immune system provides protection from disease for most people most of the time, and recent research indicates there may be techniques by which we can strengthen immune response so it can provide more protection more of the time.

One way to prevent both infectious and noninfectious disease is emphasized here rather than listed under prevention for each disease. It is something each individual can do to have less illness: Anything persons can do to achieve a more healthful lifestyle will increase their resistance to disease. The factors involved in improving resistance are shown in the illustration below.

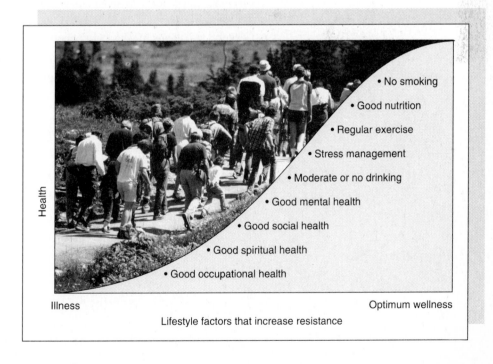

Lifestyle factors that increase resistance

Bacterial Diseases Acquired through the Respiratory Route

Chapter 4

OBJECTIVES

1 Explain the positive and negative effects that lifestyle can have on our susceptibility to disease.

2 Identify common upper respiratory infections.

3 Identify the two most common forms of pneumonia.

4 State environmental conditions conducive to Legionnaires' disease.

5 Discuss the connection between streptococcal sore throat, scarlet fever, rheumatic fever, and acute poststreptococcal glomerulonephritis (APSGN).

6 Describe the stages of whooping cough.

7 Explain why diphtheria may still be a problem today.

8 Explain the processes involved in primary and secondary tuberculosis.

9 Apply techniques to prevent the spread of bacterial diseases acquired through the respiratory route.

10 Discuss characteristics, transmission, symptoms, treatment, prevention, and control for bacterial diseases.

RESPIRATORY DISEASES AND DISORDERS

BRIEF REVIEW OF THE RESPIRATORY SYSTEM

Normal respiration requires efficient action of the diaphragm, a clear route to the lungs, healthy bronchial tubes, and effective diffusion of gases (Figure 4-1). Oxygen that is inhaled must be diffused across the alveolar-capillary membrane into the blood; at the same time, carbon dioxide is being diffused from the blood across the same membranes, into the lungs for exhalation.

Air usually enters the body through the nose. During periods of exertion, it may enter through the mouth, but the nose is a preferable point of entry for several reasons. First, the cilia (fine hairs in the nasal cavity) protect against dust and other particles from the air. Next, particles that may slip through the cilia are caught in the thick, sticky, mucous lining of the nasal cavity, allowing only clean air to pass to the lungs. Third, air is warmed in the nasal cavity, and, finally, moisture is added.

Air passes from the nose backward and downward through the pharynx to the larynx. The larynx contains the vocal cords, through which the air passes on its way to the trachea. The trachea branches into the right and left bronchial tubes, which in turn branch into bronchioles, which ultimately end in the alveolar sacs. It is here that the cycle of oxygen diffusion into the blood and CO_2 diffusion out of the blood occurs.

UPPER RESPIRATORY INFECTIONS (URIs)

Infection of the upper respiratory tract is caused most frequently by bacteria and viruses. These infections are generally superficial and may be acute, chronic, or recurrent. Pharyngitis, laryngitis, tonsillitis, and sinusitis are due to infection of the pharynx, larynx, tonsils, and sinuses, respectively (Figure 4-2). An extension into the eustachian tube of the disease agents that cause pharyngitis may lead to *otitis media* (inflammation of the middle ear). The relationship between the pharynx, eustachian tube, and middle ear can be seen in Figures 4-2 and 4-3.

The most important agents of bacterial pharyngitis and laryngitis are streptococci; *Streptococcus aureus* and other disease agents may be involved in sinusitis and *otitis media*. The incubation period for these URIs is short (1 to 2 days) when person-

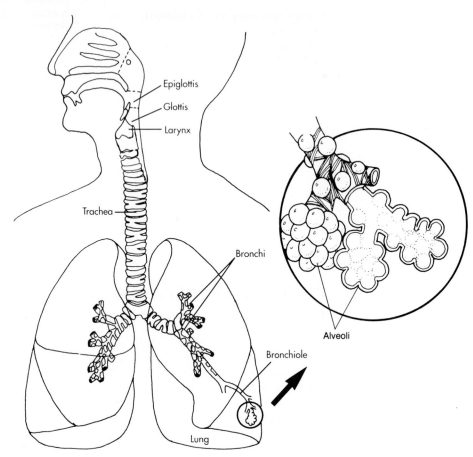

FIGURE 4-1 Respiratory system.

to-person transmission is involved. It is not known how long the infections take to develop if they are endogenous. URIs are communicable as long as they are active. Natural resistance to the disease agents that cause these infections is present in individuals whose mucous membranes are not compromised. Colds and other viral infections, inhalation of toxic vapors or smoke, excessive dryness, and pollen or dust allergies all may predispose an individual to bacterial infections.

Transmission Human beings are the reservoir for the organisms that are most often responsible for URIs. If the infection is transmitted person to person, it is generally by airborne droplets but may also be by direct or indirect contact with secretions from the nose and throat of an infected person.

Symptoms Individuals with pharyngitis experience a sore throat and slight difficulty in swallowing. Laryngitis involves pain in the area of the larynx and hoarseness or loss of voice. In sinusitis, there is pain of the sinuses involved, and otitis media causes earache. Individuals with these infections may also have a low fever, headache, and muscle and joint pain.

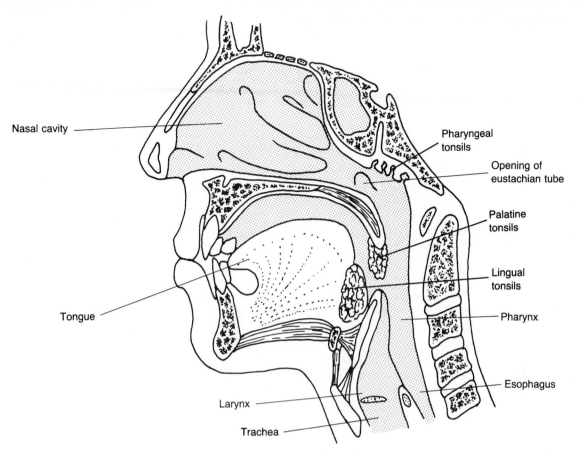

FIGURE 4-2 Upper respiratory system.

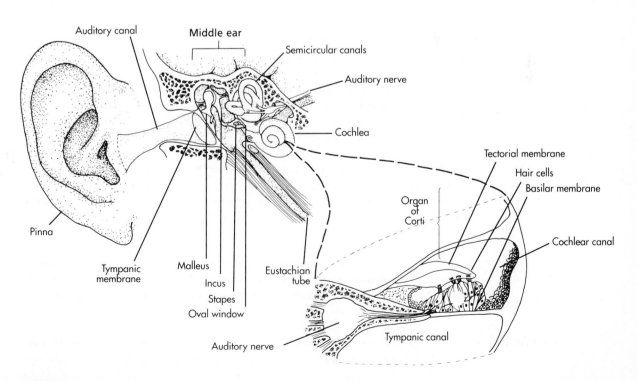

FIGURE 4-3 External, middle, and inner ear.

Prevention Washing the hands regularly, particularly after contact with people during times when these infections are known to be prevalent, is a good preventive measure along with avoidance of predisposing factors mentioned earlier.

Control Those who have an URI need to practice careful personal hygiene, disposing of any contaminated tissues in closed paper or plastic bags and washing their hands frequently and carefully. Drinking or eating utensils should be thoroughly washed.

Treatment Treatment for URIs caused by bacteria is with antibiotics.

PNEUMONIA

Pneumonia and influenza are the only communicable diseases that still hold a place among the top 10 causes of death in the United States. The two are placed together at the number six position on the chart because death from pneumonia is often preceded by influenza. Pneumonia is an acute infection of the lungs and can be caused by many infectious agents. However, bacterial pneumonia is the most common type and is the fifth leading cause of death among the elderly and debilitated.

There are three ways to classify pneumonia: (1) disease agent, (2) location, and (3) type. It may be bronchial, involving the bronchial tubes and alveoli (Figure 4-1); lobular, involving part of a lobe; or lobar, involving the entire lobe (Figure 4-1). Pneumonia is also referred to as primary, resulting from inhalation or aspiration of a pathogen, or secondary, involving spread of bacteria from another location.

Pneumococcal and mycoplasmal pneumonia will be discussed in this chapter and also a type of pneumonia that has been recognized only since 1976, Legionnaires' disease.

PNEUMOCOCCAL PNEUMONIA

Pneumococcal pneumonia, caused by *S. pneumoniae,* is the most common type of pneumonia and is more frequent among the very young and the very old. It is also commonly a cause of death among alcoholics. Pneumococci are natural inhabitants in the upper respiratory tract of healthy persons worldwide. The incubation period is uncertain but is probably 1 to 3 days. With antibiotic therapy, an infected individual will become noninfectious within 24 to 48 hours. Without treatment, the individual will be able to communicate the disease as long as discharges contain virulent pneumococci in significant numbers. Most people have good resistance to the organism, but any factor causing injury to lung tissues may lower that resistance. Viral respiratory infections, chronic lung disease, and exposure to irritants in the air are some factors responsible for lowered resistance.

Transmission Casual contact with an individual who has pneumonia does not generally lead to infection. Transmission occurs by droplet spread, direct oral contact, or indirectly through fomites (articles that have been contaminated with respiratory discharges).

Symptoms The onset of pneumococcal pneumonia is usually sudden, with chills, fever, chest pain, difficult breathing, and cough. The sputum may be bright red or rusty with blood. Pleurisy (inflammation of the external membrane surrounding the lung) may also be present, causing sharp pain during breathing or coughing. In some cases, particularly in the elderly, the onset of pneumonia is more insidious, with X-ray examination producing the first evidence. In children under 2 years of age, vomiting and convulsions may be the initial signs.

Prevention A vaccine is available and is recommended for high-risk individuals, including the elderly, the debilitated, and alcoholics.

Control Generally no measures are necessary unless an outbreak is a threat, in which case, crowding should be avoided, especially in populations with low resistance, such as pediatric wards, geriatric institutions, and military hospitals.

Treatment Penicillin is the drug of choice, but other antibiotics are also effective.

MYCOPLASMAL PNEUMONIA

It is estimated that 20% of all pneumonias are caused by *Mycoplasma pneumoniae*. This small, unusual bacterium is responsible for what has been called walking pneumonia. It is considered a primary atypical pneumonia, pneumonia that begins in the lower respiratory tract and does not produce the typical exudative (fluid-causing) response in the lungs. The disease occurs worldwide, with the greatest incidence during the fall and winter months in temperate climates. Humans are the reservoir of infection. Mycoplasmal pneumonia may be very mild or asymptomatic in children under 5 years and is more frequent among school-age children and young adults. The incubation period is usually about 2 weeks, and the disease is probably most communicable during the first week of apparent illness. Premature infants, those who have chronic debilitating diseases, and those in whom the immune system is compromised are more susceptible to mycoplasmal pneumonia.

Transmission Infection is transferred by direct and indirect contact with respiratory secretions.

Symptoms The onset of mycoplasmal pneumonia is insidious, with headache, malaise, and cough. The cough often occurs in sudden episodes (paroxysms), and there is usually substernal (under the chest bone) pain. The illness lasts from a few days to a month or more, and since symptoms are often mild, the infection may not be recognized as pneumonia. There generally are no complications, and fatalities are rare.

Treatment The mycoplasma bacteria are resistant to penicillin, but erythromycin or tetracycline is effective in treating the disease.

Prevention No vaccines are available. Avoidance of crowding in living and sleeping quarters, especially in institutions, barracks, and on shipboard can decrease the risk.

Control Investigation of contacts may identify cases of treatable disease. Proper sanitary measures including disposal of articles contaminated with respiratory secretions will help to control the spread of the infection.

LEGIONNAIRES' DISEASE

An epidemic of respiratory illness swept through a group of people attending a state convention of American Legionnaires in Philadelphia during the summer of 1976. Before it ended, the epidemic took 29 lives and hospitalized 182 people of the 5000 or more who had gathered for the convention. Epidemiologists worked around the clock in a search for the cause of the illness and death. Finally, bacteria were discovered in the cooling towers of the hotel headquarters for the convention and were identified as *Legionella pneumophila*.

Although the organism had not been named before this time, it had been described as early as 1947 and probably had been the unrecognized cause of some cases of pneumonia for many years. Other types of *L. pneumophila* have been responsible for milder forms of respiratory illness. The organism thrives in warm, moist conditions, and its reservoir is in soil and water. The disease has been diagnosed in most states in the United States, as seen in Figure 4-4, and in some foreign countries. Outbreaks are recognized more often in the summer and autumn. The incubation period is 2 to 10 days, most often, 5 to 6 days. Susceptibility to the organism is general, but the disease is uncommon in those under 20 years of age. Mortality rates in Legionnaires' disease have run as high as 15% in hospitalized patients. Generally they occur among those whose immunity is compromised.

Transmission Outbreaks of this disease have revolved around faulty air cooling systems, cooling towers, or excavation sites. In these conditions, the organism is transmitted by air from the soil or water where it resides. Humans become infected through inhalation

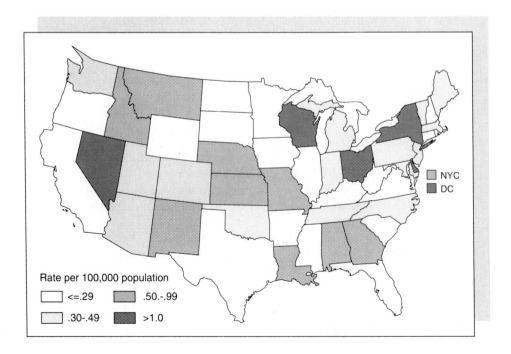

FIGURE 4-4 Legionnaires' disease—reported cases, per 100,000 population, United States, 1989.

Rate per 100,000 population

- <=.29
- .30-.49
- .50-.99
- >1.0

of the bacteria that have become airborne. There is no evidence of person-to-person transmission.

Symptoms   Onset of the disease may be gradual or sudden. Nonspecific symptoms appear first, including diarrhea, anorexia, malaise, myalgias, and generalized weakness, headache, recurrent chills, and an unremitting fever that may reach 105° F within 12 to 48 hours. After this, a nonproductive cough develops that may eventually produce grayish, blood-streaked sputum. Other characteristic symptoms include nausea, vomiting, disorientation, pleuritic chest pain, and, in 50% of patients, bradycardia (slow heartbeat). Complications include congestive heart failure, acute respiratory failure, renal failure, and shock, any of which can be fatal.

Prevention   No immunization is available. Cooling towers and water supplies that have been implicated need to be disinfected.

Control   The source of infection needs to be identified when there is a cluster of cases. Since there is no evidence of person-to-person transmission, isolation of individuals with the disease is not considered necessary.

Treatment   Penicillin is ineffective against *L. pneumophila*. Erythromycin is the drug of choice, and if it is not effective alone, rifampin can be added. Tetracycline and rifampin may also be used together.

STREPTOCOCCAL SORE THROAT

Ninety-five percent of all bacterial sore throats are caused by *S. pyogenes*. Sore throats are most common in children 5 to 10 years old and from October to April. Up to 20% of schoolchildren are thought to be carriers. Otitis media (middle ear infection) or acute sinusitis are the most frequent complications. Later sequelae include rheumatic fever, glomerulonephritis, and rheumatic heart disease.

Transmission   Transmission is by direct or intimate contact with an individual with active pharyngitis or a carrier. Ingestion of contaminated food may lead to sudden outbreaks of streptococcal sore throat.

Symptoms   A temperature of 101 to 104° F, severe sore throat, swollen glands and tonsils, malaise and weakness, anorexia, and occasional abdominal discomfort are included in the symptoms. Up to 40% of small children have symptoms too mild for diagnosis, and all symptoms that do occur tend to disappear in a week.

Prevention   Although strep sore throat is generally severe enough for the individual to seek medical attention, symptoms may be milder in children. Any child who has a sore throat that is constant, and is accompanied by fever and other signs of infection, should be seen by a doctor. The public needs to be educated about the possible sequelae of strep sore throat. Information on means of transmission should be widely published. Avoidance of close contact with infected persons and proper food handling are the best means of prevention.

Control   In an outbreak of strep sore throat, the source of infection and manner of spread should be investigated, since these can often be traced to a carrier. Milk and food supplies should be checked for contamination. In special circumstances, antibiotics may be given prophylactically.

FIGURE 4-5 White strawberry tongue symptomatic of scarlet fever.

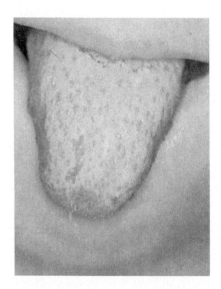

FIGURE 4-6 Red strawberry tongue symptomatic of scarlet fever.

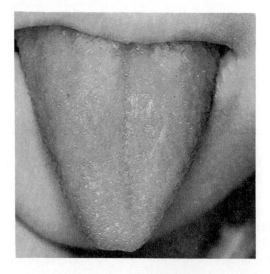

Treatment Penicillin (or erythromycin if the patient is allergic to penicillin) should be administered for 10 days. If the treatment is given within the first 24 to 48 hours, the illness may be milder, and the risk of complications is diminished. Bed rest is also recommended.

SCARLET FEVER

Scarlet fever is generally preceded by streptococcal sore throat. It occurs when the pathogenic organism *S. pyogenes* produces erythrogenic (red-causing) toxin. Many individuals are immune to this toxin, but if they are not, then scarlet fever is the result. The incidence and severity of scarlet fever have been declining, probably as a result of the frequent use of antibiotics. Penicillin and other antibiotics are extremely effective in destroying the streptococcal organisms. Humans are the reservoir for the streptococci that are responsible for scarlet fever. The incubation period is rarely more than 3 days. Communicability generally ends after 24 to 48 hours of antibiotic treatment. Almost everyone is susceptible, although some individuals may have immunity, as noted above.

Transmission Transmission is by droplet spread, direct contact, and indirect contact with temporarily contaminated environmental sources, including milk or food.

Symptoms The infected individual has a sore throat, rash, nausea, vomiting, and fever. A distinctive symptom for scarlet fever is the strawberry tongue, which at first has red papillae showing through a furry white coat (Figure 4-5). In two or three days the tongue loses the white coat and gradually becomes red (Figure 4-6). The rash is fine, blanches on pressure, and resembles sunburn with goosebumps. It usually

FIGURE 4-7 Desquamation in final stages of scarlet fever on hand and finger tips.

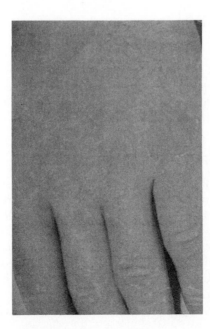
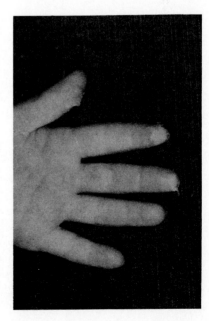

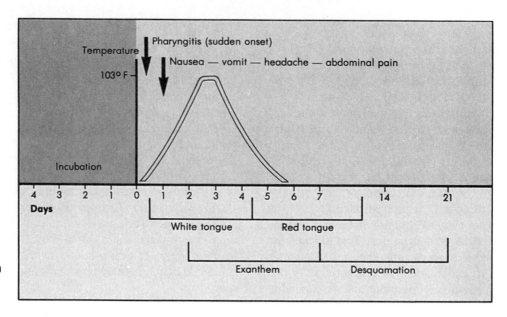

FIGURE 4-8 Evolution of signs and symptoms of scarlet fever.

appears first on the upper chest, then spreads to the neck, abdomen, legs, and arms, sparing the soles and palms. The cheeks are flushed, with pallor (paleness) around the mouth. In Figure 4–7, the desquamation (shedding of skin) that occurs during convalescence can be seen. Figure 4–8 shows how the signs and symptoms of scarlet fever develop.

Treatment   Penicillin is the drug of choice. Streptococci are also susceptible to erythromycin and clindamycin. Adequate levels of antibiotics need to be maintained for 10 days.

Prevention   Preventive methods are the same as for the other streptococcal diseases already discussed.

Control   Isolation is not necessary if antibiotics are given immediately. Disinfection of all items contaminated with purulent discharge, and other hygienic measures, will control the infection.

RHEUMATIC FEVER

Rheumatic fever is a disease of childhood that does not stand alone. It is always preceded by another streptococcal infection, often strep sore throat, and it may lead to heart or kidney disease. As with many other bacterial diseases, it is no longer as serious as it once was and is becoming rare since the availability and use of antibiotics. However, because not everyone gets treatment for a sore throat and because the symptoms of rheumatic fever may be mild enough to go unnoticed, it is still a potentially dangerous disease. It is possible for damage to be done to the heart that may not become apparent until much later in life.

Why infection with *S. pyogenes* sometimes leads from strep sore throat to rheumatic fever to rheumatic heart disease or to other tissue damage is not known. It is thought that altered host resistance and a hypersensitivity reaction (antibodies manufactured to combat the streptococci attacking the heart and joints) are factors. Rheumatic fever is more prevalent in some families and in lower socioeconomic groups, perhaps because of malnutrition and crowded living conditions. It is a disease of childhood but is often recurrent, especially without adequate treatment.

Transmission   Rheumatic fever cannot be transmitted from one person to another, since it is not a bacterial infection but a hypersensitivity reaction. If the person still harbors the streptococcal organism that preceded the rheumatic fever, then transmission of that organism could occur. (See the information on strep sore throat.)

Symptoms   Fever and migratory joint pain are most commonly the early symptoms of rheumatic fever. Some individuals have the infection but do not suffer joint pain. Other symptoms include abdominal pain, a rash, nodules under the skin, cardiac involvement, and up to 6 months later, chorea (involuntary muscular twitching of face or limbs).

Prevention   The public needs to be educated on the relationship between a streptococcal infection and rheumatic fever. The best prevention for rheumatic fever is immediate antibiotic treatment for any streptococcal infection.

Control   In recurrent episodes of rheumatic fever in a family or in epidemic situations, an investigation needs to be carried out to find all carriers and administer proper treatment. Contact investigation (finding those known to have been exposed to the disease and testing each one for possible infection) should be pursued. Any unusual grouping of cases should be investigated for the possibility of contaminated milk or foods. In some circumstances, penicillin or another antibiotic may be given prophylactically (to prevent infection).

Treatment   Immediate treatment of the primary infection with antibiotics will eradicate the organism, relieve the symptoms, and prevent development of hypersensitivity-related complications. Penicillin is the drug of choice, but for those allergic to it, erythromycin can be used.

ACUTE POSTSTREPTOCOCCAL GLOMERULONEPHRITIS (APSGN)

This inflammation of the glomeruli (Figures 4-9 and 4-10) in the kidneys follows a streptococcal infection of the respiratory tract or, less often, a skin infection such as impetigo. APSGN is most common in children ages 6 to 10 years but can occur at any age. Up to 95% of children and up to 70% of adults recover completely; the rest may progress to chronic renal failure within months. APSGN is thought to occur as a result of the deposition of circulating streptococcal antigen-antibody complexes on the membranes of glomerular capillaries. The disease usually appears 1 to 2 weeks after the streptococcal infection.

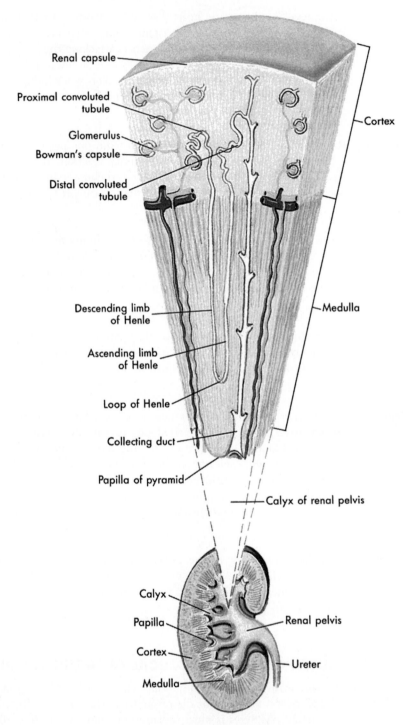

Renal capsule

Proximal convoluted tubule

Glomerulus

Bowman's capsule

Distal convoluted tubule

Cortex

Descending limb of Henle

Ascending limb of Henle

Loop of Henle

Collecting duct

Papilla of pyramid

Medulla

Calyx of renal pelvis

Calyx

Papilla

Cortex

Medulla

Renal pelvis

Ureter

FIGURE 4-9 Wedge shows position of glomeruli in kidney.

Transmission   There is no person-to-person transmission of this disease.

Symptoms   The most common symptoms are fever, nausea, cocoa-colored urine, hypertension, diminished urine output, edema (water retention), and fatigue.

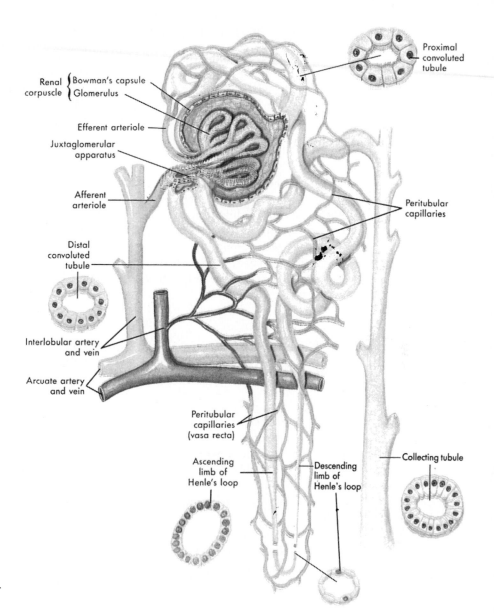

FIGURE 4-10 A glomerulus of a single nephron in the kidney.

Prevention   Avoidance of streptococcal infections by having a healthy lifestyle in order to have good resistance to disease is the only means of prevention.

Control   The source of the original streptococcal infection should be identified and measures taken to control that infection, usually streptococcal sore throat or impetigo (discussed in Chapter 6).

Treatment   Treatment to relieve symptoms and prevent complications may include bed rest, restrictions of fluid and dietary sodium, correction of electrolyte imbalance, diuretics, and an antihypertensive.

WHOOPING COUGH (PERTUSSIS)

Whooping cough is an extremely contagious respiratory infection common to children throughout the world. Since the 1940s there has been a decrease in incidence and deaths from the disease because of immunization and aggressive diagnosis and treatment. However, in some countries, the incidence has increased in recent years due to fear of vaccine-associated complications which are rare, but were given headlines in newspapers. Epidemic cycles of pertussis tend to run every 2 to 4 years, and the epidemic incidence is highest in the winter and early spring.

Bordetella pertussis, a bacillus, causes the disease. The mortality from pertussis is usually a result of secondary pneumonia in children under age 1 year, but it can also be dangerous to the elderly. Humans are the only reservoir for the organism. Whooping cough is highly communicable during late incubation and in the catarrhal stage (when mucous membranes of the head and throat are inflamed). Once the cough is present, communicability declines until in about 3 weeks there is little danger to contacts even though the cough persists. If treated with antibiotics, the communicable stage lasts only 5 to 7 days. One attack generally confers prolonged immunity.

Transmission

Transmission is primarily by direct contact with airborne droplets from respiratory discharges of infected persons. It may also be indirect from contact with contaminated objects.

Symptoms

There are three stages of whooping cough: the catarrhal (mentioned earlier), paroxysmal, and convalescent. The *catarrhal stage* has an insidious (cunning or sneaky) onset, and the symptoms resemble a cold. They may include an irritating cough, particularly at night; this may be accompanied by anorexia, sneezing, listlessness, infected conjunctiva, and sometimes a low-grade fever. The cough becomes progressively more irritating and violent and eventually paroxysmal (sudden and periodic).

This second or *paroxysmal stage* produces spasmodic and recurrent coughing that may expel tenacious mucus. The characteristic cough ends in a loud, high-pitched inspiratory whoop, and vomiting can occur because of choking on mucus. The coughing can be violent enough to cause complications such as nosebleed, detached retina, and hernias. During this stage, the individual is highly susceptible to secondary infections such as otitis media (middle ear infection), encephalopathy (brain damage), or pneumonia. The second stage lasts about 3 weeks or until the paroxysmal coughing becomes less violent and less frequent.

The third stage is the *convalescent stage*. The cough may last 1 to 2 months, and even a mild upper respiratory infection may trigger it again. A summary of characteristics of the three stages is found in Figure 4-11.

Prevention

Active immunization is available and should be administered at 2 to 3 months of age. A schedule is recommended for booster shots of the vaccine and should be followed to provide the best immunity. The vaccine for pertussis is generally given in combination with that for diphtheria and tetanus and is referred to as DTP.

Stage	Incubation	Catarrhal	Paroxysmal	Convalescent
Duration	7-10 days	1-2 weeks	2-4 weeks	3-4 weeks (or longer)
Symptoms	None	Rhinorrhea, malaise, fever, sneezing, anorexia	Repetitive cough with whoops, vomiting, leukocytosis	Diminished paroxysmal cough, development of secondary complications (pneumonia, seizures, encephalopathy)

FIGURE 4-11 Duration and symptoms for the incubation period and three stages of whooping cough.

Control   Suspected cases should be isolated, particularly from young children and infants, until antibiotic therapy has been administered for at least 5 days. Close contacts who have not received the four DTP doses or have not received a DTP dose in the past 3 years, and are under 7 years of age, should be given a dose as soon after exposure as possible. Prophylactic administration of gamma globulin may be indicated for susceptible children and adults who are exposed to whooping cough. Investigation of contacts should be performed to identify undiagnosed cases for proper treatment.

Treatment   Treatment of whooping cough is now vigorous and thorough. Infants are hospitalized, often in the intensive care unit (ICU), and fluid and electrolytes are administered. Nutritional supplements where needed, codeine and mild sedation to decrease coughing, oxygen therapy, and antibiotics may be used, depending on the case. Antibiotics are not very effective in relieving symptoms but do shorten the period of communicability.

DIPHTHERIA

At one time diphtheria was one of the leading causes of death in all parts of the world. Since the 1920s, when large-scale immunization of children began in the United States, the death rate has dropped dramatically, and the disease is uncommon in developed nations. Sporadic outbreaks continue to occur in unimmunized groups. Diphtheria is still an important cause of disease and death in developing nations, particularly among children.

Corynebacterium diphtheriae is the organism responsible for diphtheria. Unlike many of the other pathogenic organisms, this one does not invade other areas or tissues of the body but stays in the upper respiratory region. Here it produces a deadly exotoxin that irritates the tissue, producing a pseudomembrane (false membrane) which, along with swelling, may occlude the air passages, leading to death by suffocation. The toxin also spreads through the body, causing other serious symptoms, and often death, from its effects on the heart, nerves, and kidneys.

The reservoir of infection for the diphtheria organism is humans. The incubation period is generally 2 to 5 days, occasionally longer. The communicable period is variable, lasting up to 4 weeks, but the carrier state may persist for a lifetime. Infants born of immune mothers usually have passive resistance for up to 6 months. An attack of diphtheria does not always confer immunity.

Transmission   Means of transmission are by direct contact, droplet spread, and indirect contact with articles soiled with discharges from infected persons. Milk that has been contaminated after pasteurization or raw milk may serve as a vehicle also.

Symptoms   The characteristic symptom of diphtheria is the thick, patchy, grayish green membrane that forms over the mucous membranes of the pharynx, larynx, tonsils, soft palate, and nose. Other symptoms include fever, sore throat, a rasping cough, hoarseness, and other symptoms similar to croup. If the pseudomembrane causes airway obstruction, then there is difficulty in breathing and possible suffocation if the disease is untreated. Complications include myocarditis, neurologic involvement, and kidney involvement.

Prevention   The only effective means of prevention is by a community program of active immunization with diphtheria toxoid. Generally it is combined with tetanus toxoid and pertussis vaccine (DTP). Children should be fully immunized before entering school. The exact schedule is up to the physician, but the first injection is generally given 2 to 3 months after birth, with one to four more being given at intervals. Special efforts should be made to see that persons who are at higher risk, such as health workers, are fully immunized and receive a booster dose every 10 years.

Control   There should be strict isolation for anyone ill with pharyngeal diphtheria. All articles that come in contact with the individual who is sick should be disinfected. Any adult contacts who are food handlers should be screened to be sure they are not carriers. Antibiotics should be given prophylactically to nonimmunized contacts of the individual. Future control of diphtheria depends on continuing the education of people everywhere as to the necessity of adequate artificial active immunization.

Treatment   Diphtheria antitoxin is administered, antibiotics are used to destroy the organism, and measures taken to prevent complications.

TUBERCULOSIS (TB)

Tuberculosis is an ancient, worldwide disease, sometimes acute, more often chronic, caused by *Mycobacterium tuberculosis,* or tubercle bacillus. This bacillus has been found in Egyptian mummies from 4000 BC. In the year 1900, two of every 1000 Americans died of tuberculosis, and 20 were ill with the disease. Great strides have been made in the prevention and control of this disease, but today, even in the United States, there are still some 30,000 cases of TB reported annually, and the numbers are increasing. It is estimated that 10 million people are infected with the tubercle bacillus in the United States. Individuals with AIDS are very susceptible to TB, and at least one antibiotic-resistant strain has occurred. The case rate by state is shown in Figure 4-12.

TB is primarily a disease of the lungs, but if the organism invades the bloodstream, the liver, brain, urogenital tract, and bone can become infected. Illness and death rates increase with age and, in older persons, are higher in males than in females. There are much higher rates of the disease among the poor and among nonwhite races, as seen in Figure 4-13, and rates in cities are usually higher than in rural areas.

The primary reservoir is in humans, but in some areas it is also present in infected cattle. The incubation of 4 to 12 weeks is longer than for most infectious diseases. TB is communicable as long as the individual has tubercle bacilli in their sputum. The degree of communicability depends upon the intensity of infectious droplet contamination of the air. Susceptibility is general but is influenced by age, sex, race, nutrition, and general health.

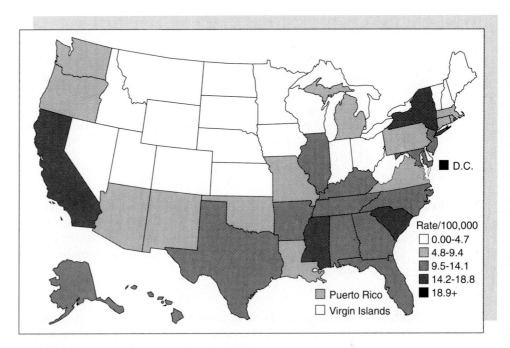

FIGURE 4-12   TB—rates by state, United States, 1989.

FIGURE 4-13   TB—percentage of cases by race and ethnicity, United States, 1989.

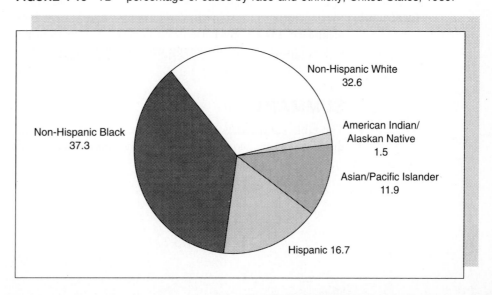

Transmission   Transmission of TB may occur by direct or indirect contact with persons who have active pulmonary lesions, but the usual route is by inhalation of airborne droplets containing the bacilli. Although TB is not as easy to catch as many communicable diseases, prolonged exposure to an unrecognized active case may lead to infection. If there is an active case in a family situation, an army barracks, a college dormitory, or other institutional living arrangement, prolonged exposure may lead to infection of contacts.

Symptoms   In primary TB, there are usually no symptoms. If symptoms do occur, they include fatigue, weakness, anorexia, weight loss, night sweats, and low-grade fever. The initial infection is generally controlled by the body defense mechanism, and the *M. tuberculosis* organisms are encapsulated or "walled up" in the lungs, where they cause no further damage unless something occurs to reduce the host's resistance. Secondary TB or reactivation TB usually occurs late in life or at a time when the adult victim's immune system is compromised. Symptoms of reactivation TB include a cough that produces sputum containing mucus and pus, chest pains, and, occasionally, bloody sputum.

Prevention   Vaccination with BCG (bacillus Calmette-Guérin) vaccine is not used routinely in the United States, since its use prevents Public Health Service tracing of TB outbreaks by skin tests. Improving social conditions that increase the risk of infection with TB and education of the public are the main means of prevention in the United States.

Control   Control of TB in the United States has evolved by a number of measures. These include finding and treating TB as soon as possible; investigation of source and contacts and application of appropriate chemotherapeutic methods; frequent community surveys by skin testing and X-ray examination; and continuing public education concerning the importance, origin, and control of TB.

Treatment   Most primary infections heal without recognition or treatment. Individuals with diagnosed TB are given isoniazid combined with rifampin or other antitubercular drugs. Nine months of therapy usually resolves an active case of TB.

SUMMARY

The table summarizes the most important facts concerning the leading infectious diseases that are acquired by way of the respiratory system.

	SUMMARY TABLE	Bacterial diseases acquired through the respiratory route		
Disease	**Special Characteristics**	**Transmission**	**Common Symptoms**	**Prevention/ Control**
URI	Pharyngitis, laryngitis, tonsillitis, sinusitis, otitis media.	Person-to-person or autoinfection, by direct or indirect contact.	Sore throat, hoarseness, loss of voice, sinus pain, earache.	Frequent hand washing.
Pneumonia	With influenza, one of top 10 causes of death in United States. Caused by all disease agents except metazoa.	See specific type.	See specific type.	See specific type.
Pneumococcal pneumonia	Most common type of pneumonia. More common among very young and very old. Common cause of death among alcoholics.	Direct or indirect contact with respiratory discharges.	Sudden onset of chills, fever, chest pain, difficult breathing, and cough. Red or rusty sputum. Pleurisy often present. Older people may be asymptomatic.	Vaccine for high-risk individuals. In an outbreak, avoid crowds.
Mycoplasmal pneumonia	"Walking pneumonia." May last a month or more.	Direct or indirect contact with respiratory discharges.	Insidious onset with headache, malaise, cough (often paroxysmal), and chest pain.	Avoidance of crowding.
Legionnaires' disease	Pneumonia-like illness. Outbreaks from faulty cooling systems or at excavation sites. Described in 1947. An unrecognized cause of pneumonia for many years. Has been diagnosed in most states and in some foreign countries.	Organism exists in soil and water. Inhalation of airborne particles results in infection. No evidence of person-to-person transmission.	Sudden or gradual onset. Diarrhea, anorexia, malaise, myalgia, weakness, headache, high fever, chills, followed by nonproductive cough that may eventually produce grayish, blood-streaked sputum.	Disinfection of source if a cooling system, control of dust if source is an excavation.
Streptococcal sore throat	Sequelae include rheumatic fever, glomerulonephritis, rheumatic heart disease, and scarlet fever.	Direct contact and ingestion of contaminated food.	Temperature, severe sore throat, swollen glands and tonsils, malaise, weakness, and anorexia.	Avoidance of close contact with infected persons and proper food handling.
Scarlet fever	Generally preceded by strep sore throat. *S. pyogenes* is the disease agent.	Direct and indirect contact with respiratory discharges or in contaminated milk or food.	Sore throat, fine rash (blanches on pressure) nausea, vomiting, fever, strawberry tongue.	Same as streptococcal sore throat.
Rheumatic fever	Childhood disease always preceded by another strep infection. May lead to heart or kidney disease.	No person-to-person transmission but possible transmission of strep organism if victim is a carrier.	Fever and migratory joint pain.	Immediate antibiotic treatment for any streptococcal infection. Contact investigation and treatment of sources (individuals or food.)

Continued

SUMMARY TABLE Bacterial diseases acquired through the respiratory route—cont'd				
Disease	**Special Characteristics**	**Transmission**	**Common Symptoms**	**Prevention/ Control**
Acute post-strepto-coccal glomerulo-nephritis.	Follows strep infec-tion of respira-tory tract or skin.	No person-to-per-son transmission.	Fever, nausea, cocoa-colored urine, hyper-tension, diminished urine output, edema, fatigue.	Avoidance of strep-tococcal infec-tion. Identifica-tion and control of source.
Whooping cough	Highly communi-cable during late incubation and prodrome. In-creased incidence in recent years.	Direct and indirect by contact with respiratory dis-charges.	Three stages: catarrhal stage resembles a cold. Paroxysmal stage produces spas-modic and recurrent coughing, sometimes expelling tenacious mucus. Cough ends in high whoop. Con-valescent stage 1-2 months with inter-mittent coughing.	Vaccination with booster shots. Isolation of sus-pected cases. In-vestigation of contacts and ad-ministration of vaccine or treat-ment when nec-essary.
Diphtheria	One of leading kill-ers in the world at one time. Still an important cause of disease and death in de-veloping nations.	Direct or indirect contact from in-fected persons. Milk can also serve as a vehi-cle.	Thick, patchy, grayish green mucous mem-branes of pharynx, larynx, tonsils, soft palate, and nose.	Vaccination and booster shots as necessary. Isola-tion of infected individuals. An-tiseptic measures, screening of con-tacts who are food handlers. Antitoxin pro-phylactically to contacts under age of 10 years.
TB	Still 30,000 cases reported an-nually. Rates much higher among poor, nonwhites, and in urban areas. Incidence in the U.S. in 1989 was 9.5 per 100,000. Many cases reac-tivated. Illness and death rates increase with age.	Usual route by air-borne droplets. Prolonged expo-sure to an active case necessary for infection.	Usually no symptoms in primary TB. In secondary TB: pro-ductive cough, chest pains, sometimes bloody sputum.	No vaccination in U.S.* Improve-ment of social conditions and education of the public. Frequent screening by skin testing and chest X-ray exams.

Treatment of bacterial disease is generally by antibiotics.

*BCG used in some countries but detection by skin test not possible after it is used.

QUESTIONS FOR REVIEW

1. What means of prevention increases resistance to all infectious disease?
2. What upper respiratory diseases are often caused by bacteria?
3. What is otitis media?
4. What conditions predispose people to URI?
5. Which organisms cause pneumonia?
6. How is pneumonia classified?
7. What factors may make a person susceptible to pneumonia?
8. What is pleurisy?
9. What is "walking pneumonia"?
10. What are the symptoms of mycoplasmal pneumonia?
11. When was Legionnaires' disease first described?
12. What conditions are conducive to Legionnaires' disease?
13. What complications may occur from Legionnaires' disease?
14. Which organism is responsible for most sore throats?
15. What are the sequelae of strep sore throat?
16. In what way does a strep infection lead to scarlet fever?
17. What are the distinctive symptoms of scarlet fever?
18. Why is it said that rheumatic fever is a disease that does not stand alone?
19. What are the early symptoms of rheumatic fever?
20. How can rheumatic fever be prevented?
21. What is thought to be the cause of APSGN?
22. What occurs during the three stages of whooping cough?
23. When is whooping cough most contagious?
24. What is the treatment for whooping cough?
25. What has caused the periodic rise in diphtheria in the United States?
26. What is the distinctive symptom of diphtheria?
27. What complications may occur with diphtheria?
28. What is the difference between a toxoid, an antitoxin, and a vaccine?
29. Why is TB increasing today?
30. What is the reservoir for TB?
31. What is reactivation TB?
32. What are the characteristics, means of transmission, symptoms, treatment, prevention, and control for
    URIs caused by bacteria?
    Pneumococcal pneumonia?
    Mycoplasmal pneumonia?
    Legionnaires' disease?
    Streptococcal sore throat?
    Scarlet fever?
    Rheumatic fever?
    Acute poststreptococcal glomerulonephritis?
    Whooping cough?
    Diphtheria?
    TB?

FURTHER READING

Boyd, Robert F. *General Microbiology*. St. Louis: Mosby, 1988.

Breiman, Robert F., et al. "Association for Shower Use with Legionnaires' Disease: Possible Role of Amoebae." *Journal of the American Medical Association,* June 6, '90, 263:2994-2926.

Cassidy, Jo "Rheumatic Fever: Going . . . Going . . . Coming Back?" *Current Health,* Feb. '90, 20-21.

Control of Communicable Disease in Man. Abram S. Benenson, ed. Fifteenth Edition, Washington, D.C.: American Public Health Association, 1990.

Chisholm, Patricia. "Global Emergency." (Tuberculosis), *Maclean's,* May 24, '93, 106:52.

Cromer, BA, et al. "Unrecognized Pertussis Infection in Adolescents." *American Journal of Disease in Children,* May 1993, 147(5):575-577.

Ezzell, Carol. "Captain of the Men of Death. (Multidrug-Resistant Strains of Tuberculosis)." *Science News,* Feb. 6, '93, 143:90-92.

Fackelmann, KA, "Vaccine Confers Pertussis Protection." *Science News,* Oct. 28, '89, 136:276.

Ferguson, GT and RM Cherniack. "Management of Chronic Obstructive Pulmonary Disease." *New England Journal of Medicine,* April 8, '93. 328(14):1017-1022.

Finegold, Sydney M., "Legionnaires' Disease—Still with Us." *New England Journal of Medicine,* Mar. 3, '88, 318:571-573.

Gantz, Nelson M., et al. "Questions and Answers on Sinusitis." *Patient Care,* Aug. 15, '88, 22:53-65.

Goldsmith, Marsha F. "Forgotten (Almost) but Not Gone, Tuberculosis Suddenly Looms Large on Domestic Scene." *Journal of the American Medical Association,* July 11, '90, 264:165-166.

Griffin, Marie R., et al. "Risk of Seizures and Encephalopathy after Immunization with the Diphtheria-Tetanus-Pertussis Vaccine." *Journal of the American Medical Association,* March 23, '90, 263:1641-1645.

"Guidelines for the Diagnosis of Rheumatic Fever. Jones Criteria, 1992 Update." Special Writing Group of the Committee on Rheumatic Fever, Endocarditis, and Kawasaki Disease of the Council on Cardiovascular Disease in the Young of the American Heart Association. *JAMA,* Oct. 21, '92, 268(15):2069-2073.

Johnson, DH and BA Cunha. "Atypical Pneumonias. Clinical and Extrapulmonary Features of Chlamydia, Mycoplasma, and Legionella Infections. *Postgraduate Medicine,* May 15, '93, 93(7);69-72, 75-76, 79-82.

Kaplan, Edward L. "A Comeback for Rheumatic Fever?" *Patient Care,* Mar. 15, '88, 22:80-88.

Kopanoff, Donald E., Dixie E. Snider, Jr. and Martha Johnson. "Recurrent Tuberculosis: Why Do Patients Develop Disease Again? A United States Public Health Service Cooperative Survey." *American Journal of Public Health,* Jan. '88, 78:30-33.

Madsen, Lorie A. "Tuberculosis Today." *RN,* Mar. '90, 53:44-51.

McCance, Kathryn L. and Sue E. Huether. *Pathophysiology: The Biologic Basis for Disease in Adults and Children.* St. Louis: Mosby, 1990.

Murray, et al. *Medical Microbiology.* St. Louis: Mosby, 1990.

O'Donnell, DE, KA Webb and MA Mcguire. "Older Patients with COPD: Benefits of Exercise Training." *Geriatrics,* Jan. '93, 48(1):59-62, 65-66.

"Outbreak of Multidrug-Resistant Tuberculosis—Texas, California, and Pennsylvania." *Journal of the American Medical Association,* July 11, '90, 264:173-174.

"Pertussis Surveillance-United States, 1986-1988." *Journal of the American Medical Association,* Feb. 23, '90, 263:1058-1059.

Purkis, Tony, Jackie Wilson, and Roger Milne. "Cleaning Up the Cooling Towers." *New Scientist,* Sept. 16, '80, 123:52-56.

Rossen, Anne E. "Comeback Diseases: They're No Joke . . . Don't Let Them Get the Last Laugh." *Current Health,* Jan, '91, 17:26-27.

Schrock, CG. "Clarithromycin vs. Penicillin in the Treatment of Streptococcal Pharyngitis." *Journal of Family Practice,* Dec. '92. 35(6):611-616.

Schwartz, Benjamin, Richard R. Facklam and Robert F. Breiman. "Changing Epidemiology of Group A Streptococcal Infection in the USA." *Lancet,* Nov. 10, '90, 336:1167-1171.

Snider, Dixie E., Louis Salinas and Gloria D. Kelly. "Tuberculosis: An Increasing Problem among Minorities in the United States." *Public Health Reports,* Nov.-Dec. '89, 104:646-653.

Stevens, Dennis J., et al. "Severe Group A Streptococcal Infections Associated with a Toxic Shock-Like Syndrome and Scarlet Fever Toxin A." *New England Journal of Medicine,* July 6, '89, 321:1-6.

"A Strategic Plan for the Elimination of Tuberculosis in the United States." *Journal of the American Medical Association,* May 26, '89, 261:2941-2942.

Turner, James C., et al. "Association of Group C Beta-Hemolytic Streptococci with Endemic Pharyngitis among College Students." *Journal of the American Medical Association,* Nov. 28, '90, 264:2644-2647.

"Update: Tuberculosis Elimination—United States." *Journal of the American Medical Association,* Apr. 18, '90, 263:2032-2033.

Wallace, Mark R. "The Return of Acute Rheumatic Fever in Young Adults." *Journal of the American Medical Association,* Nov. 10, '89, 262:2557-2561.

Watson, Traci. "A Shot in the Arm for TB Research." *Science,* Feb. 12, '93, 259:886.

"Whooping Cough: The Last Gasp?" *Harvard Medical School Health Letter,* Dec. '89, 15:3-4.

Zamula, Evelyn, "Tuberculosis: Still Striking after All These Years." *FDA Consumer,* Mar. '91, 25:18-23.

Chapter 5

Bacterial Diseases Acquired through the Alimentary Route

OBJECTIVES

1 Distinguish between food poisoning and foodborne illness.

2 State means of prevention for infections that are transmitted by food or water.

3 Recognize symptoms that might indicate foodborne illness.

4 State the ways that food and water can become contaminated with salmonella and other pathogenic bacteria.

5 Discuss characteristics, transmission, treatment, and control of the following:
Staphylococcus aureus food poisoning
Chlostridium perfringens food poisoning
Botulism
Escherichia coli food poisoning
Shigellosis
Salmonellosis
Campylobacter enteritis
Cholera
Typhoid fever
Brucellosis

INTRODUCTION

There are a number of different terms for disease acquired through ingestion, and one that is commonly used is "food poisoning." It is important to understand that the poison or toxin comes from bacteria and is not inherent in the food. In some cases, it is the ingestion of preformed toxins (poisons) from pathogenic organisms that cause the illness; at other times it is ingestion of the organisms themselves that then produces toxins in the bowel. True food poisoning occurs when a food, such as some species of mushroom or shellfish, is ingested and illness occurs because of toxins (poisons) in the mushrooms or shellfish. In this text, *food poisoning* will be used to refer to an illness that is the result of ingesting food.

There are some bacteria acquired through the alimentary route that cause only gastroenteritis (inflammation of the stomach and intestine) or only enteritis, and there are others that cause a systemic illness. Most of these are acquired from contaminated food and water. Some of the most common bacterial diseases acquired through the alimentary route will be discussed in this chapter.

The World Health Organization has developed "Ten Golden Rules for Food Preparation." They are listed here and are part of the preventive measures against all infections from contaminated food and water*:

1. Choose food processed for safety.
2. Cook food thoroughly.
3. Eat cooked food immediately.
4. Store cooked food carefully.
5. Reheat cooked foods thoroughly.
6. Avoid contact between raw foods and cooked foods.
7. Wash hands repeatedly.
8. Keep all kitchen surfaces meticulously clean.
9. Protect foods from insects, rodents, and other animals.
10. Use pure water.

When people are camping, hiking, hunting, fishing, or otherwise spending time outdoors, for any reason, they need to be sure that any water supply is safe; if there is any doubt, all water should be boiled before drinking or use in food preparation. Streams, lakes, and ponds can easily be contaminated from various sources and are a ready source of organisms that cause food poisoning.

*Beneson, Abram S., p. 171.

STAPHYLOCOCCUS AUREUS FOOD POISONING

Staphylococcus aureus is one of the most common causes of food poisoning in the United States. The illness is caused by ingesting food in which staphylococci have been multiplying and producing toxin. *S. aureus* is a natural inhabitant of the human body. Occasionally the reservoir also may be in cows with infected udders. The interval between eating the food and the onset of symptoms may be as little as 30 minutes or as long as 7 hours. Usually the incubation period is 2 to 4 hours. Most persons are susceptible to this kind of food poisoning. The illness is short lasting and rarely fatal. Victims recover within a day or two, but the intensity of symptoms may require hospitalization. Figure 5-1 shows the pattern of outbreaks; although the disease occurs year-round, it peaks during the summer and the holiday season (November and December).

Transmission   Staphylococci grow in many foods, especially precooked hams, milk, custards, cream fillings, and salad dressing. Some of the most likely sources of this food poisoning are shown in Figure 5-2. The source of food contamination is usually a person with an infected lesion on the hands, arms, or face. Milk from an infected cow may also be toxic. Figure 5-3 shows a possible sequence of transmission of *S. aureus*. This same progression could happen with some of the other organisms that will be discussed.

Symptoms   Staphylococcal food poisoning has an abrupt and sometimes violent onset, which helps to distinguish it from other types of foodborne illness. Nausea, vomiting,

FIGURE 5-1 Staphylococcal food poisoning can be seen year-round but is most common during the summer and November/December holidays.

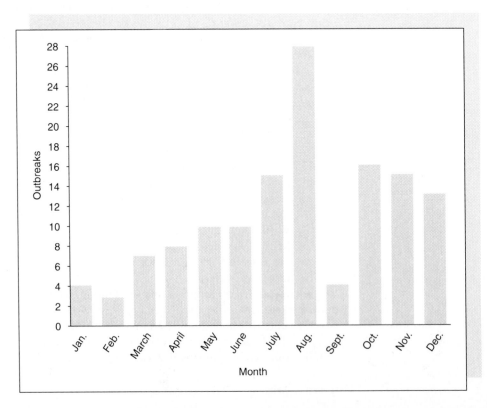

cramps, and diarrhea are the typical symptoms. The loss of fluid and violent vomiting may lead to prostration, low-grade fever, and lowered blood pressure.

Treatment   Treatment is not necessary unless the individual becomes dehydrated, in which case oral rehydration or, in extreme cases, intravenous (IV) therapy may be used to replace fluids.

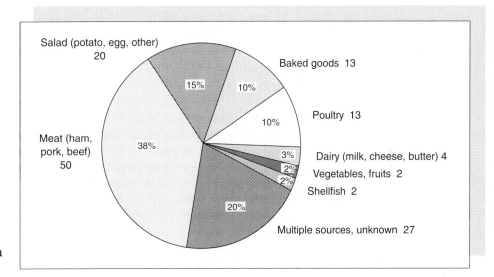

Salad (potato, egg, other) 20

Baked goods 13

15%

10%

10%

Poultry 13

Meat (ham, pork, beef) 50

38%

3%

Dairy (milk, cheese, butter) 4

2%

Vegetables, fruits 2

2%

Shellfish 2

20%

Multiple sources, unknown 27

FIGURE 5-2 Foods implicated in staphylococcal outbreaks reported to CDC during a 5-year period.

FIGURE 5-3 One possible means of transmission for *S. aureus* food poisoning.

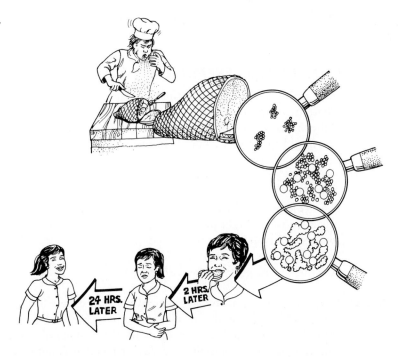

24 HRS. LATER

2 HRS. LATER

DID YOU KNOW?

Safety Tips for Cooling and Storing Food

One way to avoid contamination of cooked foods is to refrigerate them as soon as possible. In any case they should not be allowed to sit out more than 2 hours. The U.S. Food Safety and Inspection Service also recommends that food cooked in large quantities should be divided into smaller containers in order to cool more quickly. Warm food is an ideal place for some microorganisms to multiply to an infectious dose. Many outbreaks of food poisoning have been traced to food in large containers that was not cooled or stored correctly. Shallow containers, no more than 3 inches deep, are best. And if food has to be left out of the refrigerator for cooling, even for a short time, it should be covered.

Prevention   The time from the preparation of food to serving needs to be as short as possible. Proper heating or cooling procedures need to be followed, as well as using the right procedures for perishable foods. Any individual with boils, abscesses, or other infected lesions of the hands, face, or nose should be prohibited from food handling. Food handlers and others should be educated about food hygiene, sanitation and cleanliness of kitchens, proper temperature control, and personal hygiene (hand washing, cleaning fingernails, etc.). (See the preceding "Ten Golden Rules for Food Preparation.")

Control   Single cases of food poisoning are generally so mild that they are not reported. Individuals who say they have had "stomach flu" or "24-hour flu" may simply be using incorrect terms for vomiting and diarrhea. Control is only necessary when there is an outbreak, and then the source of infection needs to be identified and eliminated.

CLOSTRIDIUM PERFRINGENS FOOD POISONING

Food poisoning from *Clostridium perfringens* is generally a mild disease of short duration. It occurs worldwide wherever conditions favor increased multiplication of the organism. The incubation period is 6 to 24 hours, although the victims usually become ill in 10 to 12 hours. Improper cooking and handling methods for food provide the necessary condition for the intoxication to occur. Figure 5-4 shows confirmed outbreaks of *C. perfringens*–confirmed cases for one 5-year period.

Transmission   Food contaminated by soil or feces and then held under conditions that allow the organism to multiply provides the means of transmission. Most outbreaks are associated with inadequately heated meats and gravies. The outbreaks are usually traced to restaurants or other businesses that prepare food but do not have adequate cooking or refrigeration facilities.

Symptoms   Poisoning from *C. perfringens* generally produces much milder symptoms than those from most other food infections or intoxications. Cramps followed by diarrhea appear suddenly, and there is often nausea, but vomiting and fever seldom occur. The symptoms are present for a day or less and fatalities are rare.

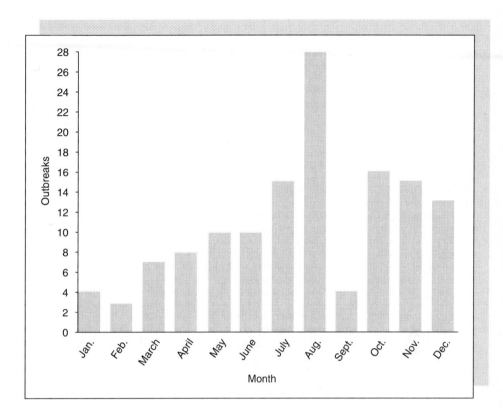

FIGURE 5-4 *C. perfringens* outbreaks.

Treatment   Treatment is unnecessary unless the victim becomes dehydrated.

Prevention   Outbreaks usually can be traced to places such as schools and restaurants where foods are prepared in large batches. Meat dishes are a common source. Food handlers should be educated concerning the dangers in large-scale cooking. Hot dishes should be served while still hot from original preparation. If stored, they must be cooled rapidly, and reheating must be thorough and rapid in order to prevent the organism from multiplying.

Control   Control is only necessary when there is an outbreak, and then the source of the poisoning needs to be identified and eliminated.

BOTULISM

Poisoning from the exotoxin produced by *Clostridium botulinum* results in a life-threatening paralytic illness. Unlike other forms of bacterial food poisoning or infection, botulism is a systemic illness. The powerful toxin, when ingested in contaminated food, is absorbed from the intestine into the system, resulting in the paralysis of cranial and peripheral nerves. Infection with *C. botulinum* also occurs in infants, in whom the toxin is produced by the organism in the intestines, and in wound botulism, when the organism enters a wound and anaerobic conditions are present. Infant botulism has been recognized only since 1976; wound botulism is rarely seen.

There were more outbreaks of botulism when home canning and preserving were common, but family outbreaks can still occur. There have also been some cases identified recently that were traced to commercially canned products. Incubation is usually 12 to 36 hours but can be longer. In shorter incubation periods, the illness is generally more severe. Everyone is susceptible to botulism if the toxin is ingested. Figure 5-5 shows the distribution of the organism in soil samples in the United States. Figure 5-6 indicates the number of confirmed cases for one 5-year period. The case fatality rate has been under 15% during the last 10 years for patients who receive adequate treatment. Without treatment, about one third of the patients may die within 3 to 7 days after onset. Recovery may be slow and take months or even years.

Transmission   Botulism generally is the result of eating foods that have been inadequately cooked, allowing the toxin to form. The foods that have been involved most often in the United States are home canned fruit and vegetables; in Europe, smoked or preserved meat and sausages; and in Japan, smoked or preserved fish. A number of the sources are pictured in Figure 5-7.

Symptoms   The first signs of botulism generally relate to the effects of the toxin on the nervous system. The person may experience dizziness, difficulty in swallowing, and double vision. Nausea, vomiting, and diarrhea may occur earlier, at the same time, or later. There is descending paralysis, and death usually occurs from respiratory paralysis.

Treatment   Treatment consists of intramuscular (IM) or IV administration of botulinum antitoxin.

FIGURE 5-5 *C. botulinum* distribution, letters refer to different types.

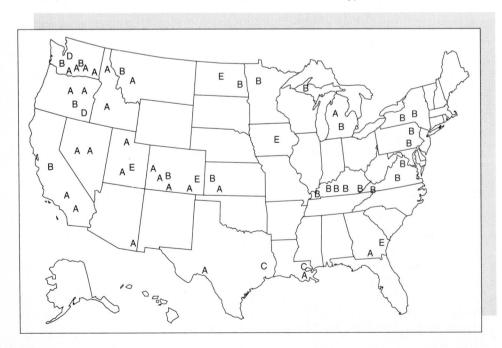

Prevention   The best means of prevention is through effective control of processing and preparation of commercially canned and preserved foods and education of everybody who prepares and serves food to themselves and others. Education must also extend to those concerned with home canning and other food preservation and must include instruction in proper techniques regarding time, pressure, temperature, storage, and

FIGURE 5-6   Botulism outbreaks.

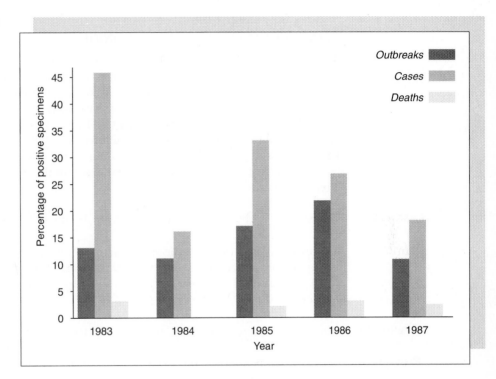

FIGURE 5-7   Bulging can and improperly stored food—possible sources of botulism.

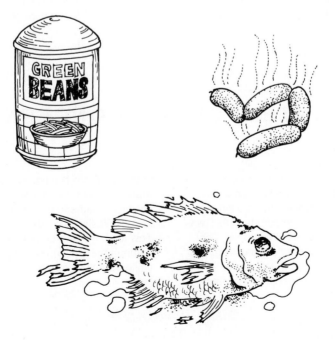

cooking. Any bulging cans or jars that do not seem sealed should not be opened or used.

Control   Early detection and identification of the source of botulism can save lives. Contaminated food should be boiled before discarding and buried deeply to keep animals from eating it. Contaminated utensils also need to be sterilized.

ESCHERICHIA COLI FOOD POISONING

The organism responsible for bacterial gastroenteritis, *Escherichia coli,* probably produces most of the illnesses called "travelers' diarrhea" or "Montezuma's revenge." Illness from infection with this organism strikes individuals who visit less-developed countries and is also the cause of infant diarrhea in these countries. See the box below for discussion of recent outbreaks of *E. coli* in the United States. There are at least four different strains and many different serotypes of *E. coli*. The incubation period ranges from 12 to 72 hours, depending on the strain. As long as the organism is being excreted, it is communicable. Immunity to the specific serotype is acquired after one attack of the disease.

Transmission   Transmission is by food or water and rarely by direct fecal contact.

Symptoms   The major symptom is diarrhea, and there may be abdominal cramps, vomiting, weakness, and dehydration. A low-grade fever may also be present. The symptoms last 3 to 5 days and are generally mild, although in babies, dehydration can lead to fatality.

Treatment   Most cases require no therapy, but fluid replacement may be necessary.

Prevention   See the aforementioned "Ten Golden Rules for Safe Food Preparation." In addition, the preventive measures given for typhoid fever on p. 126 should be followed. Sometimes prophylactic antibiotics are used for travelers going to high-risk areas.

Control   Identify and eliminate or avoid the source when an outbreak is reported.

CONTEMPORARY CONCERNS

E. Coli Outbreaks

Recent reports from both east and west coasts show that outbreaks of *E. coli* can happen wherever proper food handling procedures are ignored. An outbreak in Massachusetts in autumn, 1991 was traced to apple cider from a single cider mill. The apples used were not washed before pressing, and the cider was neither pasteurized nor treated with preservatives. Contaminated beef caused a later outbreak. From November 15, 1992, through February 28, 1993, more than 500 cases and four associated deaths from *E. coli* were reported in four states: Washington, Idaho, California, and Nevada. This time, the source of infection was undercooked hamburgers sold in branches of a restaurant franchise that all used meat from the same supplier.

SHIGELLOSIS (BACILLARY DYSENTERY)

Shigellosis, or bacillary dysentery, is an acute intestinal disease caused by the bacterium *Shigella*. *Dysentery* means diarrhea with abdominal cramping and tenesmus (straining at stools) from any cause. The term *bacillary dysentery* is reserved for infection by the four species of *Shigella: S. dysenteriae, S. flexneri, S. boydii,* and *S. sonnei.*

Shigellosis is endemic in North America, Europe, and the tropics. Figure 5-8 shows the number of confirmed cases in the United States from 1955 to 1992. The infection is more common in children ages 1 to 4 years and in the elderly, debilitated, and malnourished. Two thirds of the cases and most of the deaths are in children under age 10 years. It is unusual in children under 6 months of age.

The only reservoir for *Shigella* organisms is the human intestinal tract, and infected feces are always the source of the infection. The incubation period is usually 1 to 3 days; the disease is communicable during acute infection and until the infectious agent is no longer present in feces, which is usually within 4 weeks after the illness. Everyone is susceptible to infection with *Shigella* organisms; drinking or ingestion of as few as 10 of the organisms can lead to shigellosis. With prompt treatment, only 1% of the cases are fatal, although in epidemics caused by *S. dysenteriae,* as high as 8% of the cases may result in death. The graph in Figure 5-9 shows that *shigellosis* has moved ahead of salmonellosis and infection by *Campylobacter* in percentage of reported cases.

Transmission   Transmission of shigellosis is directly by fecal–oral transmission or indirectly through contact with contaminated objects. The widest distribution of the organism is through contaminated water or food. Transmission occurs primarily through individuals who fail to wash their hands or clean their fingernails thoroughly after defecation. They can then spread the infection to others by physical contact with them or by contaminating food or water. Food can also be contaminated by flies

FIGURE 5-8 *Shigella* confirmed cases in the United States from 1955 to 1992.

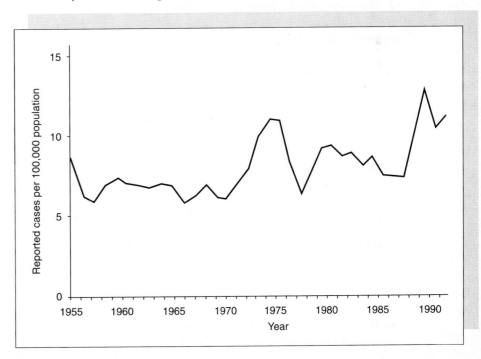

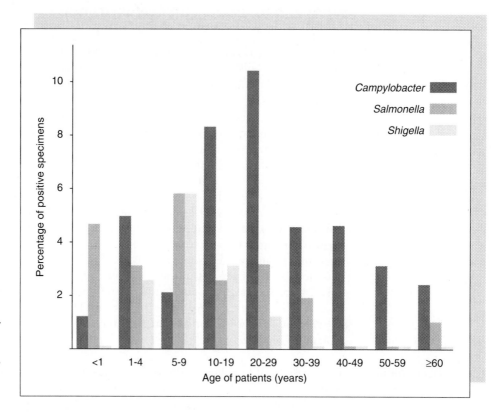

FIGURE 5-9 Age distribution for diarrheal diseases caused by campylobacter, salmonella and shigella organisms.

that carry enough of the organism for it to multiply to an infectious dose in the food. When dogs ingest human feces, the infection can be passed by them to children or other susceptible persons.

Symptoms   Shigellae invade the intestinal mucosa and cause inflammation. In children, shigellosis usually produces diarrhea with tenesmus, high fever, nausea, vomiting, abdominal pain with distention, irritability, and drowsiness. Pus, mucus, and blood may appear in the stools as a result of the intestinal ulceration typical of this infection. Shigellosis in adults produces many of the same symptoms except that adults generally do not have fever. Complications such as electrolyte imbalance and shock are rare but may be fatal in children and debilitated patients.

Treatment   Many strains of *Shigella* are resistant to antibiotics. If an effective one can be found, then the shigellae can be eliminated quickly. Antidiarrheal drugs are contraindicated, since they prolong the excretion of shigellae, fever, and diarrhea. The most important treatment is control of dehydration, with fluid and electrolyte replacement.

Prevention   There is no vaccine at present. Prevention is based on control of the human reservoir and sanitary control of environmental sources through adequate treatment of water and sewage, fly control, and protection of food, water, and milk from human or mechanical vectors.

Control   Control measures are the same as for other diseases acquired through the alimentary route.

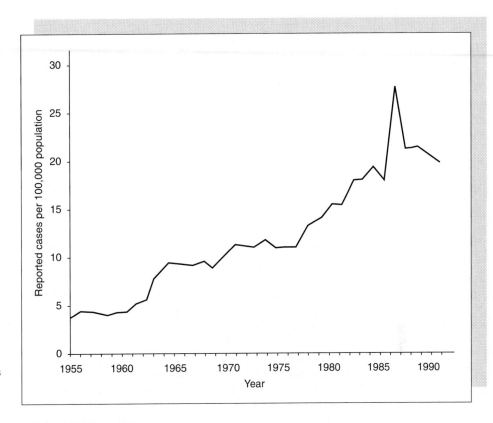

FIGURE 5-10 The number of reported cases of salmonellosis in the United States from 1955 to 1991.

SALMONELLOSIS

Salmonellosis is a medical term for infection with any species of *Salmonella*. Although over 1800 species of *Salmonella* have been recognized, only 10 commonly cause salmonellosis in the United States. Infection with *Salmonella* organisms can range from a symptomless carrier state to potentially fatal infections. The most frequent form of salmonellosis today is gastroenteritis. Salmonellae were not named after fish but after an American veterinarian, Daniel Salmon, who first isolated the organism from animals. In addition to typhoid fever and gastroenteritis, salmonellosis also occurs as bacteremia, localized infection, and parathyphoid.

FOODBORNE SALMONELLOSIS

Infection with salmonella from ingesting food is caused most often by *Salmonella enteritidis*. It has been the most common foodborne infection in the United States but is now being challenged by *Campylobacter* enteritis (Figure 5-9), which will be covered later on in the chapter. In 1985, the largest outbreak of salmonellosis to date occurred in Illinois. Over 5000 cases were confirmed by the Illinois Public Health Department. Two lots of contaminated milk were identified as the cause but not until they had been sold in supermarket chains in Indiana, Iowa, and Michigan.

The rate of infection is highest for babies and young children. It is estimated that there are 2 to 3 million salmonella infections in the United States each year. The incubation period varies but is usually about 12 to 36 hours. Communicability lasts for the duration of the infection, which can be several days to several weeks. A small percentage of infected adults and children over 5 years excrete the organism for over 1 year. Everyone is susceptible to salmonella infection from food. Figure 5-10 indicates the reported cases in the United States from 1955 to 1991.

Transmission   Salmonella infections leading to gastroenteritis are generally transmitted by ingestion of (1) food derived from an infected animal, (2) food contaminated during storage by the feces of infected animals, especially rodents, or (3) food contaminated by an infected person during its processing or preparation. Foods that are often found to be the source of salmonella infection include commercially processed meat products, inadequately cooked poultry or poultry products, raw sausages, lightly cooked foods containing eggs or egg products, and unpasteurized milk or dairy products, including dried milk. Turtles also carry salmonella and have been banned as pets because of the potential for infection.

Symptoms   When individuals become infected from eating contaminated food, there is generally a sudden onset of nausea, vomiting, abdominal pain, and diarrhea, often accompanied by fever and chills.

Treatment   There is no specific treatment indicated for salmonella gastroenteritis unless dehydration occurs. Rehydration and electrolyte replacement may be necessary in extreme cases. Since the use of antibiotics may prolong the carrier state and lead to resistant organisms, they are only given in high-risk cases such as infants under 2 months, the elderly, the debilitated, and those with continued high fever or with indications that the infection has spread beyond the intestines.

Prevention   Meats, eggs, and milk must be protected by sanitary processing. Stored foods should be safeguarded from possible contamination by rodent feces. Food handlers and methods for preparing foods in public places should be under the continuing supervision of local health departments. Carriers must be restricted from food handling. Food handlers and the public should be continuously educated as to the sources and transmission of salmonella infection. Infection in domestic animals, fowl, and pets must be controlled.

Control   Individuals with salmonella infection need to be instructed in using proper hand-washing techniques. Symptomatic individuals should be excluded from food handling. They should not be allowed to return to work until stool cultures are negative. Those who come into direct contact with individuals with salmonellosis should be checked for infection. It is required that salmonella gastroenteritis be reported to local health authorities.

CAMPYLOBACTER ENTERITIS

This disease is caused by *Campylobacter jejuni* and is responsible for 5% to 11% of all cases of diarrhea and dysentery in the United States. The organism was recognized recently as an important cause of foodborne infection and is thought to cause more illness than salmonellae. Duration of the symptoms is generally 2 to 5 days but may last as long as 10 days or more, especially in adults, and there may also be relapses. *C. jejuni* is harbored in animals, poultry, and humans; dogs are frequent carriers. The disease is communicable from several days to several weeks, depending on the length of infection. Lasting immunity develops after an initial infection.

Transmission   *Campylobacter* bacteria are transmitted in food or water and may also be contracted by contact with infected pets, wild animals, or infected children. One means of transmission has been identified as youth activities (often field trips to dairy farms) during which children drink raw milk (Figure 5-11).

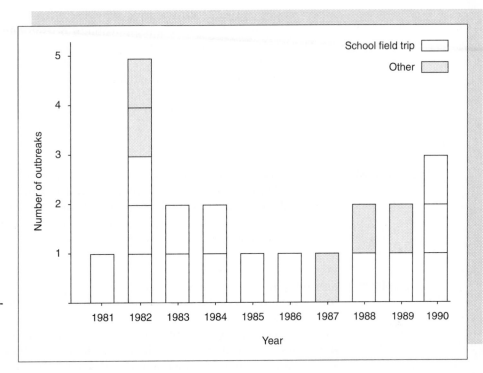

FIGURE 5-11 One means of *Campylobacter* transmission is identified as youth activities such as field trips.

Symptoms   Symptoms include diarrhea, abdominal pain, malaise, fever, nausea and vomiting, and blood in the stools. The victim can be asymptomatic or very sick. Sometimes there are symptoms resembling typhoid and, rarely, meningitis can occur.

Treatment   Generally no treatment is needed unless it is rehydration and electrolyte replacement. In special cases, antibiotics may be used.

Prevention   All food derived from animal sources and poultry should be thoroughly cooked, milk pasteurized, and water supplies purified. Recognition and control of infection in domestic pets is also necessary. Hand washing after animal contact and contact with chickens will also aid in prevention.

Control   Individuals with the infection should be excluded from any food preparation. In case of an outbreak, the source of infection needs to be identified and eliminated or isolated.

CHOLERA

Cholera is an acute gastrointestinal infection caused by *Vibrio cholerae*. The disease is caused by an exotoxin produced by the organism. Severe, untreated cases of cholera may be fatal in as many as 50% of its victims. With treatment, it is fatal in fewer than 1%. Cholera is most common in Africa, southern and Southeast Asia, and the Middle East, although isolated outbreaks have occurred in Japan, Australia, Europe, and the United States. (A small outbreak in Texas in 1978 could not be traced to any imported source.) It occurs more frequently among lower socioeconomic groups and more often during the warmer months. Humans are the only known reservoir, although there is a possibility of environmental reservoirs.

The incubation period is generally 2 to 3 days; communicability lasts as long as stools are positive, usually only a few days after recovery. A carrier state may last for months. Susceptibility to cholera varies. Attack rates, even in severe epidemics, rarely exceed 2%. In endemic areas, cholera is predominantly a disease of children. In these areas, most persons acquire antibodies by early adulthood. However, when cholera spreads to areas where it has not been endemic, adults are at least as susceptible as children.

Transmission

Cholera is transmitted through feces or vomitus of carriers or persons with active infections. Epidemic spread usually results from contaminated water supplies. Food is involved more often in sporadic cases in endemic areas. Hands, utensils, clothing, and flies may contaminate food or carry the infection directly to the mouth. Figure 5-12 pictures some of the means of transmission of cholera.

Symptoms

The symptoms of cholera are acute, painless, and profuse watery diarrhea and effortless vomiting. White flecks appear in the stools as they increase ("rice water stools"). Due to the massive loss of fluid, many symptoms occur, including thirst, weakness, wrinkled skin, sunken eyes, pinched facial expression, muscle cramps, and cardiovascular problems. Collapse, shock, and death may follow if the patient is not continuously rehydrated until the infection subsides.

Treatment

An electrolyte solution must be given immediately and continuously to replace lost fluids. In mild cases, oral fluid replacement is adequate. Tetracycline and other antibiotics are used if symptoms persist and are effective in reducing the duration and volume of diarrhea as well as speeding the elimination of the bacteria from the feces.

Prevention

Proper sanitation and vaccine are the best methods of prevention. The routine use of cholera vaccine is not recommended. However, people traveling to epidemic areas in other countries may be required to have a vaccination.

FIGURE 5-12 Possible means of cholera transmission.

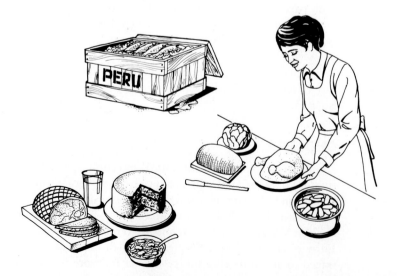

Control   Control methods are the same as they are for other diseases acquired through the alimentary route.

TYPHOID FEVER

In the last decade of the nineteenth century, it was recognized gradually that well persons who were carriers of pathogenic organisms were responsible for a significant number of new cases of disease. In 1906, the identification of an Irish cook, Mary Mallon, who had been the cause of seven epidemics of typhoid fever in 6 years, highlighted the importance of the *chronic carrier*. "Typhoid Mary" became the symbol around the world for a carrier of disease. Pictured in Figure 5-13 is one way that Typhoid Mary spreads the disease.

Salmonella typhi, the organism that causes typhoid fever, is the only species of *Salmonella* whose reservoir is only in humans. The disease has become comparatively rare in the United States since the advent of sanitation and immunization procedures. The fatality rate for untreated individuals is 10% and for those who get treatment, 3%. Typhoid results most frequently from drinking water that has been contaminated with body discharges from a carrier. The incubation period is usually 1 to 3 weeks; communicability usually lasts from the first week through the end of convalescence but can last longer. In about 10% of patients, the typhoid bacilli are discharged for 3 months after the onset of symptoms, and 2% to 5% become carriers. Susceptibility is general but usually declines with age.

Transmission   Typhoid bacilli are transmitted by food or water that has been contaminated with the fecal matter or, less commonly, urine, of an infected person or carrier. Among some of the common foods responsible for transmission of typhoid are shellfish from contaminated beds, raw fruits, vegetables, milk, and milk products contaminated by food handlers who are carriers or unidentified cases. Flies have also been known to be carriers when they infect foods in which the organisms can multiply sufficiently to cause the disease.

Symptoms   Unlike most other *Salmonella* infections that generally produce only acute gastroenteritis, typhoid is a systemic disease. If individuals ingest *S. typhi,* they may soon

FIGURE 5-13 Typhoid Mary working with food in a restaurant, unknowingly transmitted typoid fever to many customers.

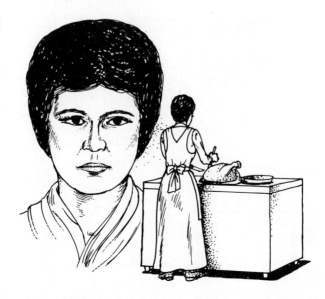

have gastric and intestinal symptoms, but these usually subside before the classic symptoms of typhoid fever begin. Within the first week, these symptoms include anorexia, myalgia, malaise, headache, and fever.

During the second week the fever rises to 104 or 105° F, usually in the evening, and it is accompanied by chills, sweating, weakness, delirium, increasing abdominal pain and distention, diarrhea or constipation, cough, moist rales (chest sounds on breathing), enlarged spleen, and rose spots, especially on the abdomen.

During the third week there is persistent fever, increasing fatigue, and weakness, as the symptoms gradually subside. Complications include intestinal perforation or hemorrhage, abscesses, blood clots in the legs and head, pneumonia, osteomyelitis, myocarditis, and acute circulatory failure.

Treatment A number of different antibiotics can be used to treat typhoid fever. Selection is based on the sensitivity of the strain of *S. typhi* involved. Symptomatic treatment includes bed rest and replacement of fluids and electrolytes. Various medications may also be used to relieve diarrhea and control cramps. Further treatment depends on the symptoms and kinds of complications that may occur.

Prevention Immunization is not routinely recommended in the United States or for travel to developed areas. Individuals at high risk because of occupation, travel to endemic areas, or living conditions where typhoid could be introduced should be given the vaccine. Prevention of typhoid depends on adequate protection of water supplies; sanitary disposal of human excreta; pasteurization of milk and dairy products; fly control; scrupulous cleanliness in preparing food at home and in public eating places; careful controls on shellfish sources and cooking; and identification and supervision of typhoid carriers. Even city water must be boiled in the wake of a flood, tornado, or hurricane if there is any chance of ruptured lines.

FIGURE 5-14 Sources of infection for brucellosis.

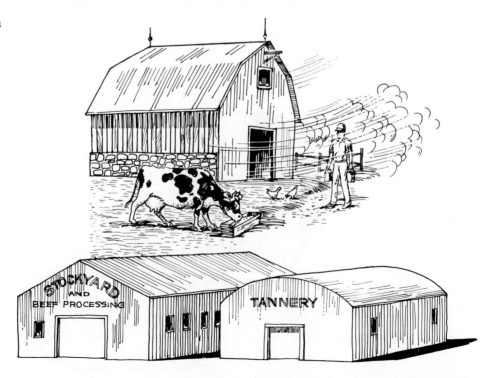

Control   Hospital care with proper sanitary precautions is recommended, particularly if the patient cannot be given adequate nursing and the necessary sanitary conditions cannot be maintained at home. An investigation should be conducted to determine the actual or probable source of infection for every case. Necessary measures should be taken to control any carriers who may be identified.

BRUCELLOSIS

Another name for brucellosis is undulant fever, a term that describes the variable nature of the disease. The word *undulant* means "rising or falling like waves," and brucellosis is a disease that does this. It is a disease that affects cattle and other animals and is transmitted to humans directly or indirectly. Brucellosis occurs worldwide but is more prevalent in other countries than it is in the United States. In North America, the most common infecting organism is *Brucella abortus,* which is found in cattle. Brucellosis is transmitted to humans from domestic animal reservoirs. The incubation period is difficult to determine because the onset of the disease is slow and insidious, but it is estimated at 1 to 3 weeks. There is ordinarily no human-to-human transmission. Individuals who recover from brucellosis acquire immunity to it, but the duration of the immunity is uncertain. Most individuals who drink contaminated milk become infected, and it is believed that a majority of human beings are susceptible to brucellosis infection.

Transmission   Humans become infected with brucellosis through direct contact with animal tissues, inhalation of contaminated dust of barns or slaughterhouses, or ingestion of unpasteurized dairy products from infected animals. Figure 5-14 shows some of the ways that brucellosis might be transmitted.

Symptoms   The onset of brucellosis is usually slow and insidious, with an irregular fever, chills and sweating, myalgia (muscle aches and pains), weakness, and malaise. If the onset is acute, the symptoms are more pronounced, and there may be severe headache, backache, and exhaustion. There may be other generalized symptoms such as gastrointestinal discomfort, enlarged lymph nodes and spleen, hepatitis with jaundice, and mental depression. These symptoms may gradually become milder and eventually disappear, but the disease often becomes chronic and recurs over the years. Some individuals develop endocarditis, osteomyelitis, or pyelonephritis (inflammation of kidney and pelvis), and endometritis (inflammation of the lining of the uterus) may occur in women.

Abscesses may also form in the testes, ovaries, kidneys, and brain. Fatality is rare, but even with recovery, there is often residual allergy or damage to bones and other tissues.

Treatment   Prolonged treatment with antibiotics is necessary to eradicate the organism in protected intracellular sites. Tetracycline and streptomycin are used for 3- and 2-week periods, respectively, and in severe cases corticosteroids may be given IV for 3 days, followed by oral corticosteroids. Bed rest is advised as long as there is a fever.

Prevention   There is no vaccine for brucellosis. Farmers and workers in slaughterhouses, packing plants, and butcher shops need to be educated as to the nature of the disease and the risk in the handling of carcasses or products of potentially infected animals. Milk should be pasteurized, and if not, boiling is effective in destroying brucella organisms.

Control Control depends on thorough investigation to find the source of the infection and setting up appropriate controls on infected animals or their products.

SUMMARY

The table below summarizes principal data regarding the most important diseases contracted through the alimentary system.

SUMMARY TABLE	Diseases acquired through the alimentary route			
Disease	**Special Characteristics**	**Transmission**	**Common Symptoms**	**Prevention/ Control**
S. aureus food poisoning	Short incubation (2-4 hr). Short duration. Rarely fatal.	Ingestion of food containing toxin.	Abrupt, violent onset, nausea, vomiting, diarrhea.	Safe food preparation.*
C. perfringens food poisoning	Mild, short duration.	Ingestion of food containing toxin.	Mild cramps, diarrhea, nausea.	Same as *S. aureus*.
Botulism	Life-threatening illness. Effects the nervous system. Fatality under 15% with treatment. Around 33% without treatment. Rare in humans.	Ingestion of food containing toxin.	Dizziness, difficulty in swallowing, double vision, nausea, vomiting, diarrhea, descending paralysis. Shorter incubation = more severe disease.	Same as *S. aureus*.
E. Coli enteritis	Causes most of "travelers' diarrhea" and "Montezuma's revenge."	Ingestion of food or water contaminated with the organism. (Rarely by direct fecal contact.)	Diarrhea.	Protection of water supplies; sanitary disposal of human excreta; pasteurization; safe food preparation; controls on shellfish; identification and supervision of carriers, education of everyone on importance of hand washing.
Shigellosis	Also called bacillary dysentery. More common in children, elderly, debilitated, and malnourished. Infected human feces only source.	Ingestion of food or water contaminated with the organism. Fecal-oral route.	Diarrhea, tenesmus, nausea, high fever, vomiting, irritability, abdominal pain and distention, drowsiness.	Same as *E. coli*.

*Benenson, Abram S. p. 171.

SUMMARY TABLE Diseases acquired through the alimentary route—cont'd				
Disease	**Special Characteristics**	**Transmission**	**Common Symptoms**	**Prevention/ Control**
Foodborne salmonellosis	Most common food-borne infection. Incubation usually 12-36 hr.	Ingestion of food or water contaminated with the organism. Gravies, sauces, custards, chicken, most likely sources.	Sudden onset of nausea, vomiting, abdominal pain, diarrhea, fever, chills.	Safe preparation of food. Eggs, meat, and milk must be protected by sanitary processing. Do not allow carriers or individuals with diarrhea to handle food. Control infections in domestic animals and pets.
Campylobacter enteritis	Recognized recently. Rivals salmonellosis as most common foodborne infection.	Ingestion of food or water contaminated with the organism.	Diarrhea, fever, abdominal pain, malaise, nausea, vomiting.	Thorough cooking of food from animal sources; pasteurization of milk; control of infection in pets. Hand washing after contact with animals and chickens.
Cholera	Fatal in up to 50% if untreated.	Ingestion of food or water contaminated with the organism.	Acute, painless, profuse watery diarrhea and effortless vomiting.	Same as *E. coli*.
Typhoid fever	"Typhoid Mary"-carrier state. Rare in U.S. today.	Ingestion of food or water contaminated with the organism.	Systemic disease: fever, anorexia, malaise, headache, myalgia, rose spots on abdomen, constipation or diarrhea.	Same as *E. coli*.
Brucellosis	"Undulant fever"	Ingestion of unpasteurized milk or milk products; contact with tissues of infected animals; inhalation of contaminated dust.	Fever, chills, sweating, muscle aches and pains, weakness and malaise.	Education of individuals who work with cows or their products. Pasteurizing or boiling milk.

Treatment for bacterial diseases is generally with antibiotics. However, many of the foodborne diseases are so mild that antibiotic treatment is not necessary. When diarrhea and vomiting are severe and prolonged, fluid and electrolytes may need to be replaced. In the case of botulism, an antitoxin is administered to counteract the poison. Prolonged treatment with antibiotics is necessary for brucellosis.

QUESTIONS FOR REVIEW

1. In what three ways can people be "poisoned" by food?
2. What foods are the most likely to become the source of staphylococcal food poisoning?
3. What distinguishes staphylococcal food poisoning from other types of foodborne illness as far as symptoms are concerned?
4. Why is fluid replacement sometimes necessary in foodborne illness?
5. What procedures should be followed in food preparation to prevent foodborne diseases?
6. Why is there sometimes a problem in the reporting and control of foodborne disease?
7. What conditions may lead to the transmission of *C. perfringens* in food?
8. Where do outbreaks of *C. perfringens* commonly occur?
9. In what way is botulism a dangerous form of foodborne illness?
10. Why have the cases of botulism decreased in this century?
11. What are the symptoms of botulism?
12. How can botulism be prevented?
13. Which organism is most often identified with "travelers' diarrhea" or "Montezuma's revenge"?
14. What measures are taken to prevent *E. coli* infection?
15. What population groups are more susceptible to shigellosis? Why?
16. What is dysentery?
17. What are the symptoms of shigellosis in children?
18. What is the most frequent form of salmonellosis in the United States today?
19. What may be the reasons for the increase in the rate of salmonellosis from 1955 to 1985 and the decrease from 1985 to 1991?
20. In what three ways are *Salmonella* infections transmitted by ingestion?
21. Which foods are often found to be the source of *Salmonella* infection?
22. What pet has been found to harbor salmonellae?
23. What precautions should be taken to prevent foodborne salmonellosis?
24. What organism has recently been recognized to cause more cases of foodborne illness than *Salmonella?*
25. What measures will aid in the prevention of *C. jejuni?*
26. What is the fatality rate for cholera when it is untreated? Treated?
27. Where and when is cholera most likely to occur?
28. What is a distinctive symptom of cholera?
29. What is the main cause of death from cholera?
30. How is cholera prevented?
31. What is the story about Typhoid Mary and why is it important?
32. How does typhoid differ from other *Salmonella* infections?
33. What are the symptoms and complications of typhoid fever?
34. Upon what does prevention of typhoid fever depend?
35. Why is brucellosis called undulant fever?
36. How is brucellosis transmitted?
37. What complications may result from brucellosis?
38. What is the best means of preventing brucellosis?

FURTHER READING

Alpers, David H., Jerry L. Greenburg and William A. Sodeman Jr. "Gastroenteritis Treatment Tips." *Patient Care,* Mar. 30, '90, 24:18-32.

Baird-Parker, A.C. "Foodborne Salmonellosis." *Lancet,* Nov. 17, '90, 336:1231-1234.

Benenson, Abram S. *Control of Communicable Diseases in Man.* Washington, D.C.: American Public Health Association, 1990.

Besser, R.E., Lett, S.M., Weber, J.T. et al. "An outbreak of Diarrhea and Hemolytic Uremic Syndrome from *Escherichia coli* 0157:H7 in Fresh-Pressed Apple Cider." *JAMA,* 269(17):2217-2220.

Birkhead, GS, et al. "Typhoid fever at a resort hotel in New York: a large outbreak with an Unusual Vehicle". *Journal of Infectious Disease,* May '93, 167(5):1228-1232.

Blumenthal, Dale. "*Salmonella enteritidis:* From the Chicken to the Egg." *FDA Consumer,* Apr. '90, 24:6-10.

Boyd, Robert F. *General Microbiology.* St. Louis: Mosby, 1988.

Carey, Catherine. "Mary Mallon's Trail of Typhoid." *FDA Consumer,* June '89, 23:18-21.

Cerrato, Paul L. "Food Poisoning Makes a Dangerous Comeback." *RN,* Oct. '89, 52:73-76.

Clemens, John D., et al. "Field Trial of Oral Cholera Vaccines in Bangladesh." *Lancet,* Feb. 3, '90, 335:270-273.

Cohen, Deni, et al. "Reduction of Transmission of Shigellosis by Control of Houseflies." *Lancet,* Apr. 27, '91, 337:993-997.

Control of Communicable Disease in Man. Abram S. Benenson, Ed. Fifteenth Edition, Washington, D.C.: American Public Health Association, 1990.

Cooke, Mary E. "Epidemiology of Foodborne Illness." *Lancet,* Sept. 29, '90, 336:790-793.

Fackelmann, Kathy. "Football players benched by foul foods." *Science News.* Dec. 12, '92, 142, 407.

Flieger, Ken, et al. "Foul Flying Subs." *FDA Consumer,* July-Aug. '89, 23:34-36.

Flowers, Russell S. "Shigella." *Food Technology,* Apr. '88, 42:185-186.

Flowers, Russell S. "Salmonella." *Food Technology,* Apr. '88, 42:182-185.

From the Centers for Disease Control and Prevention. Update: Cholera—Western Hemisphere, *Journal of the American Medical Association,* March 17, '92, 269(11):1369.

Gorman, Christine. "Death in the Time of Cholera." *Time,* May 6, '91, 137:58-60.

Hardy, Ted. "The Tortoise and the Scare." *BioScience,* Feb. '88, 38:76-79.

Hedberg, CW, et al. "An international foodborne outbreak of shigellosis associated with a commercial airline." *Journal of the American Medical Association,* Dec. 9, '92, 268(22):3208-3212.

Hunter, Beatrice Trum. "A Newly Emerging Foodborne Disease." *Consumers' Research Magazine,* May '91, 74:8-9.

Jankovic, Joseph and Mitchell F. Brin. "Therapeutic Uses of Botulinum Toxin." *New England Journal of Medicine,* Apr. 25, '91, 324:1186-1194.

Jones, Keith, David Telford. "On the Trail of a Seasonal Microbe." *New Scientist,* Apr. 6, '91, 130:36-39.

Labbe, Ronald G. "*Clostridium perfringens.*" *Food Technology,* Apr. '88, 42:195-196.

Lancaster, Miriam J. "Botulism: North to Alaska." *American Journal of Nursing,* Jan. '90, 90:60-62.

Lund, Barbara M. "Foodborne Illness: Foodborne Disease Due to Bacillus and *Clostridium* Species." *Lancet,* Oct. 20, '90, 336:982-986.

Lyks, Rick. "Typhoid Fever Stuns Catskills." *Hotel and Motel Managment,* Sept. 4 '89, 204:117-118.

MacDonald, Kristine L., et al., "*Escherichia coli* 0157:H7, an Emerging Gastrointestinal Pathogen." *Journal of the American Medical Association,* June 24, '88, 259:3567-3570.

McCance, Kathryn L. and Sue E. Huether. *Pathophysiology: The Biologic Basis for Disease in Adults and Children.* St. Louis: Mosby, 1990.

McCombie, Susan, et al. "The Epidemiology of *S. sonnei* and *S. flexneri* in Pima County: An Exploratory Study." *American Journal of Public Health,* Sept. '88, 78:1227-1229.

Murray, Patrick, et al. *Medical Microbiology.* St. Louis: Mosby, 1990.

Newsome, Rosetta L. "*Staphylococcus aureus.*" *Food Technology,* Apr. '88, 42:194-195.

"On Tap: Safe Drinking Water." *Current Health,* Apr. '88, 14:16-18.

Ostroff, Stephen, John M. Kobayashi and Jay H. Lewis. "Infections with *Escherichia coli.*" *Journal of the American Medical Association,* July 21, '89, 262:355-359.

Personnet, Julie, et al. "Shigella Dysentery Type 1 Infections in U.S. Travelers to Mexico, 1988." *Lancet,* Sept. 2, '89, 2:543-545.

Piersdon, Merle D., N.R. Reddy. "*Clostridium botulinum.*" *Food Technology,* Apr. '88, 42:196-198.

Reeve, Gordon, et al. "An Outbreak of Shigellosis Associated with the Consumption of Raw Oysters." *New England Journal of Medicine,* July 27, '89, 321:224-227.

Ronsmans, Carine, Michael L. Bennish and Thomas Wierzba. "Diagnosis and Management of Dysentery by Community Health Workers." *Lancet,* Sept. 3, '88, 2:552-555.

Ruben, Bruce, et al. "Person-to-Person Transmission of *Brucella melitensis.*" *Lancet,* Jan. 5, '91, 337:14-15.

St. Louis, Michael E., et al. "The Emergence of Grade A Eggs as a Major Source of *Salmonella enteritidis* Infections." *Journal of the American Medical Association,* Apr. 8, '88, 259:2103-2107.

"Salmonella and Food Safety." *Consumers' Research Magazine,* Mar. '89, 72:29-31.

Segal, Marian, Peter M. Sandman. "Is It Worth The Worry? Determining Risk." *FDA Consumer,* June '90, 24:7-11.

Segal, Marian and Richard Thompson. "Fish 'Delicacy' Causes Botulism Illness and Death." *FDA Consumer,* May '88, 22:33-36.

Skirrow, M.B. "*Campylobacter.*" *Lancet,* Oct. 13, '90, 336:921-923.

Tauxe, Robert V., et al. "The Persistence of *Shigella flexneri* in the United States: Increasing Role of Adult Males." *American Journal of Public Health,* Nov. '88, 78:1432-1435.

Telzak, Edward E., et al. "A Nosocomial Outbreak of *Salmonella enteritidis* Infection due to the Consumption of Raw Eggs." *New England Journal of Medicine,* Aug. 9, '90, 323:394-397.

Tranter, Howard S. "Foodborne Staphylococcal Illness." *Lancet,* Oct. 27, '90, 336:1044-1046.

"Update: Multistate Outbreak of Escherichia Coli 0157:H7 Infections from Hamburgers—Western United States, 1992-1993." *Morbidity and Mortality Weekly Reports,* April 16, 1993, 42(14):258-263.

Waites, W.M., J.P. Arbuthnott. "Foodborne Illness." *Lancet,* Sept. 22, '90, 336:722-725.

Woodruff, Bradley A., Andrew T. Pavia and Paul A. Blake. "A New Look at Typhoid Vaccination." *Journal of the American Medical Association,* Feb. 13, '91, 265:756-759.

Chapter 6

Bacterial Infections Acquired through Skin, Mucosa, and Bloodstream from Human and Endogenous Sources

O B J E C T I V E S

1 Identify common diseases that may be due to infection from endogenous sources and/or autoinfection.

2 Distinguish among folliculitis, boils, and carbuncles.

3 Indicate conditions in the host that are conducive for toxic shock syndrome.

4 Explain the importance of recognizing impetigo in children.

5 Explain the stigma attached to leprosy.

6 Discuss reasons for the rise and fall of syphilis and gonorrhea cases over the years.

7 Compare chlamydia and gonorrhea.

8 Discuss symptoms, treatment, prevention, and control for the following diseases:
Folliculitis, boils, and carbuncles
Osteomyelitis
Toxic shock syndrome
Impetigo
Conjunctivitis
Meningitis
Endocarditis
Leprosy
Syphilis
Gonorrhea
Chlamydia

FOLLICULITIS, FURUNCLES (BOILS), AND CARBUNCLES

There are three common skin infections caused by *Staphylococcus aureus* and all are easily identified. The basic difference among them is in degree of severity. The first, folliculitis, is inflammation of a hair follicle. The second, furunculosis, involves deeper layers of the skin, gland, or hair follicle. The third, carbuncle, encompasses more than one hair follicle and also invades deep tissue. *S. aureus* are pyogenic (pus-causing) bacteria and are found worldwide. They are common in children, especially in warm weather, and may also occur in places where there is poor personal hygiene and people are crowded. Also, many people who have an initial infection leading to a boil or carbuncle seem to be more susceptible and may develop further infections any time their resistance is lowered sufficiently and other conditions resulting in infection are present. Why some people are more susceptible to *S. aureus* infection than others has not been determined.

Transmission   The hands are the most important mode of transmission. The reservoir of infection is people; *S. aureus* is a natural inhabitant on the skin of many people, and 30% to 40% of the general population carry staphylococci in their nasal passages. Self-infection is responsible for at least one third of the infections. Person-to-person transmission is by contact with a person who has a purulent (containing pus) lesion or with an asymptomatic carrier.

Symptoms   The staphylococcal organism may cause an infection wherever there is a break in the skin. Sometimes the infection may occur on an eyelid, and it is then referred to as a stye. When folliculitis occurs, tiny red pustules appear. Most of the time, only one hair follicle becomes infected, but there are conditions under which the result is pustules over a wide area of skin, as seen in Figure 6-1. Boils appear as hard, painful nodules, commonly on the neck, face, axillae (armpits), and buttocks (Figure 6-2). Boils will generally enlarge and rupture, discharging the pus. A carbuncle is marked by an extremely painful, deep abscess that drains through multiple openings, usually around several hair follicles.

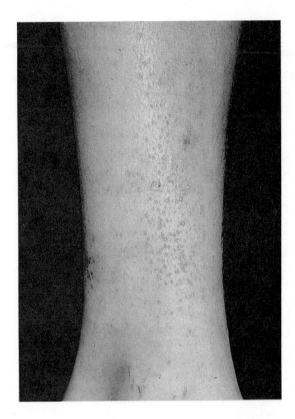

FIGURE 6-1   A case of staphylococcal folliculitis caused by occlusion of the area by a topical steroid and a plastic dressing for 24 hours, allowing the organisms to flourish.

FIGURE 6-2   A boil.

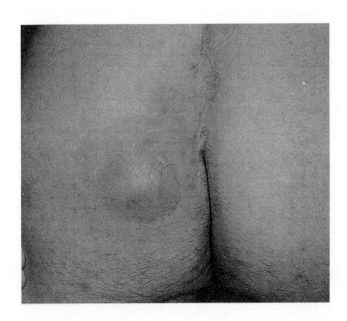

Treatment   Folliculitis generally needs no treatment other than keeping the area clean. Use of an antibiotic ointment may aid in healing. For boils and carbuncles, in addition to keeping the area clean, and use of antibiotic ointments, pressure should be kept off the site. Hot compresses will facilitate healing. Possible sites of reinfection should be identified and treated. If the infection is severe, it may require antibiotics and surgical drainage, which can be performed in a doctor's office.

Prevention   Good personal hygiene and maintaining a high level of resistance through a positive lifestyle are the best means of preventing staphylococcal infections. Children need to be educated in hand washing and the importance of avoiding common use of toilet articles.

Control   Infants, the ill, and the elderly are the most susceptible to *S. aureus,* and infected persons should avoid contact with them. Education in personal hygiene, with special emphasis on not sharing personal items, even in the family, will help to keep the infection from spreading. Boils are teeming with bacteria, and particular care should be taken in discarding dressings from lesions that are draining. Anyone having a boil needs to be cautioned not to try and squeeze it to get the pus out. If the wall of the boil breaks, it can lead to bacteremia (blood poisoning) and deep-tissue infections such as osteomyelitis, which will be discussed next.

OSTEOMYELITIS

Osteomyelitis is an infection of the bone and bone marrow that may be chronic or acute. The most frequent cause of the infection is *S. aureus.* Bone infections are not as common today as they once were, and with the advent of antibiotics, they are much easier to treat.

The infection occurs more often in children than in adults and more in boys than in girls. The most common sites in children are the lower end of the femur and the upper end of the tibia, humerus, and radius. In adults, osteomyelitis occurs most frequently in the bones of the pelvis and vertebrae. With prompt treatment, the prognosis (outcome) for the acute form is good, but the prognosis for chronic osteomyelitis is poor. The massive bone destruction and reactive sclerosis (hardening of tissue) shown in Figure 6-3 occurred more with osteomyelitis before the advent of antibiotics. Drug users and individuals undergoing trauma to the bone, or surgery, are more susceptible.

Transmission   Because osteomyelitis is an internal infection, person-to-person transmission is un-likely. However, individuals who have the infection may carry *S. aureus* on their skin or mucous membranes or may have a boil or carbuncle from which the infection has traveled to the bone.

Symptoms   Osteomyelitis has an abrupt onset with sudden pain in the affected bone, tenderness, heat, swelling, and restricted movement over the bone. There may also be sudden fever, tachycardia (fast heartbeat), nausea, and malaise.

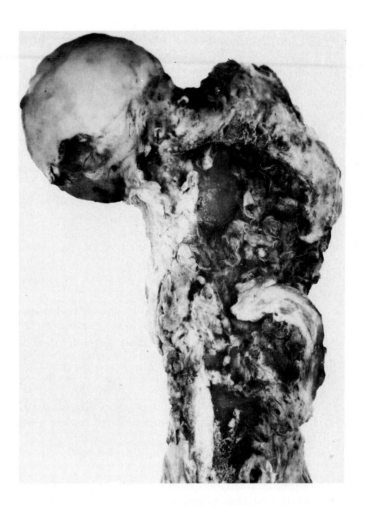

FIGURE 6-3 Osteo-
myelitis of upper femur
with massive bone de-
struction and reactive
sclerosis.

Treatment Four to 8 weeks of antibiotic therapy, surgical debridement (removal of dead tissue), and drainage are generally necessary for healing. Analgesics are administered for the pain, which may be severe.

Prevention Individuals with boils or other pus–containing lesions must refrain from squeezing them to release the pus. As was stated before, this action can break the protecting wall and allow the pus containing the pathogenic organisms to enter the bloodstream.

Control The individual with osteomyelitis should be checked for a penetration wound from which the organism originated to see whether it is presently infected. Sterile procedures need to be followed in disposal of any bandages from a draining wound.

TOXIC SHOCK SYNDROME

Toxic shock syndrome (TSS) is an acute bacterial infection that usually affects menstruating women under age 30. When cases of the disease suddenly emerged in the early 1980s, an intense investigation took place in an effort to determine the cause of the potentially fatal illness. The infecting organism was identified as *S. aureus*. Unfortunately, the strains that were identified were penicillin resistant, making the infection more difficult to treat. The use of tampons, particularly those that were super absorbent, was soon linked to the majority of cases. There have been a few cases in boys and men and also among nonmenstruating women. Of those cases not occurring in association with menstruation, some have been linked to a cervical cap, diaphragm, sponge, or an infection in another part of the body.

Transmission Since staphylococcal bacteria are commonly present in the vagina, an infection may occur whenever the right conditions are present to allow the toxin access to the circulatory system. As indicated above, these conditions include use of a tampon during the menstrual period and possibly use of certain birth control methods. There is no person-to-person transmission.

Symptoms The symptoms of toxic shock syndrome include fever (generally over 104° F), headache, vomiting, sore throat, diarrhea, muscle aches, sunburnlike rash, low blood pressure, bloodshot eyes, disorientation, reduced urination, and peeling of the skin on the palms and soles of the feet.

Treatment Although the causative organisms are penicillin resistant, other antibiotics such as oxacillin, nafcillin, and methicillin are effective. Fluid replacement may be necessary to reverse shock.

Prevention TSS during menstruation can be avoided by not using tampons. The risk can be reduced by switching to less absorbent tampons and by changing them frequently. Contraceptive devices, which have also been implicated, should not be left in place more than 30 hours or beyond the directions on the package.

Control Since there is no person-to-person transmission, control is a matter of educating women about safe usage of contraceptive methods and tampons.

IMPETIGO

Impetigo is especially common in the newborn and children, particularly during hot, humid weather. It is highly contagious and spreads rapidly in families and crowded conditions such as schools. It may be caused by *S. aureus* or *Streptococcus pyogenes*. Poor skin hygiene and skin conditions such as an abrasion or draining wounds are predisposing factors. The infection occurs worldwide and is especially prevalent in warm weather. People are the reservoir of infection. The incubation period is variable, usually 4 to 10 days. As with other staphylococcal skin infections, communicability lasts as long as there is a discharge of pus or the carrier state is present.

Transmission   Impetigo can be spread quickly through direct and indirect contact. The hands are the main method of transmission, although fomites such as damp towels and other moist objects can also be a means of transmission. As in other staph and strep infections, autoinfection is responsible for about one-third of the cases.

Symptoms   Impetigo starts as a small reddish spot on the skin that develops into a vesicle (a blisterlike small elevation containing fluid) and then becomes pustular (filled with lymph or pus). Figure 6-4 is an example of impetigo caused by *S. pyogenes*. The fluid is straw colored, and the pustule ruptures and becomes crusted. Impetigo occurs principally on the face. It is generally localized but can lead to more serious infections deeper in the system.

Treatment   Systemic antibiotics are not used unless fever, malaise, or secondary complications are present. An antibiotic ointment such as bacitracin is generally prescribed. After the crusts are removed and the skin cleansed, the ointment is applied to the lesion.

Prevention   Education in personal hygiene and a positive lifestyle are the best means of prevention.

Control   Because impetigo is highly contagious, children who have it should be excluded from school or day-care centers and not allowed contact with infants and the

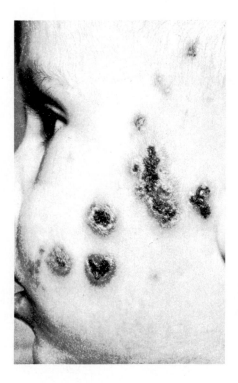

FIGURE 6-4 Impetigo on the face of a child.

chronically ill. Individuals with diabetes and the elderly are also more susceptible and should be protected from infection. There should be an emphasis on frequent hand washing by all who live with or come in contact with the infected individual, and common use of toilet articles should be avoided.

CONJUNCTIVITIS

Conjunctivitis is commonly known as "pink eye" from the redness (inflammation) that develops in the white of the eye. The conjunctiva is the mucous membrane that lines the eyelids and also covers the eyeball (Figure 6-5). The condition may be due to allergy or infection by bacteria, viruses, or chlamydia. Most often, conjunctivitis is caused by bacteria or viruses. The most important bacterial agents seem to be *Haemophilus influenzae* and *Streptococcus pneumoniae*. Incubation is 24 to 72 hours, and the infection is communicable as long as it is active. People are the reservoir of infection, and children under the age of 5 years are most susceptible, although those whose resistance is low are also at risk. Although conjunctivitis is usually a mild infection in the United States, other bacteria and also enteroviruses have caused it in other countries, and in Brazil a form known as Brazilian *purpuric* fever, or BPF, has resulted in a 70% fatality rate.

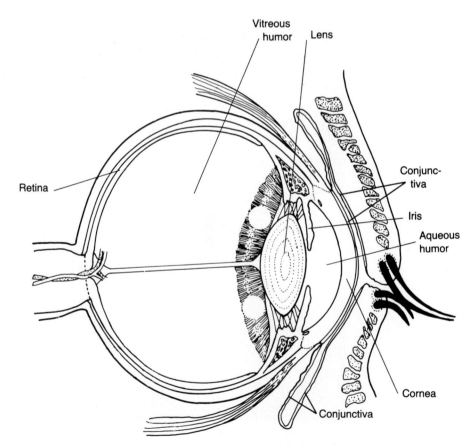

FIGURE 6-5 Longitudinal section through eyeball and eyelids showing the conjunctiva. Conjunctiva line the posterior surface of the eyelids and cover the cornea.

Transmission   There are many ways by which an infection of the eye can be transmitted. These include contact with discharges from an infected person, contaminated fingers, fomites, and insect vectors.

Symptoms   Redness, itchiness, purulent discharge, and occasionally photophobia (sensitivity to bright lights). Sometimes when the discharge is purulent, the eyelids are stuck together in the morning.

Treatment   Warm water will wash away discharge and crusts on the eyelids. An antibiotic ointment and/or eye drops may be applied, and, depending on the infecting organism, an oral antibiotic may also be used.

Prevention   Attention to personal hygiene is necessary. Sanitary conditions where children play, including the home and day-care centers, need to be enforced at all times.

Control   In addition to preventive methods above, individuals with conjunctivitis should be treated promptly, and contacts watched for possible infection. If an insect vector is involved, then insect control is called for.

MENINGITIS

The meninges are the membranes surrounding the brain and spinal cord, or central nervous system (CNS). Meningitis occurs when these membranes become inflamed as a result of infection with a pathogenic organism. Many times it is a complication of bacterial infection at some other location in the body. There are three organisms that are responsible for most cases of bacterial meningitis: *H. influenzae, Neisseria meningitidis,* and *S. pneumoniae. H. influenzae* infections (hemophilus meningitis), tend to occur more in children; *N. meningitidis* infections (meningococcal meningitis), occur more in young adults, particularly where there are close quarters such as dormitories or army barracks; and *S. pneumoniae* infections (pneumococcal meningitis) are more frequent in infants, older adults, and alcoholics. Viruses, fungi, and parasitic worms can also cause meningitis.

Transmission   The mode of transmission varies, depending upon which organism is responsible for the infection. Most forms are transmitted by direct contact with respiratory secretions from the nose and throat of infected persons.

Symptoms   Symptoms of meningitis also may vary with the infecting agent but generally include fever, chills, malaise, headache, and vomiting. As the meninges become more irritated, other problems occur, such as stiff neck, problems in leg extension after flexion, exaggerated deep tendon reflexes, and back spasm in which the back arches backward so that the body rests on the head and heels. In babies, signs are not so apparent, and the infant may just be fretful and refuse to eat. The infant may vomit a great deal, leading to dehydration. This reduces fluid in the system and keeps the fontanelle (soft spot on top of head) from bulging, which is one of the signs of intracranial pressure. As the disease progresses, twitching, seizures, or coma may develop. Children who are older generally have the same symptoms as adults. The onset may be acute or insidious.

Treatment Usually antibiotics are administered intravenously (IV) for at least 2 weeks, followed by oral antibiotics. Ampicillin is the drug of choice. However, due to resistant strains of bacteria, ampicillin may not be effective, and it is recommended that Ceftriaxone or another cephalosporin be used concurrently or by itself until it is known whether or not the infecting organism is resistant to ampicillin.

Prevention Antibiotics may be used prophylactically when trauma or surgery invade the area of the brain or spinal cord because infection is always a possibility. A vaccine is available that is effective against *H. influenzae* type B and is recommended for children under 15 months. Day-care centers and other places where there is close contact between children need to be monitored when cases are present among those attending. Vaccines are also available for some forms of *N. meningitidis*.

Control Individuals with meningitis should be isolated for 24 hours after start of treatment with antibiotics. Some physicians advise use of rifampin prophylactically for all household contacts and in day-care centers when a case has occurred among children.

ENDOCARDITIS

Endocarditis is inflammation of the endocardium (inner lining) of the heart, particularly the valves. Figure 6-6 shows the three layers of the heart. The infection

FIGURE 6-6 Section of the heart wall showing the components of the outer heart sac (pericardium), muscle layer (myocardium) and inner lining (endocardium).

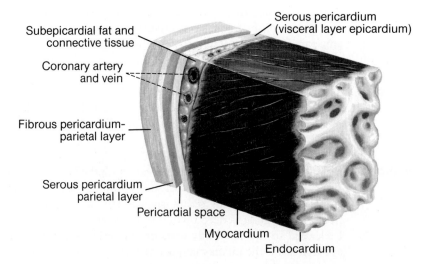

Subepicardial fat and connective tissue

Coronary artery and vein

Fibrous pericardium-parietal layer

Serous pericardium parietal layer

Pericardial space

Myocardium

Endocardium

Serous pericardium (visceral layer epicardium)

that causes the inflammation may occur by itself or as a complication of another disease. The disease agent is most often staphylococcal or streptococcal. It occurs when bacteria or other organisms are able to enter the bloodstream and infect the heart. There are two types of bacterial endocarditis, acute and subacute. Dental and surgical procedures predispose an individual to this infection, and in those whose hearts have been damaged by some other condition there is greater risk. Drug addicts who inject the drugs are also at risk. Fungal and nonbacterial endocarditis occur, but they are rare. Before antibiotics, 95% of individuals with bacterial endocarditis died. Today, 65% to 80% recover.

Transmission   Bacteria may be introduced into the bloodstream during cardiac surgery, by shared needles, as a result of any kind of intravenous injection, or through a penetrating wound. Since bacteria are common inhabitants on the skin of many people, autoinfection is also possible.

Symptoms   In the subacute form, the infection may be present for months, causing serious damage to the heart but only general and nonspecific symptoms. There may be feverishness, night sweats, vague aches and pains, fatigue, and weakness. Sometimes there is a change in an already present murmur or a new murmur. The symptoms for acute bacterial endocarditis are sudden chills, high fever, shortness of breath, and rapid or irregular heartbeat. It is a rapidly progressing infection and may lead to heart failure. Clots may break off from the initial site of the infection and travel to other organs, causing blocking or infection there.

Treatment   High doses of antibiotic drugs are given IV and continued for as long as 6 weeks. If a heart valve is damaged, surgical repair or prosthetic replacement may be necessary.

Prevention   Prophylactic treatment with antibiotics is prescribed as a preventive measure for people with heart valve defects. This is especially important before surgical or dental procedures. Those at risk need to be educated as to the signs of endocarditis.

Control   The source should be identified, if possible, in order to avoid further incidents. The individual does not need to be isolated since endocarditis is not communicable.

LEPROSY

Many people are familiar with the stories of lepers in the Bible and the isolation that was imposed upon them. If it had not been for the unsightly disfigurations caused by the disease, this segregation of the lepers would not have occurred. There must have been some fear that spread of the disease could be caused by contact with those who had it, even though the true means of disease transmission would not be discovered for centuries. It is now known that although leprosy can be spread through person-to-person contact, it is much less contagious than was once thought.

DID YOU KNOW?

Victims of Leprosy Today

An estimated 10 to 20 million people in the world still have leprosy. One percent to 2% of the population in tropical countries have the disease. Twenty percent of the cases are in children under the age of 10. In treating the disease, early identification is most important so that medical therapy can begin before deformities have developed.

Leprosy, also known as Hansen's disease, is found all over the world. Up to 80% of the individuals suffering with the disease have no access to treatment. There are now more than 4000 known cases in the United States, mainly in California, Florida, Hawaii, Louisiana, New York, and Texas; three quarters were born outside the United States. The infectious organism is *Mycobacterium leprae,* which causes two forms of leprosy, lepromatous and tuberculoid; as far as is known now, humans are the only significant reservoir. The incubation period is from 9 months to 20 years, and the disease is rarely seen in children under 3 years of age. It is estimated that only 3% of the population is susceptible to the disease.

Transmission The exact means of transmission is unknown. Only living in prolonged close contact with an infected person puts anyone at risk of contracting the disease. The organisms are present in nasal secretions and probably enter through the upper respiratory tract or a break in the skin.

Symptoms The organism attacks the peripheral nervous system. In tuberculoid leprosy, there are raised, large erythematous (red) plaques or macules (discolored spots on skin) with clear borders (Figure 6-7). These spots become larger, rough, hairless, and gradually colorless, finally leaving painless scars. The disease process occurs particularly on the face, arms, legs, and buttocks. Some typical characteristics of lepromatous leprosy are seen in Figure 6-8. Lepromatous leprosy also causes damage to the upper respiratory tract, eyes, and testes. The lesions eventually form nodules called lepromas on the earlobes, nose, eyebrows, and forehead. Claw hand, pictured in Figure 6-9, is another characteristic feature of leprosy due to involvement of the ulnar nerve.

Because individuals with leprosy lose sensation, they are subject to a number of problems. They are unable to tell when something they touch is too hot. An infection may go unnoticed until it has spread so far that amputation is necessary. In undeveloped countries where sanitation is lacking and people sleep on dirt floors, there have been cases of lepers having toes gnawed at by a rat during sleep and actually losing a toe without waking up.

Treatment Because of increased resistance of *M. leprae* to antibiotics, a number of different drugs are used to treat the disease. Early treatment, before damage has occurred,

FIGURE 6-7 Tuberculoid lesions on a man's face.

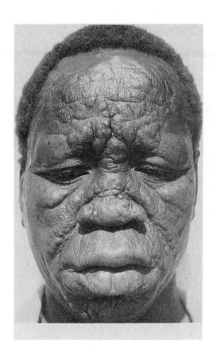

FIGURE 6-8 Nodules of lepromatous lesions on the face and hands. These photographs show early (top) and late stages of the disease in the same person.

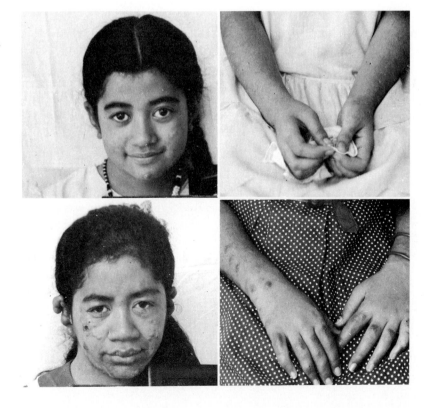

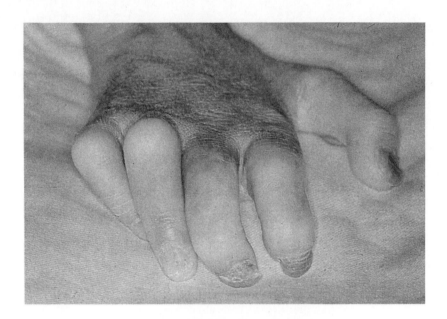

FIGURE 6-9 Claw hand of person with leprosy.

can lead to a cure. Later treatment cannot reverse damage to the skin and other organs that may be involved but can halt the disease. However, increased resistance of the organism to the most effective drugs is causing an intense search for others to be used in treating the disease.

Prevention   Treatment centers are available so that infected individuals can be away from the family until they are cured. Education of the public concerning the availability of treatment is necessary.

Control   Investigation of contacts to determine other cases and contact isolation in the case of lepromatous leprosy are the main means of control.

SYPHILIS

Syphilis was present in early Egyptian days; it was described by Hippocrates in 460 BC; the Bible refers to syphilis; it was described by a Roman physician in AD 25; syphilis is still a problem today. Plagues of syphilis have been the cause of millions of the world's crippled, blind, insane, and dead. It has infected young and old, rich and poor, prince and pauper.

Syphilis has played an important part in shaping the course of history. It is believed that Columbus and his men spread the disease in Spain after their return from the New World. Columbus himself died of the disease. Vasco da Gama carried it to India in 1498, and by 1501 it was in China. It has traveled with armies throughout history. Charles VIII of France died of syphilis, and all his heirs were born dead of syphilis, ending a dynasty. Other kings and emperors acquired syphilis that affected their minds and consequently their actions.

DID YOU KNOW?

Pause for Thought

Animals are susceptible to syphilis too, and for a long time it was thought that shepherds got the disease from their sheep, thereby causing its occurrence and transmission in humans. Now, because of a discovery in 1987 of the remains of a bear over 11,000 years old that showed signs of having syphilis, it is thought that humans got the disease from the bite of a bear or through contact with the bear's meat after killing it for a meal.

In the United States, syphilis became a very serious problem in the War of 1812. More than 77,000 Union soldiers contracted syphilis during the Civil War. In World War I, about 3 million cases of syphilis were contracted by the soldiers of all armies. One million men in the U.S. armed services were found to have syphilis between 1940 and 1945.

With the discovery and use of penicillin in the late 1940s, new cases of syphilis began to drop sharply. Almost everyone believed the end of syphilis was in sight, and programs for its control began to be curtailed. Then, in 1958, with the advent of the female contraceptive pill, penicillin-resistant strains, curtailment of programs for control, and a general feeling that the "cure" had been found, the incidence of syphilis began to rise again (Figure 6-10). In 1982, a sharp decrease in the number of cases began, probably as a result of less and "safer" sex because of the acquired immune deficiency syndrome (AIDS) scare, but by 1986, a new epidemic of syphilis had begun. According to the Centers for Disease Control (CDC), three factors have contributed to the latest epidemic. First, the use of cocaine and other drugs tends to promote high-risk sexual behaviors, and those who use it are hard to find (their illegal activity means they do not want to be found). Second, the individuals with the highest risk do not have access to health care, do not know where or when to find help, or do not consider health care a high priority. Third, those most involved with drug use are often jobless, uneducated, come from dysfunctional families, and have many sex partners.* Figures 6-11, 6-12, and 6-13 indicate the increasing rates of syphilis in genders, races, and states.

Syphilis and other diseases transmitted mainly through sexual relations were initially called venereal diseases after Venus, the Roman goddess of love. As it became clear that there were other means of transmission of these diseases, and in order to erase some of the stigma attached to the term venereal disease, a new term, *sexually transmitted diseases* (STDs), has come into use.

Syphilis is caused by a spirochete, *Treponema pallidum,* which is capable of entering the body through the mucous membrane. The infection spreads throughout the body in progressive stages: primary, secondary, latent, and late, or tertiary, syphilis. The incubation period for syphilis can run from 10 days to 3 months but is usually 3 weeks. The disease is communicable during the first three stages and

*"Primary and Secondary Syphilis—United States, 1981-1990." *MMWR,* May 17, '91, 40:19, 314+.

can be transmitted to the fetus in the womb. Susceptibility is general, although only 30% of those exposed become infected.

Transmission   Direct contact with body fluids containing the organism, during sexual or other intimate contact, is the major means of transmission. Infection of the fetus occurs through the placental membrane. The organism can be transmitted through blood transfusion from a victim in the early stages. It is possible to contract syphilis by contact with contaminated articles but highly unlikely since the organism can only exist in moist body fluids. Exposure to air, drying, and soap and water will all destroy *T. pallidum*.

Symptoms   The first sign of syphilis is a painless sore or chancre at the point at which the organism invaded the body (Figure 6-14). This sore is teeming with spirochetes, but because it is painless, because it may be in the rectum or on the cervix, and because it disappears in 4 to 6 weeks, it generally goes untreated and undiagnosed. This is the primary stage.

     The secondary stage, which may develop within a few days to 8 weeks, most often includes a rash, lymph node enlargement, headache, aches and pains in the bones, loss of appetite, fever, and fatigue. Hair may fall out in clumps, and meningitis may occur. An example of a rash from secondary syphilis can be seen in Figure 6-15. Secondary syphilis disappears without treatment in a matter of weeks or months. This is the beginning of the latent stage.

FIGURE 6-14 Syphilis chancre on the penis.

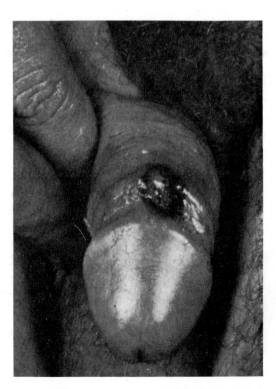

For many, there will be no more symptoms, but about 30% will go on into the late, or tertiary, stage. It is at this time, after traveling deep within the body and into many areas that the spirochete does its great damage. The first symptoms appear in 1 to 25 years. The basic lesion of tertiary syphilis is known as a gumma (Figure 6-16). There are no spirochetes in this lesion, and it is painless.

Among the more serious effects in the late stages are cardiovascular syphilis, which affects the aorta and leads to aneurysms and heart valve disease; neurosyphilis, leading to progressive brain damage and general paralysis; and tabes dorsalis, which

FIGURE 6-15   Syphilis rash.

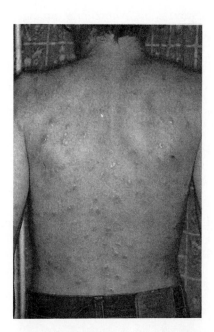

FIGURE 6-16   The basic lesion of syphilis, a gumma.

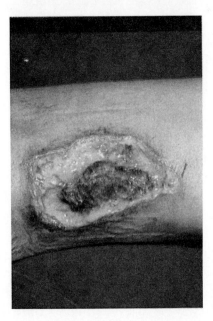

affects part of the spinal cord. The disease is no longer communicable in the late stage.

Treatment   Syphilis can be cured with penicillin in all three stages, but organ damage caused by the disease cannot be reversed. The fetus can be cured in the womb if the mother is treated soon enough.

Prevention   The best means of prevention is by maintaining monogamous relationships. Condoms offer some protection. Immunity develops slowly after infection with *T. pallidum,* but if treatment occurs early, in the first or second stage and/or human immune deficiency virus (HIV) is present, the amount of immunity is reduced.

Control   Contact investigation is the most important feature of syphilis control. Interviews with diagnosed cases by professional interviewers and a concerted effort to track down and screen all reported contacts help to control the disease.

GONORRHEA

Gonorrhea, like syphilis, is a very old disease. It was described nearly 5000 years ago by the Chinese and later by the Egyptians. There are also references to it in the Bible. Gonorrhea is caused by the gonococcus *Neisseria gonorrhoeae,* and Galen gave it its name, which means "flowing seed." The most common nickname is *the clap.*

FIGURE 6-17 Gonorrhea cases by 4-week period of report—United States, 1984-1991.

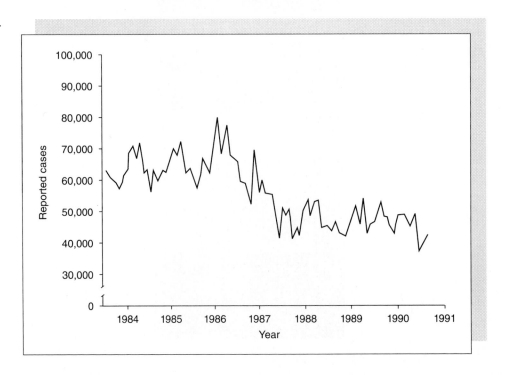

Not long ago, gonorrhea was the most common sexually transmitted disease, but it is now second to chlamydia. The incubation period is 2 to 7 days. In the last 20 years, the number of cases have increased all over the world; in the United States, the number of cases has decreased since 1985 (Figure 6-17). Communicability may be present for months, and there is general susceptibility to the disease.

Transmission

Transmission is by contact with body fluid of an infected individual and almost always through sexual activity. In children older than 1 year, it is generally a result of sexual molestation.

Symptoms

In 80% of women, there may be no symptoms until the disease has infected the fallopian tubes. If there are symptoms, they usually consist of a vaginal discharge or a burning sensation on urination.

Figure 6-18 shows a sign of gonorrhea in men, a purulent urethral discharge. There is also redness and swelling at the site of infection, and many have painful urination. Men may also be asymptomatic. If the disease is untreated, other symptoms occur, depending upon the site of infection. These may include frequent urination, itching and pain of the vulva, redness, swelling, and discharge from the vagina.

Infection through anal sex causes inflammation of the rectum and anus; gonococcal pharyngitis may result from oral sex. Babies may acquire a severe eye infection during childbirth. If they are born in a hospital, silver nitrate drops in their eyes to prevent infection are required.

Untreated gonorrhea may lead to inflammation of the prostate or testes in men, affecting fertility, and to pelvic inflammatory disease (PID) in women, leading to the possibility of ectopic pregnancy and infertility.

For both sexes, there is the chance of gonococcal arthritis, septicemia, and heart disease.

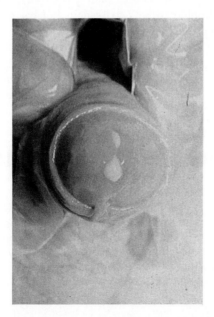

FIGURE 6-18 A purulent urethral discharge is the commonest presentation of gonorrhea in males.

Treatment   Gonorrhea is usually treated with penicillin or ampicillin. Three strains of *N. gon-orrhoeae* are resistant to antibiotics. These are penicillinase-producing *N. gonorrhoeae* (PPNG), chromosomally mediated resistance to penicillin (CMRNG), and plasmid-mediated high-level tetracycline resistance (TRNG). Although treatment has become more difficult because of these resistant bacteria, it still can be cured by other antibiotics, sometimes in combination. However, if damage has occurred (scar tissue and/or sterility) it may not be possible to correct.

Prevention   The best means of prevention is to have sex in a monogamous relationship only. Condoms offer some protection. There is no immunity after infection with gonorrhea, and no vaccine is available to date.

Control   Contact investigation and treatment of infected individuals are the best means of control. No vaccine has been developed.

CHLAMYDIA GENITAL INFECTIONS

With the improvement of laboratory equipment has come the discovery of new organisms and strains. When chlamydiae were first discovered, there was a question as to what class of microorganisms they were, since, like viruses, they multiply in cells or other organisms but otherwise have many of the characteristics of bacteria, including susceptibility to antibiotic treatment. At present, they are generally classified as bacteria. Chlamydiae are a cause of nonspecific urethritis (NSU), sometimes called nongonococcal urethritis (NGU). Chlamydia causes more STD in the United States than any other organism. In addition to causing urethritis in men and cervicitis in women, *Chlamydia trachomatis* is also responsible for trachoma and lymphogranuloma. Chlamydial infections can be found all over the world, and recognition of them has been increasing in the United States, Australia, Canada, and Europe. The incubation period is thought to be 7 to 14 days but has not been clearly identified yet. Everyone is susceptible to the chlamydia organism.

Transmission   *C. trachomatis* is transmitted by sexual intercourse and during childbirth to babies in the birth canal, causing eye infection and pneumonia in the newborn.

CONTEMPORARY CONCERNS

Stealthy Advance of STD

Chlamydia has replaced gonorrhea as the most prevalent sexually transmitted bacterial infection. It is sometimes called the silent disease because 75% of women and 20% of men with the disease have few or no symptoms. However, the organism may cause scarring and blockage leading to sterility in men and women that is not discovered until they attempt to have children. By then, it may be too late.

Symptoms   Both men and women may be asymptomatic. When there are symptoms, these may include a discharge from the penis or vagina, swelling of the testes for men or painful urination for women. If the disease is not treated, it can lead to infertility in men and women.

Treatment   Antibiotics are usually very successful for treatment of chlamydia.

Prevention   The best method of prevention is to have sexual relations only within a monogamous relationship. Condoms offer some protection.

Control   Testing of partners and other contact investigation are the means of control.

SUMMARY

The table summarizes the principal information related to infectious diseases acquired through the skin, mucous membranes, and bloodstream.

SUMMARY TABLE   Bacterial diseases acquired through skin, mucosa, and bloodstream from human and endogenous sources

Disease	Special Characteristics	Transmission	Common Symptoms	Prevention/ Control
Folliculitis, furuncles, and carbuncles	All caused by *S. aureus*. Boil or carbuncle—pressure or squeezing can lead to complications.	Person-to-person or autoinfection.	Inflammation, pain. Boils—hard, painful nodule, discharge of pus, one opening. Carbuncle—extremely painful deep abscess, discharge of pus, multiple openings.	Good personal hygiene, education of children in hand washing. Healthful lifestyle.
Osteomyelitis	Infection of bone and bone marrow. May be caused by a blow. *S. aureus* is the disease agent.	No person-to-person transmission.	Abrupt onset, sudden pain in bone, tenderness, heat, swelling, and restricted movement.	None known.
Toxic shock syndrome	Usually affects menstruating women under 30.	No person-to-person transmission.	Fever, headache, vomiting, sore throat, diarrhea,	Use no tampons, or less absorbent tampons, and change frequently.

Treatment: Antibiotics used topically (in an ointment), orally, or intravenously are the primary treatment for bacterial infections.

Continued.

SUMMARY TABLE Bacterial diseases acquired through skin, mucosa, and bloodstream from human and endogenous sources—cont'd

Disease	Special Characteristics	Transmission	Common Symptoms	Prevention/Control
Toxic shock syndrome, cont'd	S. aureus is the disease agent. Super-absorbent tampons implicated.		Muscle aches, rash, bloodshot eyes, low blood pressure, disorientation, reduced urination, peeling of skin on palms and soles of feet.	Do not leave contraceptive devices in place more than 30 hours or beyond directions on package. If tampons are used, use low absorbency ones and change frequently.
Impetigo	Especially in newborn and children, highly contagious.	Direct and indirect contact.	Fluid-filled vesicles that rupture and become crusted. Mostly around mouth and nose.	Good personal hygiene and a positive lifestyle.
Conjunctivitis	"Pink eye." More common in children under 5. May be caused by staph, strep, gonococci, others.	Direct and indirect contact.	Redness, itchiness, purulent discharge.	Good personal hygiene and a positive lifestyle.
Meningitis	Caused by several different bacteria and other organisms.	Direct and/or indirect, depending on infecting organism.	Fever, chills, malaise, headache, vomiting, stiff neck, back spasms. Twitching, seizures, coma.	Prophylactic antibiotics for high-risk individuals. Vaccine for children less than 18 months. Isolation for 24 hours after antibiotic treatment begins.
Endocarditis	Two types: acute and subacute. Risk in dental and surgical procedures, drug addicts. Caused by different strains of bacteria and other organisms. Before antibiotics, 95% died.	Bacteria introduced into bloodstream by IV, surgery, shared needles, wound. No person-to-person transmission.	Acute: Sudden chills, high fever, shortness of breath, rapid or irregular heartbeat.	Prophylactic treatment with antibiotics for those at risk.
Leprosy	Hansen's disease, low contagion, incubation 9 months to 20 years. Two types: tuberculoid and lepromatous. More common in rural tropics. Most cases in the U.S. are imported.	Exact means unknown. Probably through upper respiratory system or break in skin. Prolonged, close contact with infected individual necessary.	Large red plaques or macules on skin that become nodules. Affects the nervous system.	Organism resistant to antibiotics. Other drugs being used.

SUMMARY TABLE   **Bacterial diseases acquired through skin, mucosa, and bloodstream from human and endogenous sources—cont'd**

Disease	Special Characteristics	Transmission	Common Symptoms	Prevention/ Control
Syphilis	Has caused much suffering and death for thousands of years. Has affected history. *T. pallidum,* a spirochete, causes the disease. Survives only in body fluids. Fetus infected through placenta. All stages, mother and fetus can be cured with penicillin; damage irreparable.	Direct contact with body fluids containing the spirochete; 99% of time syphilis is transmitted through sexual intercourse.	Primary: Chancres swarming with spirochetes. Secondary: More chancres, rash, enlarged lymph nodes, headache, aches and pains in bones, fever, fatigue, loss of hair. Latency: none. Tertiary: cardiovascular; brain damage, paralysis, and much more. Last stage may not appear for months or years. Body exudates then free of organism.	Monogamy, condoms, contact investigation, and treatment of infected individuals.
Gonorrhea	Ancient disease. Second most common STD. Babies may acquire eye infection passing through birth canal. Causes more damage in women than in men. Very common among homosexual men with many sexual partners.	By contact with infected body fluids, generally through sexual activity.	Women often, men sometimes, asymptomatic. If there are symptoms, they usually include a discharge from the vagina or urethra, painful urination, redness and swelling at site of infection. If not treated, ectopic pregnancy may occur in women, heart disease, arthritis, and sterility in both sexes.	Treatment of sexual partners, contact investigation, and treatment of infected individuals. Monogamy and tampons.
Chlamydia	*C. trachomatis* is an intracellular organism, but other characteristics resemble bacteria. Susceptible to antibiotics. Causes more STD than any other organism.	By sexual intercourse; to babies in birth canal.	Both men and women may be asymptomatic. A discharge from the penis or swollen testicles may be present in men and painful urination in women. If present in a pregnant woman, baby can have eye infection and pneumonia.	Monogamous sexual relations and use of condoms.

QUESTIONS FOR REVIEW

1. What are the differences among folliculitis, furuncles, and carbuncles?
2. Why does autoinfection play such a big part in contracting folliculitis, furuncles, and carbuncles?
3. What dangers are there in squeezing a boil?
4. What increases susceptibility to osteomyelitis?
5. What conditions seem to predispose an individual to TSS?
6. What are the symptoms for TSS?
7. How can TSS be avoided?
8. What causes "pink eye"?
9. How is an eye infection transmitted?
10. Describe the lesion caused by impetigo.
11. What treatment is effective for impetigo?
12. How does meningitis usually occur?
13. What are some specific symptoms of meningitis?
14. What factors predispose an individual to endocarditis?
15. What is the difference between acute and subacute endocarditis?
16. In what states has leprosy been reported?
17. What is one of the main problems with eradication of leprosy?
18. What is the difference between tuberculoid and lepromatous leprosy?
19. In what way has syphilis affected history?
20. Why has the incidence of syphilis fluctuated so over the years?
21. Identify the four stages of syphilis and symptoms for each stage.
22. Why is syphilis sometimes not identified until the late stage?
23. What happens to the baby in the womb if the mother has syphilis?
24. Why is it unlikely that syphilis will be contracted by means other than sexual intercourse?
25. What are the most important ways to prevent and control syphilis?
26. Why has treatment of gonorrhea become difficult?
27. What is generally the cause of gonorrhea in children?
28. What are the symptoms and complications of gonorrhea?
29. In what ways can chlamydia be transmitted?

FURTHER READING

Aquavella, James V., et al. "Better Eye-Infection Care." *Patient Care,* Sept. 30, '89, 22:69-79.

Aral, Sevgi O. and King K. Holmes. "Sexually Transmitted Diseases in the AIDS Era." *Scientific American,* Feb. '91, 264:62-69.

Aral, Sevgi O., et al. "Gonorrhea Rates: What Denominator Is Most Appropriate?" *American Journal of Public Health,* June '88, 78:702-703.

Boyd, Robert F. *General Microbiology.* St. Louis: Mosby, 1988.

Burden, Larry L. and Judy C. Rodgers. "Endocarditis: When Bacteria Invade the Heart." *RN,* Dec. '88, 51:38-46.

"Chlamydia: Cloak and Dagger." *Harvard Medical School Health Letter,* Oct. '88, 13:7-8.

Chow, Joan M., et al. "The Association Between *Chlamydia trachomatis* and Ectopic Pregnancy." *Journal of the American Medical Association,* June 20, '90, 283:3184-3187.

Cierny, George III, et al. "Outlook on Osteomyelitis." *Patient Care,* Sept. 15, '89, 23:95-105.

Cohen, Ilan, Jean Claude Veille and Beverly M. Calkins. "Improved Pregnancy Outcome following Successful Treatment of Chlamydial Infection." *Journal of the American Medical Association,* June 20, '90, 203:3180-3183.

Cohn, Jeffrey P. "Leprosy: Out of the Dark Ages." *FDA Consumer,* Sept. '89, 23:24-27.

Colachis, Sam O., et al. "Prevention of Bacterial Endocarditis." *Journal of the American Medical Association,* Apr. 3, '91, 265:1686-1688.

Control of Communicable Disease in Man. Abram S. Benenson, Fifteenth Edition, Washington, D.C.: American Public Health Association, 1990.

Dajani, Adnan S., et al. "Prevention of Bacterial Endocarditis." *Journal of the American Medical Association,* Dec. 12, '90, 264:2919-2922.

Emond and Rowland, A Color Atlas of Infections Disease 2nd ed, Chicago. Wolfe, 1987.

Farley, Dixie. "Preventing TSS: New Tampon Labeling Lets Women Compare Absorbencies." *Consumer,* Feb. '90, 24:6-9.

Finch, Roger. "Skin and Soft-Tissue Infections." *Lancet,* Jan. 23, '88, 1:164-168.

Folkenberg, Judy. "Pet Ownership Risky Business?" *FDA Consumer,* Apr. '90, 24:28-31.

Gibbons, Wendy. "Clueing in on Chlamydia: Microbial Stealth Leads to Reproductive Ravages." *Science News,* Apr. 20, '91, 138:250-252.

Goldsmith, Marsha F. "'Silent Epidemic' of 'Social Disease' Makes STD Experts Raise Their Voices." *Journal of the American Medical Association,* June 23, '89, 261:3509-3510.

"Gonorrhea and Syphilis Pose Renewed Threats." *Patient Care,* Apr. 30, '88, 22:23-24.

Hammerschlag, Margaret R., et al. "Efficacy of Neonatal Ocular Prophylaxis for the Prevention of Chlamydial and Gonococcal Conjunctivitis." *New England Journal of Medicine,* Mar. 23, '88, 320:788-791.

Hanssen, Pal Wolner, et al. "Decrease Risk of Symptomatic Chlamydial Pelvic Inflammatory Disease Associated with Oral Contraceptive Use." *Journal of the American Medical Association,* Jan. 9, '90, 283:54-61.

Hillis, S.D., et al. "Delayed Care of Pelvic Inflammatory Disease as a Risk Factor for Impaired Fertility." *American Journal of Obstetrics and Gynecology,* May '93, 168(5):1503-1509.

Hoge, C.W., et al. "The Changing Epidemiology of Invasive Group A Streptococcal Infections and the Emergence of Streptococcal Toxic Shock–Like Syndrome. A Retrospective Population-Based Study." [Published erratum appears in *Journal of the American Medical Association,* Apr. 7, 1993;269(13):1638] *Journal of the American Medical Association,* Jan. 20, '93, 269(3):384-9.

Huminer, David, et al. "Family Outbreaks of Psittacosis in Israel." *Lancet,* Sept. 10, '88, 2:815-818.

Johnson, Betty A., et al. "Derivation and Validation of a Clinical Diagnostic Model for Chlamydial Cervical Infection in University Women." *Journal of the American Medical Association,* Dec. 20, '90, 264:3181-3185.

Kahn, R.M. and E.J. Goldstein. "Common Bacterial Skin Infections. Diagnostic Clues and Therapeutic Options." May 1, '93, 93(6):175-82.

Kaplan, Beth. "Tick Borne Diseases." *Current Health,* May 2, '90, 10:20-21.

Katz, Alan R. "The Hawaii Chlamydia Network Project." *American Journal of Public Health,* Apr. '89, 78:505-507.

Langley, Joanne M., et al. "Poker Players' Pneumonia." *New England Journal of Medicine,* Aug. 11, '88, 318:354-356.

Malotte, C. Kevin, Edward Wiesmeier and Kristin J. Celineu. "Screening for Chlamydial Cervicitis in a Sexually Active University Population." *American Journal of Public Health,* Apr. '90, 80:488.

Maurice, John. "Leprosy: Liberation From the Colonies." *New Scientist,* Feb. 4, '89, 121:48-52.

McAuliffe, Kathleen. "The Killing Fields: Latter-Day Plagues." *Omni,* May '90, 12:50-58.

McCance, Kathryn L. and Sue E. Huether. *Pathophysiology: The Biologic Basis for Disease in Adults and Children.* St. Louis: Mosby, 1990.

McElhose, Priscilla. "The 'Other' STDs: As Dangerous as Ever." *RN,* June '88, 51:52-59.

"Meningitis-Encephalitis: Pains in the Neck." *Current Health,* May '88, 14:14-15.

Miday, Robert K. and E. Royce Wilson. "Toxic Shock Syndrome." *American Journal of Public Health,* May '88, 78:578-580.

Moraga, Fernando A., et al. "Invasive Meningococcal Conjunctivitis." *Journal of the American Medical Association,* July 18, '90, 264:333-334.

Moran, John S., et al. "The Impact of Sexually Transmitted Disease on Minority Populations." *Public Health Reports,* Nov.-Dec. '89, 104:560-565.

Murray, Patrick, et al. *Medical Microbiology.* St. Louis: Mosby, 1990.

Nettina, Sandra L. "Syphilis: A New Look at an Old Killer." *American Journal of Nursing,* Apr. '90, 90:68-70.

Nunley, D.L. and P.E. Perlman. "Endocarditis. Changing Trends in Epidemiology, Clinical and Microbiologic Spectrum." *Postgraduate Medicine,* Apr. '93, 93(5):235-8, 241-4, 247.

Otten, M.W., Jr., et al. "Changes in Sexually Transmitted Disease Rates after HIV Testing and Posttest Counseling, Miami, 1988 to 1989." *American Journal of Public Health,* Apr. '93, 83(4):529-33.

"Rocky Mountain Spotted Fever—United States 1987." *Journal of the American Medical Association,* July 22, '88, 200:405.

Rolfs, Robert T. and Allyn K. Nakashima. "Epidemiology of Primary and Secondary Syphilis in the United States." *Journal of the American Medical Association,* Sept. 19, '90, 264:1432-1437.

Rolfs, Robert T. Martin Goldberg and Robert G. Sharrar, "Risk Factors for Syphilis." *American Journal of Public Health,* July '90, 80:853-857.

Roueche, Barton. "The Poker Room." *New Yorker,* Sept. 4, '88, 85:100-107.

Salgo, Miklos P., et al. "A Focus of Rocky Mountain Spotted Fever within New York City." *New England Journal of Medicine,* May 20, '88, 318:1345-1348.

Schwarcz, Sandra K., et al. "National Surveillance of Antimicrobial Resistance in *Neisseria gonorrhoeae.*" *Journal of the American Medical Association,* Sept. 19, '90, 264:1413-1417.

Simon, Pamela A. "Allergic Rhinitis and Conjunctivitis." *Drug Topics,* Aug. 6, '90, 134:61-69.

Strovas, Jane. "Boils: Unsafe in Numbers." *Physician and Sports Medicine,* May '90, 18:39.

Toomey, Kathleen E., Alisa G. Oberschelp and Joel R. Greenspan. "Sexually Transmitted Diseases and Native Americans." *Public Health Reports,* Nov.-Dec. '89, 104:566-572.

Vetter, R.G., R. Iverson and M.D. Kuzel. "Adult Meningitis. Rapid identification for prompt treatment." *Postgraduate Medicine,* Jan. '93, 93(1):99-102, 105-106, 109-112.

Zimmerman, Helen L., et al. "Epidemiologic Differences Between Chlamydia and Gonorrhea." *American Journal of Public Health,* Nov. '90, 80:1338-1342.

Zole, Judith C. "Topical Impetigo Antibiotic Reduces Side Effects." *Drug Topics,* June 20, '88, 132:20-21.

Bacterial Diseases Acquired through Skin and Mucosa from Arthropod Vectors, Animal Sources, and the Soil

O B J E C T I V E S

1 State ways by which disease is transmitted to humans from animals.

2 Identify some of the arthropod vectors responsible for disease transmission.

3 Recognize the importance of pest control and sanitation.

4 Describe preventive measures to be taken in order to avoid infection with zoonoses.

5 Explain why tetanus shots and boosters are important.

6 Distinguish between epidemic typhus and endemic typhus.

7 Compare Rocky Mountain spotted fever and Lyme disease.

8 Discuss characteristics, transmission, symptoms, prevention, and control for the diseases in this chapter.

PATHOGENIC BACTERIAL RESERVOIRS AND ZOONOSES

Humans are the chief reservoir for most pathogenic bacteria. Animals, insects, and the soil also serve as reservoirs for these disease agents. Arthropod vectors (insects that carry disease) are often involved in the transfer of organisms from one reservoir to another. Most of these arthropod vectors are parasitic (living on other species) and, while securing a blood meal from an animal or human, may pick up infectious microorganisms and later infect another animal or human by inoculation. Some of these arthropods act only as mechanical carriers and are not true reservoirs, since the vector does not maintain the organism. Other arthropods become reservoirs for an organism if it infects them and is able to develop and multiply.

Infection by arthropod vector is not the only way that bacterial and rickettsial diseases of animals can be transmitted to humans. They may also be transmitted through other direct and indirect means, depending upon the nature of the disease and the animal involved. The mode of transmission will be discussed with each disease.

The infectious diseases of animals that can be transmitted to humans are called zoonoses. Animals also carry other pathogenic organisms in addition to bacteria that can cause disease in humans. In this chapter we will discuss only the zoonotic diseases caused by bacteria and rickettsia and acquired through the skin and mucosa.

ANTHRAX

Anthrax is a disease of domestic animals, mainly sheep, cattle, goats, and horses. It has been known since antiquity and was described in Homer's *Iliad*. Anthrax is caused by *Bacillus anthracis,* which Robert Koch identified in 1876. Human anthrax thus became the first human disease proved to be of bacterial origin. Human anthrax occurs in workers who process animal products or in farmers or veterinarians who work directly with infected animals. The spores of *B. anthracis* can survive for years after the infected animal has died, in soil and in the hide, hair, and wool.

Immunization and other measures to protect workers who might be exposed have made anthrax infrequent and sporadic in the United States, but it is endemic

DID YOU KNOW?

Germ Warfare—Anthrax

During the height of the Persian Gulf conflict, there were reports that Saddam Hussein was preparing capsules laden with the anthrax bacillus to drop on the U.N. troops. Anthrax develops quickly and if the the bacteria are inhaled, death occurs quickly. For-tunately the war was comparatively brief, and either the Iraqis decided not to break international laws against germ warfare or the mechanism for releasing the bacteria was not in place.

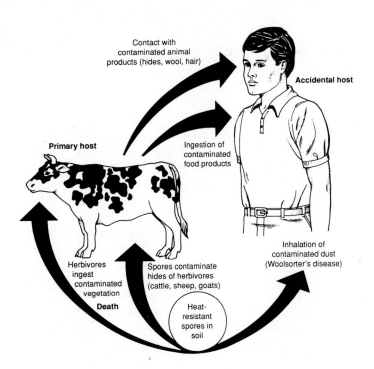

FIGURE 7-1 Transmission of anthrax.

in areas of the Middle East, Asia, Africa, and South America. The disease usually appears within a week after exposure. Indications are that animals and humans surviving an attack of the disease are resistant to reinfection. Some individuals have inapparent infections and may have some natural resistance.

Transmission   Figure 7-1 shows the way in which anthrax is transmitted. *Infection of the skin (cutaneous infection)* is caused by contact with tissues of animals dying of the disease, or by a great variety of animal products, including bone meal, shaving-brush bristles, hair or wool used in textile industries, and hides processed for leather goods. Cutaneous anthrax also may result from contact with soil associated with infected animals. An additional source of skin infection may be biting flies that feed on a

FIGURE 7-2 Early lesion of anthrax on neck.

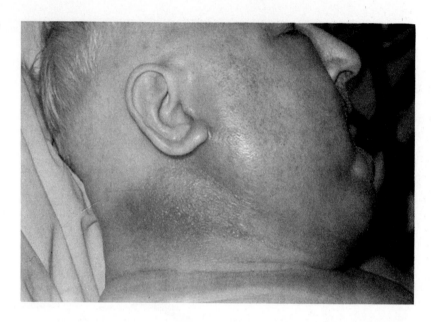

diseased animal. *Intestinal anthrax* is caused by eating undercooked, contaminated meat. There is no evidence that the spores are transmitted by milk from infected animals. Inhalation of the spores leads to *inhalation anthrax*. The spore source can remain infective for years. There is no person-to-person transmission.

Symptoms   In cutaneous anthrax, itching begins first at the site of entry. A papule (red, elevated area) appears within a day or so and quickly becomes a vesicle. Figure 7-2 shows the lesion and vesicles of anthrax in the early stages. There is generally no pain in the early stages. In a few days, the vesicle becomes larger and turns black and is referred to as a malignant pustule (Figure 7-3). There is swelling around the ulcer, caused by the multiplication of the bacilli and production of a cell-damaging toxin.

If untreated, the infection spreads to nearby lymph nodes and to the bloodstream, causing overwhelming septicemia (blood poisoning), that leads to shock and death in a few days. The case fatality rate is 5% to 20% when untreated. Inhalation anthrax produces only mild symptoms at first, similar to those of an upper respiratory infection. In 3 to 5 days, the symptoms become more severe, with respiratory distress, fever, and shock. Death occurs soon after the symptoms become worse in almost every case of inhalation anthrax. Intestinal anthrax is rare and difficult to recognize, with typical symptoms of abdominal distress, fever, and signs of septicemia. Death occurs in most cases.

Treatment   Because anthrax develops so quickly, early diagnosis and treatment are essential. Penicillin is the drug of choice, and tetracycline has also been found to be effective.

Prevention   A vaccine is available that provides active immunization to animals and persons at high risk. Education in sanitary measures, in means of anthrax transmission, and

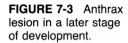

FIGURE 7-3 Anthrax lesion in a later stage of development.

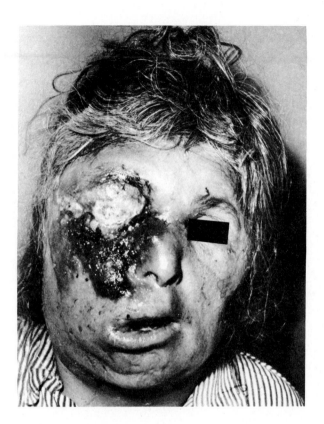

in care of minor abrasions for those working with the animals or animal products also help to prevent infection.

Control Special precautions need to be taken with dead or dying animals. Animal products for commercial processing should be sterilized whenever possible. Protective clothing and gloves should be used by workers in the at-risk occupations. Dust control may also be necessary in contaminated areas.

TULAREMIA

A number of wild animals harbor the bacterium *Francisella tularensis,* the cause of tularemia, but hares and rabbits are the main source for the infection in humans. The disease received its name from Tulare, California, where it was first discovered. Figure 7-4 shows the counties where cases were reported in 1989. The number of cases has generally been decreasing in the United States as seen in Figure 7-5. The incubation period may range from 2 to 10 days, but in most cases it is 3 days. All ages are susceptible to the disease, and cases of reinfection are rare. With appropriate treatment, there are few fatalities.

Transmission Humans may become infected with *F. tularensis* by inoculation while cleaning or working with the skins of infected animals; by fluid from infected flies, ticks, or

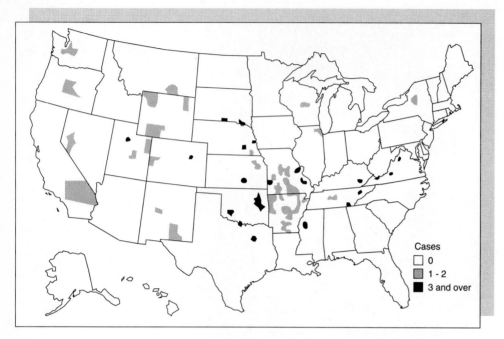

FIGURE 7-4   Reported cases of tularemia in the United States, 1989 (by county).

FIGURE 7-5   Reported cases of tularemia in the United States by year, 1955 to 1990.

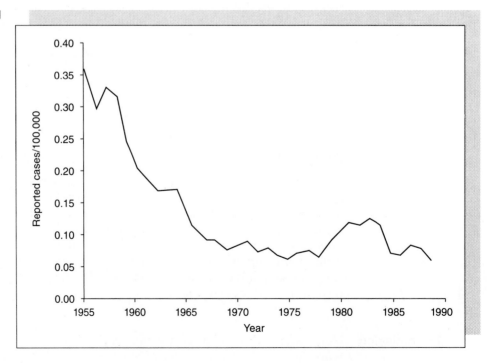

other animals; by the bite of insects carrying the organism; by eating insufficiently cooked rabbit or hare meat; by drinking contaminated water; or by inhalation of dust from contaminated soil, grain, or hay. There is no person-to-person transmission.

Symptoms   The infection may be limited to tissues surrounding the portal of entry, with the formation of an ulcer and involvement of regional lymph glands. If the infectious material is inhaled, this may be followed by a pneumonic or typhoidal disease. If infection comes from eating meat containing the organism, there may be pharyngitis, intestinal pain, diarrhea, and vomiting. Some strains of the organism are more virulent than others. Occasionally the disease begins with a fever and systemic illness.

Treatment   Tularemia can be treated with any number of antibiotics, including streptomycin. Early treatment leads to a cure, but antibiotics are administered until the temperature of the victim has been gone for several days in order to avoid a chronic low-grade infection that may occur.

Prevention   Gloves should be used when skinning or handling wild animals, especially rabbits. The meat of rabbits and wild rodents must be cooked thoroughly. In areas where there is known infection among the rodent population, people need to be educated in methods that will protect them. Vaccines are available, but their use in the United States is restricted to high-risk populations, particularly laboratory workers.

Control   There is no need to isolate individuals who have been infected, since tularemia is not a communicable disease. Open lesions need to be protected, and any materials contaminated with discharge from ulcers disinfected.

LEPTOSPIROSIS

There are many different types of *Leptospira,* the spirochete responsible for leptospirosis. The infection with these organisms is more common in parts of the world other than the United States, with the exception of an infection caused by *Leptospira interrogans,* which is quite widespread in the United States. When the infection caused by *L. interrogans* is severe, it is called Weil's disease, after a German physician. Weil's disease is an acute infection in which the organisms localize in the kidneys, producing kidney dysfunction. The spirochete may spread through the blood to other parts of the body such as the liver and nervous system. Fatalities may occur due to hepatorenal (liver and kidney) failure or because of myocardial involvement. The reservoir for leptospirosis is in domestic and wild animals, including rats and other rodents. The average time for developing symptoms is 10 days after exposure, with a range of 4 to 19 days. Excretion of the spirochete in the urine may continue up to 11 months after the illness. Human susceptibility appears to be universal, but immunity follows infection.

Transmission   Transmission is by contact of the skin, especially if the surface is broken by abrasion or a cut, and by water, moist soil, or vegetation contaminated with the excreta of infected animals. Infected animals secrete large numbers of the spirochete in their urine and may contaminate water used for drinking, swimming, or irrigation. Some individuals such as sugarcane workers, those who work in rice fields, sewer workers, and miners are at higher risk of contracting the infection. Veterinarians, farmers, and slaughterhouse workers are also at greater risk. Children have been known to contract this infection after swimming in farm ponds.

Symptoms   Symptoms are variable and include fever, headache, chills, malaise, vomiting, muscle aches, and watery eyes. A comparison of the symptoms for the mild and severe forms of leptospirosis is shown in Figure 7-6. Sometimes, meningitis, rash, jaundice, renal insufficiency, anemia, and hemorrhages in the skin and mucous membrane occur. Deaths are rare, but increase with age, particularly among individuals who have jaundice and untreated kidney insufficiency. Death is generally due to liver failure, kidney failure, and/or heart problems.

Treatment   Several forms of penicillin and other antibiotics are effective in destroying the organisms. Kidney dialysis may have to be performed in some cases.

Prevention   Workers in hazardous professions need to be educated to the danger of infection. Protective clothing should be worn, particularly on the hands and feet. The public needs to be educated about the dangers of swimming in potentially contaminated

FIGURE 7-6 Stages and symptoms for leptospirosis.

	Mild Leptospirosis		Severe Leptospirosis	
Fever	STAGE 1	STAGE 2	STAGE 1	STAGE 2
	3-7 Days	0-30 days	3-7 Days	10-30 days
Other symptoms	Myalgia, headache, abdominal pain, vomiting, conjunctival suffusion	Meningitis, uveitis, rash	Jaundice, hemorrhage, renal failure, myocarditis	

waters, such as farm ponds. Infected animals need to be kept out of human living, working, and recreational areas. Any rat or rodent population should be exterminated. Vaccines are available for livestock and dogs but are strain specific.

Control   The source of infection, such as a swimming pool or farm pond, needs to be found and the contamination eliminated or use prohibited if decontamination is not possible.

TETANUS

Clostridium tetani is one of the strains of bacteria sometimes found in the intestinal tract of humans and other mammals, where it does no harm. Folklore has attributed the cause of tetanus to a rusty nail, and since the type of deep-puncture anaerobic wound caused by a rusty nail provides the best growing conditions for the bacteria, tetanus may well develop from this source. However, the spores of *C. tetani* can be introduced into any wound, and if anaerobic conditions prevail, then the spores will germinate, multiply, and produce the deadly tetanus toxin.

The organism is found worldwide, but the disease is more common in agricultural regions and in underdeveloped areas. The number of cases in the United States has decreased steadily since 1955 (Figure 7-7). Tetanus is a significant cause of death in many countries where contact with animal excreta is more likely and immunization is inadequate. It is one of the most common causes of neonatal (newborn) death in these countries. In these deaths, the unhealed umbilical cord is the portal of entry. The reservoir of infection is the intestine of animals, including man.

FIGURE 7-7 Reported cases of tetanus in the United States by year, 1955 to 1990.

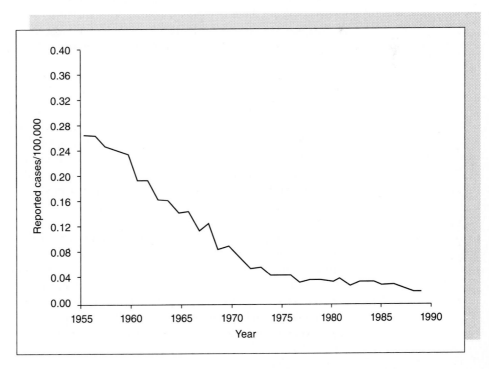

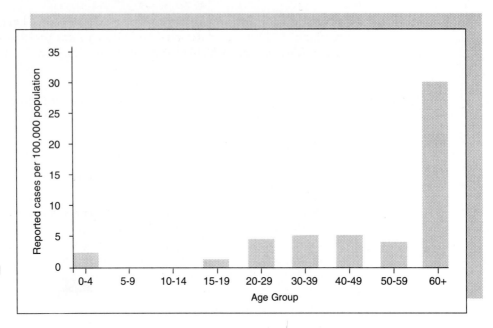

FIGURE 7-8 Reported cases of tetanus by age group, United States, 1991.

The incubation period is influenced by the type of wound and the numbers of infecting organisms. With the right conditions, tetanus toxin can be produced within a few days, but incubation sometimes requires 3 weeks or longer. The average is 10 days. Nonimmunized individuals are all susceptible to tetanus. As people get older and are no longer protected by the shots (see Prevention), they become more susceptible (Figure 7-8). Individuals who recover from tetanus may not have immunity. The fatality rate ranges from 30% to 90% depending on age, length of incubation, and treatment. In the United States, in experienced intensive care centers, the mortality rate has dropped from 60% to 30%.

Transmission   Spores of the tetanus bacillus are found everywhere and are common in the dust of streets as well as in soil. Anything or any place that has been contaminated with fecal matter may contain spores. When tetanus spores are introduced into the body, usually through a puncture wound, but also through lacerations, burns, and trivial or unnoticed wounds, and begin to multiply, then the deadly toxin is produced. The presence of dead tissue and/or foreign bodies favors the growth of the pathogen in the wound. There is no person–to–person transmission.

Symptoms   The first symptom may be rigidity in the abdomen or the area of the wound. The tetanus toxin attacks the central nervous system and results in painful, involuntary muscle contractions. These contractions affect the neck and facial muscles, leading to locked jaw (lockjaw is another name for tetanus), and a grinning expression known as *risus sardonicus* (Figure 7-9). Somatic muscles may become involved, leading to arched back rigidity and boardlike abdominal rigidity (Figure 7-10). Other symptoms include tachycardia, profuse sweating, and low-grade fever.

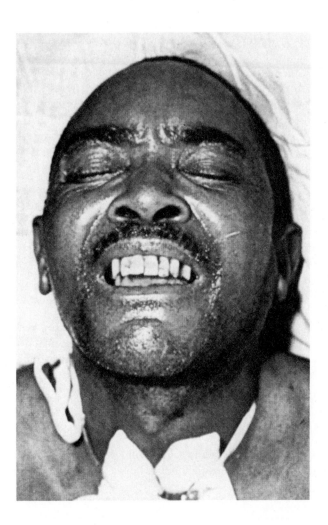

FIGURE 7-9 *Risus sardonicus* in tetanus.

FIGURE 7-10 Muscle rigidity and spasm in a child with tetanus.

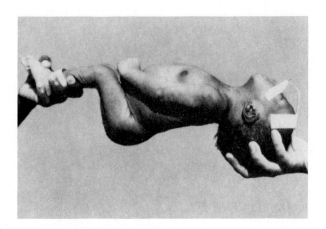

Treatment   If tetanus antitoxin is administered before the toxin becomes attached to nerve tissue, the toxin will be neutralized. If a nonimmunized individual receives a puncture wound, tetanus antitoxin or tetanus immune globulin (TIG) must be given as soon as possible (within 72 hours). After this, they need active immunization with the tetanus toxoid. If the patient has not had tetanus immunization for 5 years, a booster injection needs to be given. If tetanus develops, then the individual will require airway maintenance and a muscle relaxant. Tracheotomy and mechanically assisted respiration may also be used. High-dose antibiotics are administered, preferably penicillin, for 10 to 14 days.

Prevention   Active immunization with tetanus toxoid gives certain and durable (10-year) protection. Infants should be immunized at 2 to 3 months with the DTP vaccine, which protects against diphtheria, tetanus, and pertussis (whooping cough). Booster doses are given at regular intervals. After the initial series, boosters are recommended at 10-year intervals.

Control   Identification of the source of infection (in a situation where others could become infected because of lack of sanitary conditions or some environmental hazard) is the only measure necessary for control. Cases of tetanus should be reported to the local health authority (required in most states and countries).

LYME DISEASE

In 1975 a group of children in Lyme, Connecticut, developed symptoms of an infection that was identified as tickborne, spirochetal, and zoonotic. It was called

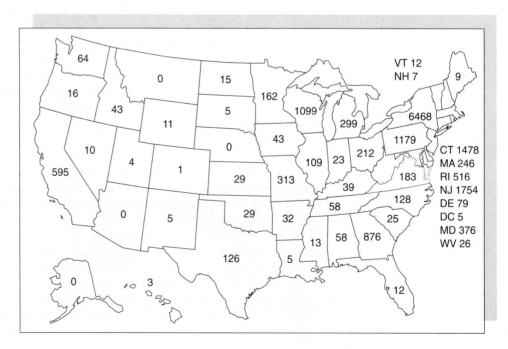

FIGURE 7-11 Reported Lyme disease cases—United States, 1989-1990.

Lyme disease, and since that time it has appeared in all but four states, Alaska, Arizona, Montana, and Nebraska (Figure 7-11). The increase in cases in the United States in recent years can be seen in Figure 7-12.

The disease agent is a spirochete called *Borrelia burgdorferi,* which is carried by the tiny tick, *Ixodes dammini,* pictured in Figure 7-13. This tick is found on deer, wild rodents, and other animals. These animals can act as secondary reservoirs. The incubation period is 7 to 32 days after exposure to the tick. All people are probably susceptible to Lyme disease, and indications are that immunity does not result from one infection, since repeated infections have occurred.

Transmission The disease is acquired through the bite of an infected tick. The spirochete can also be transmitted to the fetus if a pregnant woman gets the disease. There is no evidence of person-to-person transmission.

FIGURE 7-12 Reported Lyme disease cases, United States, 1982 to 1990. Data for 1990 are provisional.

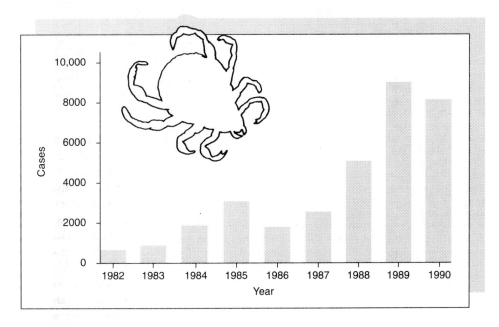

FIGURE 7-13 The deer tick *(I. dammini),* partly engorged (left) and unengorged (right).

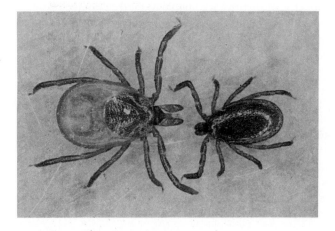

CONTEMPORARY CONCERNS

Vaccine for Lyme Disease?

Scientists believe it may be possible to eradicate Lyme disease with a vaccine that not only protects laboratory animals but also eliminates the bacteria from the tick vector. Human clinical trials are expected to start in 1993. The researchers have already demonstrated that mice in the wild can be immunized by leaving out baits that contain the Lyme disease protein used in the vaccine. Once the mice have been orally vaccinated, any ticks feeding on them would be killed and the chain of infection broken. In theory, this could cause Lyme disease to disappear.

Symptoms   There has been great difficulty in diagnosing Lyme disease in the early stages since the symptoms are variable and sometimes not noticed. Most patients do not remember being bitten nor seeing a tick.

Lyme disease typically occurs in three stages. The first is marked by a distinctive lesion, erythema chronicum migrans (ECM), which appears as a red macule or papule, often at the site of the tick bite (Figure 7-14). This lesion may expand to over 50 cm in diameter and often feels hot and sticky. Similar lesions may erupt within a few days if there was more than one tick bite. The lesion or lesions are accompanied by malaise, fatigue, fever, headache, stiff neck, muscle aches, aching in various joints, rash, and swollen lymph glands. Preceding the appearance of ECM, the victim sometimes has a persistent sore throat and dry cough. The second stage appears weeks to months later, with neurologic abnormalities that may last days or months. Cardiac abnormalities may also develop. In the third stage, which may be weeks to years later, swelling and pain in the knees and other large joints occurs, which may lead to the development of chronic arthritis.

Treatment   Lyme disease can be cured by antibiotics in all three stages. If arthritis has become established, symptoms are reversed only half of the time. In the ECM stage, penicillin is the treatment of choice for children, tetracycline for adults. Other antibiotics are also effective if victims are unable to take or do not respond to the initial treatment. Ten to 20 days of treatment with antibiotics in the early stages will minimize later symptoms. In the later stages, antibiotics given in high doses intravenously may be effective.

Prevention   Individuals who camp, hunt, or walk in areas inhabited by deer need to take special precautions. Long-sleeved shirts and long pants should be worn, with the pants tucked into socks or boots. Wearing light-colored clothing will make it easier to see the ticks. Insect repellants should be used. After leaving the areas, individuals should shower and towel down briskly, since the tick is so tiny and difficult to see (Figure 7-15). Inspect each person for ticks, and if you are alone, use a mirror to inspect yourself. If a tick is discovered, it should be grasped gently, at the head,

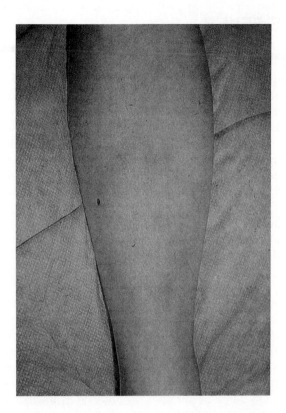

FIGURE 7-14 Erythema chronicum migrans. Broad oval area of erythema has slowly migrated from the central area.

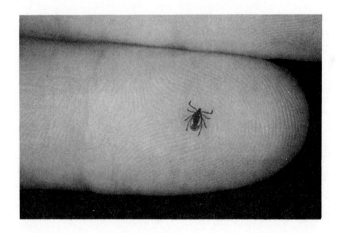

FIGURE 7-15 The deer tick *(I. dammini).* Its tiny size is demonstrated when shown in its unengorged stage on the tip of a finger.

with tweezers, and pulled off firmly but gently. Removing it promptly may prevent transferral of the bacteria. Domestic animals that have been in deer-inhabited areas should also be checked for ticks.

Control   When cases occur in areas where the disease is not endemic, studies should be conducted to determine the source of the infection.

TYPHUS FEVER

There are several types of typhus fever with similar symptoms, caused by rickettsiae, and spread by insects. The type that has caused the biggest problem historically is epidemic typhus, which is spread by body lice. Although today it is a rare disease, it once caused epidemics that killed hundreds of thousands during times of war, famine, and other disasters. Outbreaks still occur in other countries, but in the United States the last outbreak was in 1921. Murine fever or endemic typhus is also rare in the United States with less than 50 cases per 10,000 population reported annually (Figure 7-16). It is transmitted by fleas. The other types are not present in the United States, and Rocky Mountain spotted fever, which is a similar disease, will be discussed separately. The incubation period for epidemic and endemic typhus is the same, usually about 12 days. The reservoir of infection for epidemic typhus is humans and for endemic typhus it is rats and other small mammals. The infection is not spread person to person. Susceptibility to infection with these rickettsiae is general, and one attack confers life-long immunity.

Transmission Epidemic typhus is spread when lice feed on the blood of infected people and ingest the rickettsiae. The lice deposit feces, which contain the microorganisms, on the skin of other hosts while feeding. When feces or crushed lice are rubbed into the bite or any skin abrasion, then the new host is infected. Endemic typhus is a disease of rats and other animals. As with the lice in epidemic typhus, the pathogenic agents are in the feces of the fleas and transmitted to humans when deposited on the skin and rubbed into a bite or abrasion. In both cases, inhalation of dried feces in dust may account for some infections.

FIGURE 7-16 Reported cases of typhus fever (endemic, or murine) by year in the United States from 1955-1990.

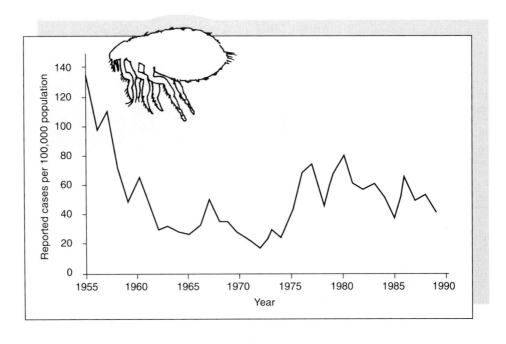

Symptoms   The symptoms are similar for epidemic and endemic typhus but endemic typhus is milder. There is a sudden onset of headache, myalgia, coughing, and constipation. These are followed by high fever, confusion, rash, prostration, weak heart beat, and delirium. Without treatment, death may occur from septicemia, heart failure, renal failure, or pneumonia.

Treatment   Antibiotics are effective in treating typhus fevers.

Prevention/Control   The best means of prevention and control is the eradication of lice and fleas by maintaining sanitary conditions and the use of insecticides. Good personal hygiene and education of the public are also important.

ROCKY MOUNTAIN SPOTTED FEVER (TICKBORNE TYPHUS)

This typhus infection was initially identified in the Rocky Mountain region of the United States but is now found in many parts of the country as seen in Figure 7-17. The number of reported cases rose sharply in the 1970s but has been declining in recent years (Figure 7-18). The disease can be fatal without proper treatment. The reservoir of infection is in ticks. The incubation period is from 3 to about 14 days. The infection is not spread person to person. Susceptibility is general, and one attack confers immunity for life.

FIGURE 7-17 Reported cases of Rocky Mountain spotted fever by county, in the United States in 1990.

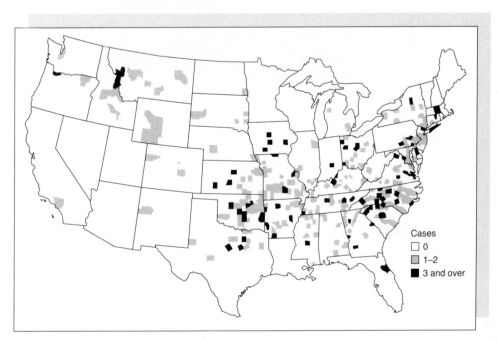

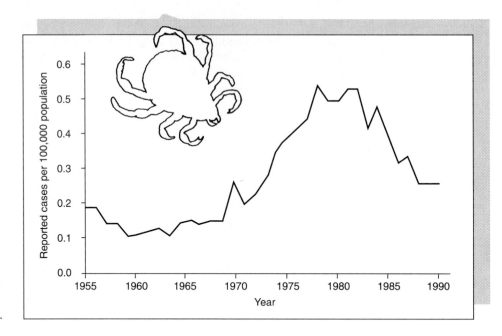

FIGURE 7-18 Reported cases of Rocky Mountain spotted fever by year in the United States from 1955-1990.

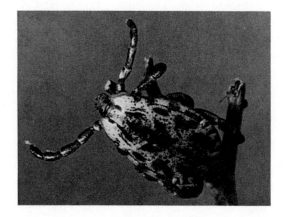

FIGURE 7-19 The Rocky Mountain wood tick, carrier for Rocky Mountain spotted fever.

Transmission   Figure 7-19 is a picture of the tick that transmits Rocky Mountain spotted fever. The tick needs to be attached for several hours before the rickettsiae become infective. Individuals may also become infected if crushed tissues or feces of the tick are rubbed into a bite or an abrasion.

Symptoms   Mild fever, loss of appetite, and a slight headache may develop gradually about a week after the bite, or there may be a sudden onset of severe symptoms including high fever, prostration, aching, tender muscles, severe headache, nausea, and vomiting. In about half the cases, small pink spots appear on the wrists and ankles and spread over the body. The spots darken, enlarge, and may bleed. They even occur on the soles of the feet and palms of the hands. The individual in Figure 7-20 has a well-developed rash on the legs and feet.

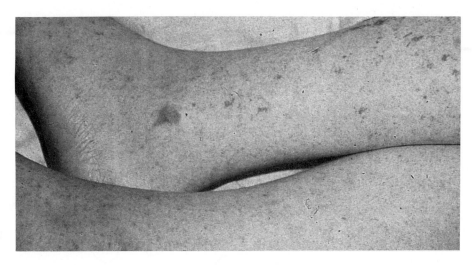

FIGURE 7-20 The rash of Rocky Mountain spotted fever.

Treatment Antibiotics are effective as treatment.

Prevention/Control Prevention and control is the same as for the other typhus infections with the addition that people who live or go into tick-infested areas should examine their bodies and their pets regularly for the presence of ticks (see Lyme disease).

PLAGUE

Bubonic plague, or the Black Death, spread through Europe and Asia during the Middle Ages and came closer to annihilating the human race than any other disease in the history of the world. The disease is caused by a bacillus, *Yersinia pestis,* which resides in wild rodents. In areas where famine exists, rodents move closer to humans to find food. When they die, the infected fleas leave the rodents and move to humans, thus spreading the disease.

Plague is still dangerous today, existing in rodent populations in the western third of the United States, large areas of South America, north-central, eastern, and southern Africa, the Near East, and other parts of the world. Figure 7-21 shows the number of reported cases per year from 1955 to 1990 in the United States.

Plague comes in several forms. *Bubonic plague* is the most common. *Pneumonic plague* can occur as a primary infection but often is an extension of the bubonic form. *Septicemic plague* may develop as a progression of bubonic or pneumonic plague but also manifests as a severe, rapid, systemic infection with no apparent signs of bubonic or pneumonic plague. Pneumonic plague is highly communicable from person to person, while the other two forms are not generally communicable except in unusual circumstances. The incubation period varies from 2 to 6 days. Without treatment, bubonic plague has a mortality rate of about 60%. The mortality rate for both pneumonic and septicemic plague approaches 100% without treatment. With treatment, the mortality rate for all three forms of plague is approximately 18% and is dependent on the victim's age, physical condition, and the time between onset and treatment. There is general susceptibility to plague, with the immunity acquired from infection offering the only form of resistance to the disease.

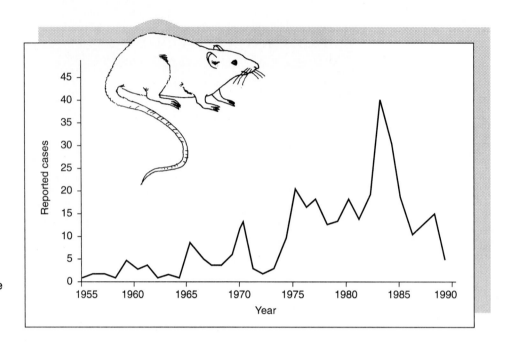

FIGURE 7-21 Plague in humans, by year, United States, 1955-1990.

Transmission   Plague is usually transmitted to humans through the bite of a flea from an infected rodent host (Figure 7-22). Rats, squirrels, prairie dogs, and hares are common carriers, and domestic pets may carry plague-infected fleas into homes. Other sources of exposure resulting in human infection include the handling of tissues of infected animals, airborne droplets from humans or pets with pneumonic plague, and careless handling of laboratory cultures.

Symptoms   Symptoms vary for the three forms of plague. The symptoms for bubonic plague include fever, chills, headache, and exhaustion, and swelling, pain, and hemorrhage in the lymph nodes. The swellings are called buboes, and the dark color from the hemorrhaging led to the term Black Death. Primary pneumonic plague generally has an acute onset, with high fever, chills, severe headache, fast heartbeat, rapid, labored breathing, and a productive cough. The sputum is at first yellowish and later turns to frothy pink or red. A cough producing bloody sputum is the first sign of secondary pneumonic plague. Primary and secondary pneumonic plagues rapidly cause severe distress and may lead to death. When septicemic plague occurs, the symptoms include extreme elevation of temperature (above 106° F), convulsions, prostration, shock, and blood clotting. Septicemic plague is rapidly fatal unless promptly treated.

Treatment   Streptomycin has proved to be the most effective drug against *Y. pestis*. Penicillin is ineffective against plague. Treatment must begin within 8 to 24 hours of onset, and, in the case of septicemic and pneumonic plagues, treatment must start within 18 hours to prevent death. Other drugs are used as supportive therapy, depending on symptoms.

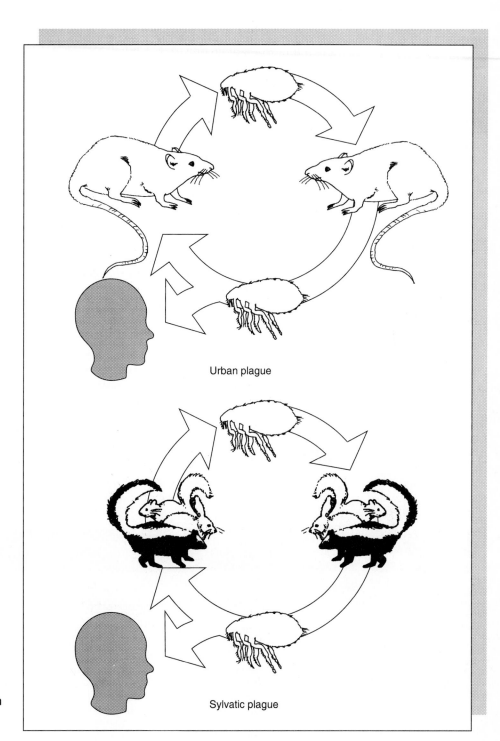

Urban plague

Sylvatic plague

FIGURE 7-22   Transmission of plague from fleas to animal hosts and to humans.

Prevention The most effective measure for preventing plague is the destruction of rats and their fleas. Elimination of unsanitary conditions that encourage rat breeding is necessary. The elimination of rats and their fleas must take place simultaneously in order to keep the hungry insects from invading human populations in the vicinity. People who live in or near plague areas should be warned not to camp near rodent burrows and to report dead or sick rodents to authorities. Seaports and buildings nearby are of particular concern because of the possibility of infected animals being brought in from other countries.

A killed bacteria vaccine is available but lasts only a few months and is not always effective. Some countries use live attenuated vaccine, but the side effects are worse, and there is no evidence that they provide better coverage. Individuals in high-risk areas and those who work in laboratories and have to handle the bacillus should be vaccinated, but other preventive methods should be taken also.

Control International health regulations require the reporting of suspected or confirmed cases of plague. The report first goes to the local health authority and from there on up. Isolation of victims and destruction of all insects on their person or clothing or in their baggage are necessary. Any soiled articles (from sputum or infected discharge) need to be disinfected. In the case of pneumonic plague, contacts should be given prophylactic treatment and isolated for 7 days. In an epidemic of bubonic plague, contacts need to be protected. Contact investigations should take place to identify the source of the infection and measures taken to eliminate any rat and flea population so identified.

SUMMARY

The table summarizes relevant data on bacterial diseases acquired through the skin and mucosa from arthropod vectors, animal sources, and soil.

SUMMARY TABLE Bacterial diseases acquired through skin and mucosa from arthropod vectors, animal sources, and the soil

Disease	Special Characteristics	Transmission	Common Symptoms	Prevention/Control
Anthrax	Spores survive for years after animal is dead.	Contact with tissues or products of an infected animal, contaminated soil, and biting flies may produce cutaneous anthrax. Eating undercooked, infected meat causes intestinal anthrax. Inhalation of spores leads to inhalation anthrax. No person-to-person transmission.	Cutaneous: itching at site of entry, vesicle that turns black. Inhalation: mild at first, like upper respiratory infection; 3-5 days— severe respiratory distress, fever, shock. Intestinal: abdominal distress, fever, septicemia.	Vaccine for animals and people at high risk. Education of those working with animals. Special precautions with dead or dying animals, sterilization of animal products when possible, protective gloves and clothing for workers in at-risk occupations, dust control in contaminated areas.

SUMMARY TABLE   Bacterial diseases acquired through skin and mucosa from arthropod vectors, animal sources, and the soil—cont'd

Disease	Special Characteristics	Transmission	Common Symptoms	Prevention/ Control
Tularemia	Hares and rabbits main source of infection in humans.	Inoculation while working with infected animal or from flies or ticks. Ingestion of insufficiently cooked meat or contaminated water. Inhalation of dust from contaminated soil, grain, or hay. No person-to-person transmission.	Formation of sore at site of entry and swollen lymph glands in region. If inhaled, pneumonic or typhoidal disease. If from ingestion, sore throat, intestinal pain, diarrhea, and vomiting.	Should use gloves when skinning or handling wild animals. Thorough cooking of meat of wild rodents. Vaccination for high-risk groups.
Leptospirosis	Also called Weil's disease. Excretion of spirochete in urine may continue up to 11 months after the illness.	Skin contact with water, moist soil, or vegetation contaminated with excreta of infected animals.	Fever, headache, chills, malaise, vomiting, muscle aches, and watery eyes.	Education of workers in hazardous areas, education of public about swimming in contaminated waters, such as farm ponds; control of infected animals.
Tetanus	Puncture wounds provide best growing conditions. Spores will produce toxin in any wound with anaerobic conditions.	Anything contaminated with fecal matter may contain spores. If they are introduced into the body and begin to multiply, the deadly toxin is produced.	Rigidity in abdomen, painful, involuntary muscle contractions.	Active immunization with tetanus toxoid with periodic boosters.
Lyme disease	Identified originally in Lyme, Conn. Found in other parts of country and spreading. Disease agent is a spirochete.	Transmitted by the bite of an infected tick. Can be transmitted to fetus if a pregnant woman gets the disease.	Three stages: First (ECM)—malaise, fatigue, muscle aches, fever, stiff neck, joint aches, rash, swollen lymph glands. Sore throat and dry cough may precede ECM. Second—neurologic and cardiac abnormalities. Third—arthritis.	Special clothing precautions need to be taken by individuals who camp, hunt, or walk in areas inhabited by deer. Inspection of animals and humans for ticks after being in such areas and prompt removal of any found.
Typhus fever	No longer common in U.S. Two types, epidemic and endemic typhus have been a problem in the past. Humans are the only known reservoir. 40% fatal if not treated. More in colder areas.	Epidemic typhus by lice, endemic typhus by fleas. Louse feces rubbed into lesion.	Similar symptoms, endemic milder. Sudden onset of headache, myalgia, cough, constipation. Followed by high fever, confusion, rash, prostration, weak heart beat, delirium. Fatal if not treated.	Eradication of lice and fleas by maintaining sanitary conditions and insecticides. Good personal hygiene and education of public.

Continued.

SUMMARY TABLE Bacterial diseases acquired through skin and mucosa from arthropod vectors, animal sources, and the soil—cont'd

Disease	Special Characteristics	Transmission	Common Symptoms	Prevention/ Control
Rocky Mountain spotted fever	Initially found in Rocky Mountains, now in many parts of country. Few cases in fall or winter. Men infected most often in West, children in eastern part of U.S.	Tick that attaches itself and injects rickettsiae. Also feces of tick rubbed into bite or abrasion.	Fever, anorexia, slight headache about a week after bite or sudden fever, prostration, myalgia, severe headache, nausea and vomiting. In 50% of cases small pink spots on wrists and ankles that spread over body. Spots darken, enlarge, and may bleed.	Same as other typhus diseases and Lyme disease.
Plague	Bubonic known as "The Black Death." Also Pneumonic and Septicemic forms. Mortality 60%-100% without treatment.	Transmitted to humans by bite of a flea from an infected rodent. Pneumonic by air borne droplets from pets to humans of person to person.	Bubonic: headache, fever, chills, and exhaustion; swelling, pain, and hemorrhage in the lymph nodes. Pneumonic: high fever, chills, severe headache, fast heart beat, rapid, labored breathing, productive cough. Septicemic: Chills, fever, prostration, convulsions, shock.	Destruction of rats and fleas. Elimination of unsanitary conditions. Isolation of victims and destruction of all fleas on person, clothes or baggage. Soiled articles disinfected. Vaccine for one year available. Contact investigation.

QUESTIONS FOR REVIEW

1. What is an arthropod vector?
2. What is the difference between an insect vector that is a reservoir for an organism and an insect vector that acts as a mechanical carrier?
3. What term is used to denote infectious diseases of animals that can be transmitted to humans?
4. Explain what is meant by saying that anthrax is an occupational disease.
5. Name and describe the means of transmission for the three kinds of anthrax.
6. What is distinctive about the anthrax lesion?
7. What are the symptoms for each type of anthrax?
8. Discuss the control methods suggested for anthrax.
9. What is the main source of tularemia?
10. In what ways can *F. tularensis* be transmitted?
11. How and why do the symptoms of tularemia vary?
12. What measures need to be taken in order to prevent tularemia?
13. What dangerous complications may occur in leptospirosis?
14. Where might children easily be exposed to leptospirosis? Why?
15. What occupations pose the greatest risk for being infected with leptospirosis?

16. What are the methods for control of leptospirosis?
17. Where does the highest rate for tetanus occur and why?
18. Why are rusty nails a possible cause of tetanus?
19. What is the procedure for treating tetanus?
20. What regimen is recommended for tetanus shots?
21. What hosts are used by *Ixodes dammini*?
22. What will happen to the fetus if a pregnant woman gets Lyme disease?
23. Describe the three stages of Lyme disease.
24. What treatment is generally used for Lyme disease?
25. What are the similarities and differences between epidemic typhus and endemic typhus?
26. What are the means of transmission for epidemic typhus, endemic typhus, and Rocky Mountain spotted fever?
27. In what part(s) of the country is Rocky Mountain spotted fever found?
28. How can Rocky Mountain spotted fever be avoided?
29. Identify three forms of plague and the symptoms for each.
30. How is plague transmitted?
31. What is the most effective way to prevent plague?
32. How is plague controlled?

FURTHER READING

Benzaia, Diana, "Is It Lyme Disease?" *Health,* June '89, 21:72-75.

Bobo, J.K., et al. "Risk Factors for Delayed Immunization in a Random Sample of 1163 Children from Oregon and Washington." *Pediatrics,* Feb. '93, 91(2):308-314.

Boyd, Robert F. *General Microbiology.* St. Louis: Mosby, 1988.

Clark, Matt. "Plagues, Man and History." *Newsweek,* May 9, '88, 111:65-66.

Control of Communicable Disease in Man. Abram S. Benenson, ed. Fifteenth Edition, Washington, D.C., American Public Health Association, 1990.

Daniels, Thomas J. and Richard O. Falco. "The Lyme Disease Invasion." *Natural History,* July '89, 98:4-7.

Gambino, Raymond, et al. "Diagnostic Tests for Lyme Disease," *Journal of the American Medical Association,* Aug. 8, '90, 264:692-693.

Hale, Marion. "Elderly Women: A High-Risk Group for Tetanus." *American Journal of Nursing,* Apr. '90, 90:83-84.

"Human Cutaneous Anthrax—North Carolina, 1987." *Journal of the American Medical Association,* Aug. 5, '88, 260:616.

Jacobs, Richard F. "Fever, Arthralgias, and a Rash." *Patient Care,* Nov. 15, '90, 24:166-168.

Kaplan, Beth. "Tick-Borne Diseases." *Current Health,* May '90, 16:26-27.

Logigian, Eric, Richard F. Kaplan and Allen C. Steere. "Chronic Neurologic Manifestations of Lyme Disease." *The New England Journal of Medicine,* Nov. 22, '90, 323:1438-1444.

"Lyme Disease—Connecticut." *Journal of the American Medical Association,* Feb. 26, '88, 259:1147-1148.

"Lyme Disease." *Harvard Medical School Health Letter,* July '89, 7-8.

McCance, Kathryn L. and Sue E. Huether. *Pathophysiology: The Biologic Basis for Disease in Adults and Children.* St. Louis: Mosby, 1990.

McEvedy, Colin. "The Bubonic Plague." *Scientific American,* Feb. '88, 258:118-123.

Mee, Charles L. Jr. "How a Mysterious Disease Laid Low Europe's Masses," *Smithsonian,* Feb. '90, 20:66-77.

Murray, Patrick, et al. *Medical Microbiology.* St. Louis: Mosby, 1990.

Nordahl, S.H., et al. Tularemia: a Differential Diagnosis in Oto-rhino-laryngology. *Journal of Laryngology and Otology,* Feb. '93, 107(2):127-129.

Paparone, Pamela. "The Summer Scourge of Lyme Disease." *American Journal of Nursing,* June '90, 90:44-47.

Patlak, Margie. "Ticks Carry Lyme Disease Across U.S." *FDA Consumer,* July-Aug. '88, 22:20-23.

"Rocky Mountain Spotted Fever—United States 1987." *Journal of the American Medical Association,* July 22, '88, 200:405.

Roueche, Berton. "The Foulest and Nastiest Creatures that Be." *The New Yorker,* Sept. 12, '88, 64:83-89.

Salgo, Miklos P., et al. "A Focus of Rocky Mountain Spotted Fever Within New York City." *The New England Journal of Medicine,* May 20, '88, 318:1345-1348.

Sorvillo, F.J., et al. "A Suburban Focus of Endemic Typhus in Los Angeles County: Association with Seropositive Domestic Cats and Opossums." *American Journal of Tropical Medical Hygiene,* Feb. '93, 48(2):269-273.

Stanek, Gerold, et al. "Isolation of Borrelia Burgdorferi from the Myocardium of a Patient with Longstanding Cardiomyopathy." *The New England Journal of Medicine,* Jan. 25, '90, 322:249-252.

Steere, Allen C. "Current Understanding of Lyme Disease." *Hospital Practice,* Apr. 15, '93, 28(4):37-44.

Steere, Allen C. "Lyme Disease." *The New England Journal of Medicine,* Aug. 31, '89, 321:586-596.

Steere, Allen C. "The Overdiagnosis of Lyme Disease." *Journal of the American Medical Association,* Apr. 14, '93, 269(14):1812-1816.

Taylor, J.P., et al. "Indigenous Human Cutaneous Anthrax in Texas." *Southern Medical Journal,* Jan. '93, 86(1):1-4.

"Tetanus—United States, 1987 and 1988." *Journal of the American Medical Association,* Mar. '90, 263:1192-1193.

"Update on Lyme Disease." *Patient Care,* July 15, '89, 23:23-24.

Voelker, Rebecca. "For Years, Physicians Thought I Was a Hypochondriac." *American Medical News,* Sept. 22, '89, 32:9-10.

Watt, George, et al. "Placebo-Controlled Trial of Intravenous Penicillin for Severe and Late Leptospirosis." *Lancet,* Feb. 27, '88, 1:433-445.

Weiss, Rick. "Anthrax Outbreak: The Soviet Scenario." *Science News,* Apr. 23, '88, 133:261.

Wickelgren, Ingrid, and Rich Weiss. "At the Drop of a Tick." *Science News,* Mar. 25, '89, 135:184-187.

Wickens, Barbara. "A Life of Pain." *Maclean's,* Feb. 6, '89, 102:540-541.

Chapter 8

Viral Diseases Acquired through the Respiratory Route

THE COMMON COLD

This most common of all communicable diseases has been responsible for more lost days on the job and has had more time and effort spent on it to find a cause than all the other communicable diseases in history. For all the misery a cold can cause, it will end without treatment and is never fatal. However, if an individual's resistance is compromised for some reason, it can lead to serious illness. Some of the more common complications are laryngitis, bronchitis, sinusitis, and otitis media. Over 100 different types of rhinovirus cause colds, and nearly 100 other "cold–causing" viruses have been identified. The incubation period for a cold is usually about 48 hours, and symptoms generally last 2 to 7 days. Colds occurs in all parts of the world. They are more frequent in children, becoming fewer with age. However, there is a greater chance for complications when an older person gets a cold. The infection is communicable from at least 24 hours before the onset of symptoms to 5 days or more after onset. Everyone seems to be susceptible to colds.

Transmission Colds are transmitted by direct or indirect contact (Figure 8-1). Recent studies conducted at the Cold Laboratory in Salisbury, England, have indicated a greater chance of infection by handling contaminated articles and then rubbing the eyes than by droplet spread. The organism is capable of entering the mucous membrane of the eyes.

DID YOU KNOW?

Running with the Flu?

If you are a runner, it is all right to run when you have a runny nose, sneezing and/or a scratchy throat, but if you have fever, aches "all over," and/or a hacking cough, you should take it easy because you could have influenza and strenuous activity will make it worse. The "flu" can be a killer, so use common sense and, in any case, if you have to push yourself to work out, don't.

Symptoms   Most colds start with a tickle in the throat, a watery discharge from the nose, and sneezing. Many times the nasal discharge is copious and causes irritation to the nose and skin around it. Some colds will gradually clear up at this point, but others produce more severe symptoms usually caused by a secondary bacterial infection. The discharge thickens and becomes yellowish or green, eyes water, and fever, sore throat, headache, malaise, myalgia, and a nonproductive cough occur. Included in the secondary infections that can occur are laryngitis, tracheitis, acute bronchitis, sinusitis, or otitis media.

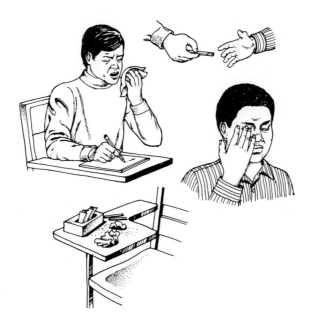

FIGURE 8-1 Transmission of the common cold.

DID YOU KNOW?

Cold Laboratory—Salisbury, England

For over 40 years experiments have been going on in the "cold lab" in Salisbury, England. The common cold has been the object of more and longer-lasting research than any other disease and still, less is known about it than most diseases. Most mothers warn their children that they will "catch" cold if they are not dressed warmly enough or get their feet wet or go outside with wet hair. However, one of the first experiments in the cold lab demonstrated that these warnings are not always based on truth.

In the experiment, a control group and an experimental group were exposed to a cold virus. The control group was just monitored for a week, but those in the experimental group sat in a puddle of water and had fans turned on them for the first few hours of the experiment and then were monitored. The result? There were no more colds in the experimental group than in the control group. Since that time other controlled experiments have reinforced the results. It is still not wise to under-dress or over-dress or get wet in cold weather, since there are several factors that could affect your resistance (see the text), and if your resistance is low, cold and wet and chilling can lower it more and make you more susceptible to viral or bacterial infection.

Treatment   There is no known cure for the common cold. Treatment is for symptoms only. Drinking plenty of liquid and getting extra rest can help the victim feel better but will not shorten the duration of the cold. Because of the possibility of Reye syndrome*, analgesics and cold remedies should not be used for children unless prescribed by the doctor. Although OTC remedies may alleviate some of the symptoms temporarily, overuse may be counterproductive. Most antibiotics have no effect on a viral disease but may be used prophylactically for individuals at risk for developing a secondary bacterial infection.

Prevention   There is no scientific evidence that extra vitamins, orange juice, or avoiding drafts and chilling will prevent colds. A high degree of fitness, socially, mentally, physically, and spiritually, may help to limit the number of colds a person has. Also good hygiene, particularly frequent handwashing, around infected individuals will help decrease a person's degree of exposure. But sooner or later, most people develop one or more colds a year. Individuals who are over 65 or at risk because of heart or respiratory problems may be counseled by their doctor to have a "cold shot," but the protection given is for only a few of the 200 or so viruses that can cause a cold.

Control   Education of the public in personal hygiene, sanitary disposal of tissues used in control of discharges from mouth or nose and in frequent handwashing will help in the control of colds. Individuals with a cold should be isolated from patients in a children's hospital. Ill persons should avoid direct and indirect contact with young children, the debilitated or aged, and people with another illness.

INFLUENZA

Most people refer to influenza as the flu. The only problem with this term is that it is used to cover so many different illnesses, some of which are not even upper

---

*Because of the danger of Reye syndrome, only acetaminophen or ibuprofen (Tylenol or Advil/Nuprin) should be given to an infant or child who is ill. Reye's syndrome is a very serious illness involving the liver and central nervous system. It has been a rare complication in children who are given salicylates (aspirin) for upper respiratory viral infections. Although this complication has occurred mostly in influenza or chickenpox, young children should not be given aspirin for any upper respiratory infection unless recommended by a physician.

DID YOU KNOW?

What and Why?

Why do more colds begin on Monday than any other day of the week?
What illnesses are mistakenly called the "flu?"
Why are high school and college-age people more likely to get infectious mononucleosis?

What does the "chicken" in chickenpox refer to?
Why is rubeola sometimes called "hard" measles?
Why is herpes zoster called "shingles?"
Why is rubella called "German" measles?
What does the "small" in smallpox refer to?

respiratory, as influenza is. Influenza can be a very dangerous disease, developing rapidly, spreading quickly, and leading to complications, most often pneumonia, which can be fatal (Figure 8-2). Influenza occurs in all parts of the world, and the greatest death toll from the disease, 20 million, was a result of the pandemic of 1918. In the last 100 years, pandemics also occurred in 1957 and 1968. Epidemics occur in the United States almost every year, principally in the winter, while in the tropics they often occur in the rainy season (Figure 8-3). The incubation period is 1 to 5 days, and the disease is communicable for 3 to 5 days from the first sign of symptoms in adults but up to 7 days in children.

Influenza viruses change all the time, and for this reason everyone is susceptible to new forms. The viruses are classified into three groups. Type A is the most prevalent and responsible for most epidemics of influenza. Type B has been associated with widespread or regional epidemics and pandemics every 2 to 3 years. There are also "mixed" A and B epidemics. Type C is endemic and has been identified in scattered cases and minor localized outbreaks. The different strains of A and B have been named according to where they were first identified, so there is Hong Kong flu, Russian flu, etc. (The forms of influenza also have identifying numbers and

FIGURE 8-2 Diseases associated with influenza virus infection.

Symptoms and Diseases Associated with Influenza	
Adults	Rapid onset of fever, malaise, myalgia, sore throat, nonproductive cough
Children	Similar to adults, but with higher fever, abdominal pain and vomiting, otitis media, myositis, and croup more frequently
Complications	Primary viral pneumonia Secondary bacterial pneumonia Myositis and cardiac involvement Neurologic syndromes: Guillain-Barré syndrome; encephalopathy; encephalitis; Reye syndrome

FIGURE 8-3 Occurrence of influenza by month in temperate regions.

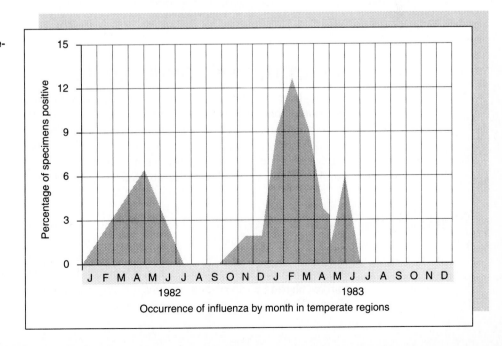

Occurrence of influenza by month in temperate regions

letters.) Infection with one strain results in immunity to that strain but not to others that develop.

Transmission

The influenza virus is spread through the air from person to person, particularly in places where a lot of people are in close quarters. It is also transmitted by airborne droplets and indirect contact with contaminated objects. The virus is able to survive for hours in dried mucus.

Symptoms

Typical symptoms for influenza are sudden onset of chills, temperature from 101 to 104° F, headache, malaise, muscle aches, and a nonproductive cough. Sometimes other symptoms develop, such as sore throat, hoarseness, conjunctivitis, and inflammation and congestion of the nasal mucosa. The symptoms generally last 3 to 5 days, but cough and weakness may last for several weeks.

Treatment

Bed rest, analgesics (acetaminophen for children), and plenty of liquid are the best treatment. For individuals in a high-risk category for developing pneumonia, a new drug, amantadine, can be used to reduce the severity of the disease if given within 24 hours. Antibiotics may also be given to combat secondary bacterial infections.

Prevention

For people over 65 and those with respiratory disease or circulatory diseases vaccination is recommended. It must be given every year and is 60% to 70% effective. Even if it does not keep the individual from getting the disease, it will lessen the severity of the symptoms.

Control

Closing of schools generally occurs too late to do any good. Education of the public in basic personal hygiene is the best means of control.

INFECTIOUS MONONUCLEOSIS

Epstein-Barr virus (EBV), a member of the herpes group, is the infecting agent for infectious mononucleosis, which mainly affects young adults and children. Only a laboratory test can determine whether a person has the disease, since the symptoms are all nonspecific. Incubation is 4 to 6 weeks, and mononucleosis may be communicable for a year or more after infection. "Mono" occurs worldwide. Most people are susceptible, but infection confers a high degree of immunity.

Transmission

Since the victim carries the EBV in the throat, transmission is generally by the oral-pharyngeal route. It has been called the kissing disease or the college disease because spread often occurs among courting teenagers and frequently in colleges. It may also be spread by transfusion, but apparent disease rarely develops from this source. Sharing a can of pop or other beverage is a possible means of transmission (Figure 8-4).

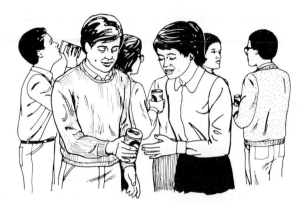

FIGURE 8-4 Transmission of mononucleosis.

Symptoms   Typically, there are prodromal symptoms of headache, malaise, and fatigue. After 3 to 5 days, fever, swollen lymph glands, and sore throat develop. Figure 8–5 shows an individual with slightly puffy eyelids and a pinkish flush to the cheeks that may appear with infectious mononucleosis. There may also be an enlarged spleen, liver involvement, and tonsillitis or pharyngitis. A rash and jaundice occur in a small percentage of victims. Complications may include ruptured spleen, meningitis, encephalitis, hepatitis and anemia.

Treatment   Treatment is symptomatic. Individuals with the disease are restricted from any contact sports because of the danger of a ruptured spleen. Individuals with mono should also be restricted in activity because their resistance is low. Fatalities have been recorded of people dying of a blow to the spleen when they participated in sports before complete recovery from mono. If a secondary bacterial infection is present, then antibiotics may be used. In severe cases, steroids may be used.

FIGURE 8-5 Appearance of the face of a girl with mononucleosis. Many who have mono have puffiness of eyelids and a pinkish flush to cheeks.

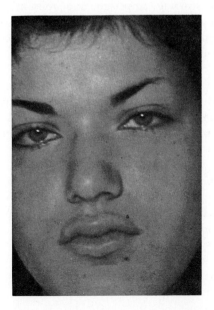

Prevention   There is no known way to prevent mono, but basic personal hygiene and avoidance of close contact with infected individuals will decrease the risk.

Control   There is also no way to control the infection except for education of the public concerning the means of transmission.

VARICELLA (CHICKENPOX)

Most people throughout the world have had chickenpox by 10 years of age. It is a mild but very contagious disease of childhood. In adults, the disease can have severe effects. Congenital chickenpox may cause birth defects. Chickenpox is caused by human herpes virus 3 (varicella zoster). Incubation period may be 2 to 3 weeks but is generally 13 to 17 days. The disease may be communicable from 5 days before to 5 days after the appearance of the first vesicles. Infection confers long immunity. The organism stays in the body after the disease has run its course and years later may cause herpes zoster, or shingles.

Transmission   Chickenpox can be spread by direct contact with respiratory secretions and fluid from lesions of the infected person or by indirect contact with fomites.

Symptoms   The first symptoms are fever, malaise, and anorexia. Within 24 hours, the rash typically begins as small red spots on the trunk or scalp that eventually become clear vesicles on a red base. This has been referred to as the dewdrop on a petal. The vesicles are extremely pruritic (itchy) and break easily, forming a scab. The rash spreads to the face and sometimes to the extremities. New vesicles develop every 3 or 4 days, so there are different stages of development present—red spots, vesicles, and scabs—at the same time. Some children even have lesions on the mucous membranes of the mouth, conjunctivae, and genitalia. If a child scratches the rash persistently, infections, scarring, impetigo, and boils may occur. In some cases, symptoms are so mild and the lesions so few that they escape notice. Figures 8-6 and 8-7 show the different lesions that can occur in chickenpox, while Figure 8-8 shows the distribution of rash on one child.

Treatment   Relief of symptoms is the main goal of treatment because there is no cure for chickenpox. Bicarbonate of soda baths or calamine or antihistamine lotions help to relieve the pruritis. In severe cases, an antiviral agent, acyclovir, may be used.

Prevention   Varicella-zoster immune globulin (VZIG) is effective in decreasing the severity of symptoms or preventing the disease if given within 96 hours after exposure. It is available for high-risk individuals. A vaccine for chickenpox has been licensed in Japan, and trials are under way in the United States.

Control   Children should be excluded from school for at least 5 days after the first lesion appears or until all vesicles are dry.

FIGURE 8-6   The evolution of the lesion in chickenpox. **A,** "Dew drop" on a rose petal: a thin-walled vesicle with clear fluid forms on a red base. **B,** Vesicle becomes cloudy and depressed in the center, the border is irregular. **C,** A crust forms in the center and eventually replaces the remaining portion of the vesicle at the periphery.

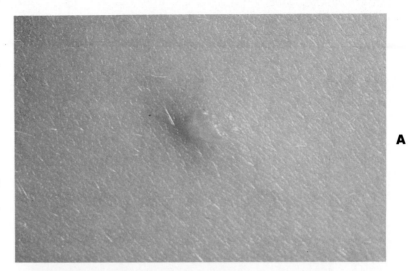

A

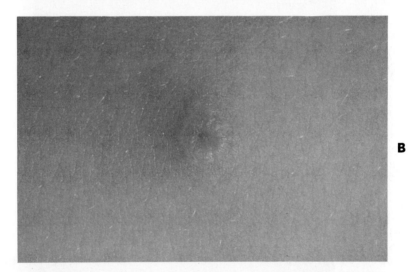

B

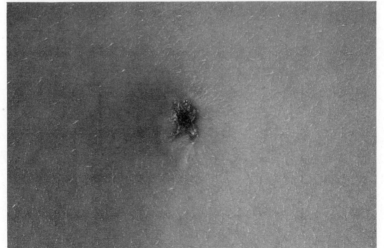

C

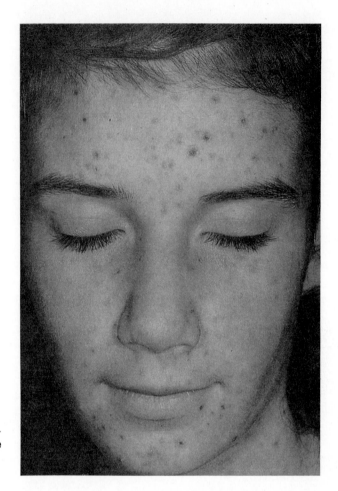

FIGURE 8-7 Chicken-pox lesions on the face in all stages of development.

FIGURE 8-8 The "pox" in children generally occur without prodromal (earlier) symptoms. The lesions occur on the body first.

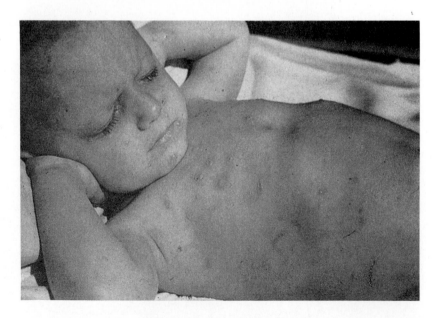

HERPES ZOSTER (SHINGLES)

There are few infectious diseases capable of causing the excruciating pain of herpes zoster. This infection usually occurs in adults and is caused by reactivation of the chickenpox virus, which has lain dormant in sensory nerves for years. It is believed that a decline in the defenses of the immune system allows the virus to reemerge and cause shingles. The attack often follows a stressful incident that also lowers resistance. It is a very common disease in older people and others whose immune systems have been weakened. Herpes zoster is communicable to individuals who have not had chickenpox, but they get chickenpox—not shingles. The disease lasts from 10 days to 5 weeks.

Transmission

Herpes zoster is not as easily transmitted as chickenpox, but nonimmune individuals can be infected by contact with fluid from the vesicles.

Symptoms

The prodromal symptoms are fever and malaise. Within 2 to 4 days, severe deep pain, pruritis, and paresthesia (numbness or tingling) or hyperesthesia (increased sensitivity) in the area affected. The eruptions usually occur on the trunk or arms or legs, along a nerve pathway (Figure 8-9). The rash generally occurs about 5 days after the pain and other symptoms appear and sometimes not at all. When it does appear, it begins as small, slightly raised red spots that turn into blisters. Within three days, the blisters turn yellow, flatten, and scab over, sometimes leaving a pitted scar (Figure 8-10). Pain following the attack can be very severe but varies in different individuals from none at all to intermittent attacks for months or years. It is generally worse in older patients.

Treatment

Treatment can be palliative only, and although many different measures have been tried, none is consistently effective. Analgesics provide temporary partial relief.

FIGURE 8-9 The lesions of shingles often follow a nerve pathway in an irregular pattern around the waist.

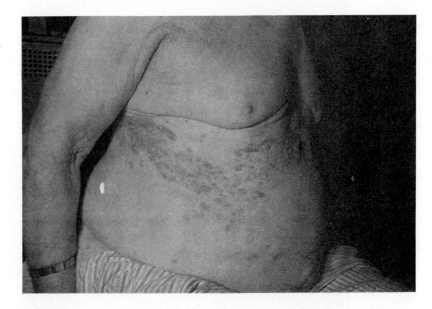

FIGURE 8-10 A, Evolution of rash—vesicles. The rash from shingles can be mild or severe. Fresh vesicles emerge for several days. They may join together to form larger lesions, some of which may hemorrhage.
B, Evolution of rash—pustules. Vesicles begin to dry up within a week, but some go through a pustular stage. **C,** Evolution of rash—crusts. If the rash is heavy, a thick plate of scabs may form, which does not separate for several weeks. If someone attempts to remove them before enough time has passed, fresh scabs will form and the skin will be harmed.

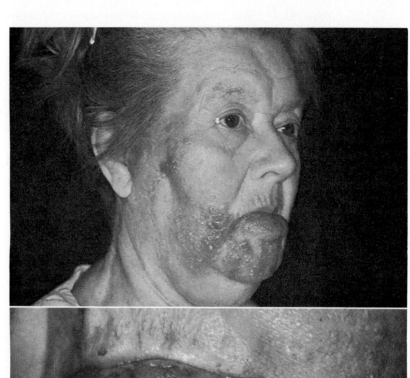

A

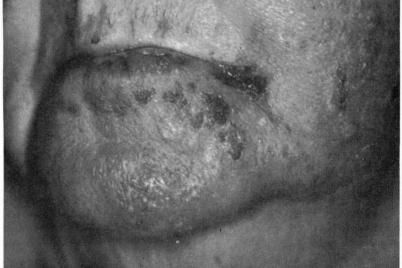

B

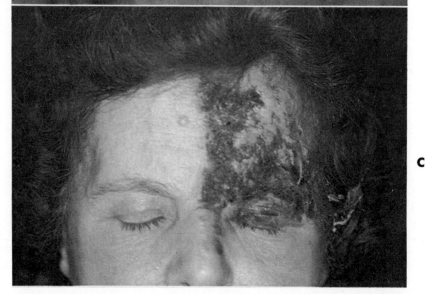

C

Prevention   None known.

Control   None necessary except for personal hygiene and avoidance of those at risk.

MEASLES (RUBEOLA, RED MEASLES, HARD MEASLES)

Before the advent of the vaccine in 1963, measles was one of the most common communicable diseases throughout the world. The incidence in developed countries has dropped considerably, and in the United States, where vaccination is now required for children before they enter school, the number of cases dropped from over 450,000 in 1960 to fewer than 3000 in 1988. However the numbers began to increase rapidly in 1988, and in 1990 over 27,672 cases were reported, a 52.1% increase over the 18,193 cases reported in 1989 (Figure 8-11). This increase has been attributed to failure to vaccinate children at the appropriate age. Measles, although most of the time comparatively mild, has the potential for complications that can be fatal. For this reason, it is a disease that needs to be controlled. In developing nations it is responsible for more than 1 million deaths each year. The incubation period is 7 to 18 days, usually 14 days to onset of the rash. The disease is communicable from slightly before symptoms appear until 4 days after the rash appears. Everyone who has not had the disease or been immunized is susceptible. Rubeola does not cause congenital defects as rubella (German measles) does. Rubella will be covered later in the chapter.

Transmission   Measles is one of the most communicable of all diseases. It is spread through airborne droplets, direct contact with nasal or throat secretions of infected individuals, and by articles that have been freshly contaminated.

FIGURE 8-11   Measles cases by year—United States, 1960-1990.

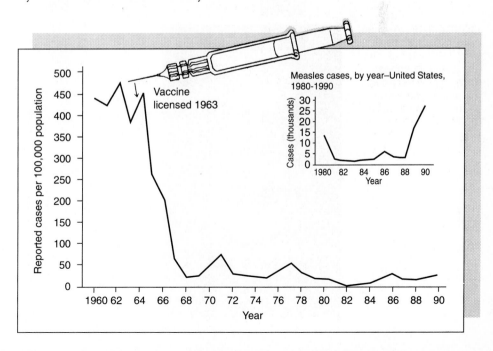

Symptoms   Early symptoms of measles include fever, photophobia (light sensitivity), malaise, anorexia, conjunctivitis, runny nose, and cough. A unique characteristic of the disease, Koplik's spots, appears 4 to 5 days after the initial symptoms. Koplik's spots are on the oral mucosa opposite the molars and look like tiny, bluish grey specks surrounded by a red halo (Figure 8-12). About 5 days after these spots appear, the temperature rises sharply, and a slightly itchy rash appears. This rash starts behind the ears and gradually spreads over the whole body (Figures 8-13 and 8-14). Once the rash reaches the feet, it begins to fade in the same order it appeared, leaving a brownish discoloration that disappears in 7 to 10 days. During the worst

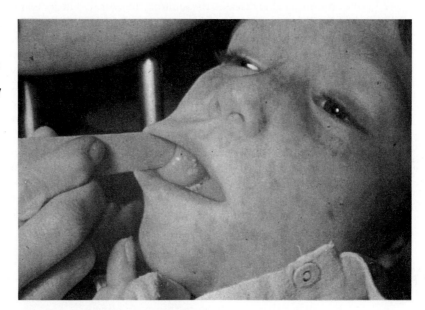

FIGURE 8-12 Koplik's spots (on tongue) and exanthem (rash) of measles. Koplik's spots are almost always present during the early stage of measles but disappear after the first or second day of the rash.

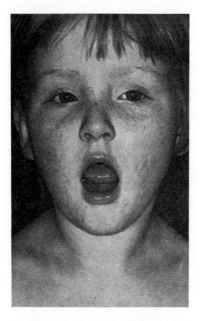

FIGURE 8-13 Appearance of face in measles. The face has an unmistakable appearance, with watery eyes, the mouth and throat a deep red, and a dusky red blotchy rash on the skin.

of the disease, about 2 to 3 days after the rash appears, there is a temperature of 103 to 105° F, severe cough, puffy red eyes, and runny nose. The face has a distinctive appearance as seen in Figure 8-14. Encephalitis is the most serious complication.

Treatment   Plenty of fluids, acetaminophen for fever, and other remedies to relieve symptoms are usual treatment. Antibiotics are only used in case of secondary bacterial infection. Aspirin is no longer recommended for children because of the chance of developing Reye syndrome.

Prevention   Routine vaccination during the second year of life.

Control   If live vaccine is given with 72 hours of exposure, it may provide protection. IG may be used for individuals in the household or who have had contact if they are at risk for complications. There should be contact investigation to determine source and to vaccinate those who have not been vaccinated.

RUBELLA (GERMAN MEASLES, THREE-DAY MEASLES)

This normally mild disease in children and adults is extremely dangerous for an unborn child when a pregnant woman is infected during the first trimester of pregnancy. Rubella was once common worldwide, but since the vaccine was developed, it is less prevalent in most developed countries. In the United States, reported cases dropped from over 12,000 in 1976 to 221 in 1988 (Figure 8-15). Figure 8-16 shows the reported incidence rate by states for 1988 to 1990.

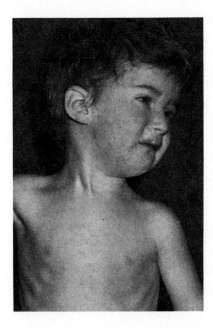

FIGURE 8-14 Measles rash on first day. This rash could be confused with scarlet fever, but Koplik's spots will usually be in the mouth if it's measles (see Figure 8-12).

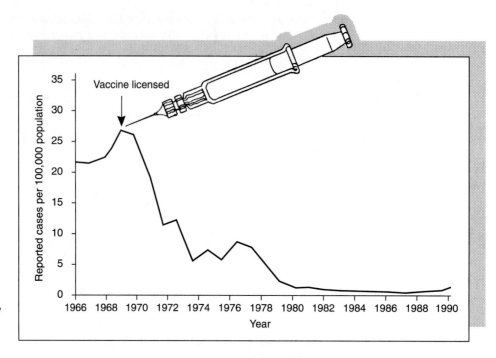

FIGURE 8-15 Rubella (German measles)—by year, United States, 1966-1990.

The incubation period is 14 to 23 days, and the disease is communicable for about 1 week before and at least 4 days after onset of the rash. Active immunity is acquired by having the infection or by vaccination. Infants receive antibodies from immune mothers, which protect them for 6 to 9 months.

Transmission   Droplets or direct contact with throat and nasal secretions of infected individuals leads to infection. Infants who have acquired rubella congenitally shed the virus in their pharyngeal secretions and urine for months after birth and are a source of the infection for their contacts.

Symptoms   In children, symptoms are mild, with a rash on the face that spreads to the body. After a few days the rash disappears. There may also be a slight fever and enlargement of the lymph nodes. In up to half of the cases the symptoms are inapparent, and the infection is never recognized. Adolescents and adults may have more pronounced symptoms.

Treatment   No specific treatment is available. Acetaminophen may be used to reduce fever.

Prevention   Vaccination of infants is highly effective in preventing the disease.

Control   Any known cases of rubella should be isolated from pregnant women. Contact investigation and identification of pregnant contacts is necessary in order to test for infection and to advise them regarding the possibilities for the unborn infant.

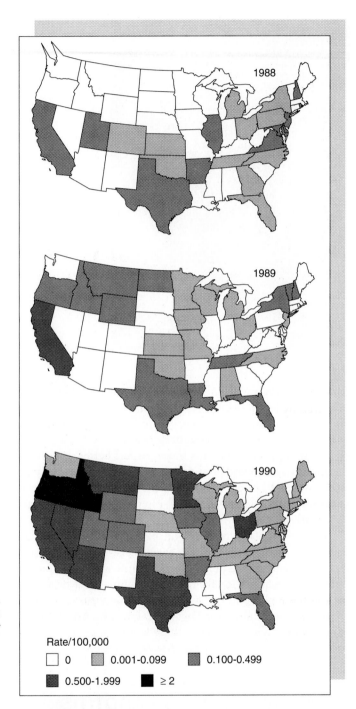

FIGURE 8-16 Incidence rates per 100,000 population of reported rubella—United States, 1988-1990. (Provisional data for 1990 from weeks 1-52 in MMWR. Mississippi requires reporting of congenital rubella syndrome but not rubella cases.)

SMALLPOX

Smallpox is included in this text because of its historical significance as the first communicable disease recognized officially as eradicated. On October 26, 1979, the World Health Organization declared smallpox eradicated 2 years after the last reported case, which was in Somalia. A case has not been reported in the United States since 1949. Smallpox was a highly infectious viral disease that was extremely

FIGURE 8-17 Characteristic rash appears on woman with smallpox.

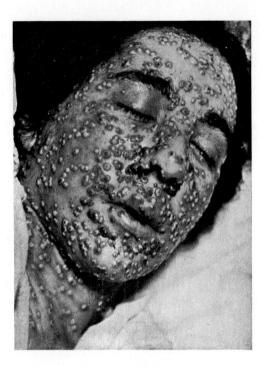

common in the nineteenth century and before. It was spread by respiratory discharges and less often by contact with lesions. The symptoms began with chills, high fever, headache, backache, severe malaise, and vomiting. Sometimes symptoms were more severe, with convulsive seizures, delirium, or coma. Two to 3 days after symptoms appeared, victims began to feel better, but then lesions appeared around the mouth and throat, and a rash spread over the body and eventually developed into pus-filled blisters (Figure 8-17). These "pox" ruptured, became crusted, and sometimes left deep, pitted scars. No treatment was available, and the disease killed up to 40% of those affected.

Cooperation in a vaccination program by countries all over the world led to eradication. There were certain characteristics of smallpox that aided in eradication. First, although spread person to person, it was infectious for only a short period of time. Second, it was easily recognized. Finally, it occurred only in humans. There are only two places in the world where the virus exists at the present time as far as is known: the Centers for Disease Control in Atlanta and at a research institute in Moscow. The virus is kept in these laboratories so that it will be available to make vaccine on the chance that the disease could break out again.

MUMPS (INFECTIOUS PAROTITIS)

Before the development of the mumps vaccine, it was commonly believed that male children should be exposed to the virus and allowed to get mumps. The belief had good reason behind it because, in the adult male, mumps could be an excruciatingly painful disease because of orchitis (inflammation of the testes). Today, with the vaccine, the wisest course of action is for everyone to be protected from the disease because, at any age, there can be serious complications. Figure 8-18 shows the occurrence of mumps for 1968-1990. Mumps is most prevalent in the 5- to 9-year-old age group. Mumps is caused by *paramyxovirus,* which infects the parotid gland. The incubation period is commonly 18 days, and it is communicable from 6 days before symptoms appear and up to 9 days after they appear. Many individuals have inapparent infections, but they can still communicate the disease. Immunity to the disease (lasting about 1 year) is transferred from mother to baby. Having the disease confers lifelong immunity. Most adults born before 1967 (when vaccine became available) were probably infected and had the disease even though there were no recognizable symptoms.

Transmission   Mumps is spread by airborne droplets and by direct contact with the saliva of an infected person.

Symptoms   It is estimated that about 30% have no symptoms. When symptoms do occur, they vary widely and may include myalgia, anorexia, malaise, headache, and low-grade fever, followed by an earache that's aggravated by chewing, and parotid gland tenderness and swelling (Figure 8-19). The temperature is 101 to 104° F, and there is pain during chewing or drinking sour or acidic liquids. In addition to orchitis, which has already been mentioned, complications include epididymitis, meningitis, and, rarely, a number of other serious illnesses. All complications occur more frequently in males.

Treatment   As with most viral diseases, antibiotics are ineffective. Analgesics, plenty of fluids, and rest are the main forms of treatment. Antipyretics may be used if the fever remains high, and intravenous fluid replacement if the victim has difficulty swallowing.

FIGURE 8-18
Mumps—by year, United States, 1968-1990.

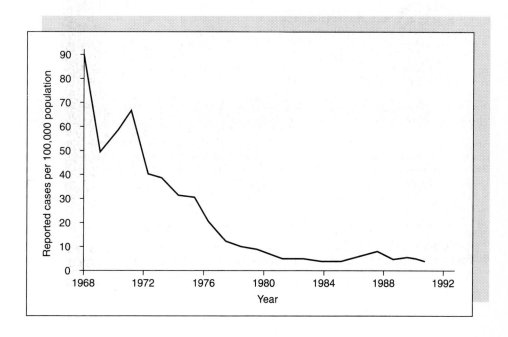

FIGURE 8-19 Mumps (infectious parotitis) in a child. In 70% of patients with mumps, both sides become infected. For this child, only the right side is involved.

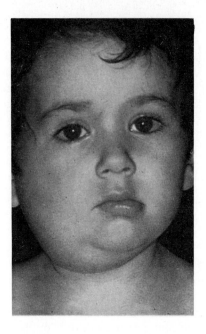

Prevention   A safe, effective vaccination is available and should be administered to all children. Fifteen months is the recommended time for the vaccination along with that for measles and rubella.

Control   Individuals with mumps should be excluded from school for 9 days after the onset of the disease. Contact investigation and immunization of any contacts is advised.

SUMMARY

The table summarizes relevant data on viral diseases acquired through the respiratory route.

SUMMARY TABLE	Viral diseases acquired through the respiratory route			
Disease	**Special Characteristics**	**Transmission**	**Common Symptoms**	**Prevention/ Control**
Common cold	Caused by close to 200 different viruses. Most common communicable disease.	Direct or indirect. Hand to eye, droplets.	Runny nose, watery eyes, headache.	Personal hygiene, frequent washing of hands, general fitness.
Influenza	Upper respiratory disease. Fatalities from complications, often pneumonia.	Direct or indirect contact. Airborne droplets.	Sudden onset of chills, temperature, headache, malaise, muscle aches, cough.	Vaccination for at-risk individuals.

Disease	Special Characteristics	Transmission	Common Symptoms	Prevention/ Control
Infectious mononucleosis	Epstein-Barr virus, herpes group. Lab test necessary to confirm diagnosis. Serious complications.	Oral-pharyngeal route.	Headache, malaise, fatigue, fever, swollen glands, sore throat.	Basic personal hygiene and avoidance of close contact with infected persons.
Varicella (chickenpox)	Herpes virus. Mild in children, severe in adults. Virus stays in body, may cause herpes zoster years later.	Direct or indirect contact, airborne droplets from respiratory tract, discharge from vesicles.	Fever, malaise, anorexia, rash, vesicles.	IG for high risk individuals; vaccine in Japan. Exclusion of children from school.
Herpes zoster	Reactivation of chickenpox virus in adults. Occurs with lowered resistance from stress or other causes.	Communicable through fluid from vesicles.	Fever, malaise; severe pain, pruritis, numbness, tingling, increased sensitivity in affected area; blisters, scab, pitted scar; may be intermittent severe pain for years.	Palliative only. No remedy has proved to be consistently effective.
Measles	A comparatively mild disease with potentially fatal complications.	Direct and indirect transmission through airborne droplets, nasal or throat secretions, fomites.	Fever, photophobia, malaise, anorexia, conjunctivitis, coryza, cough, Koplik's spots, temperature, rash.	Vaccination. IG for at-risk household contacts. Contact investigation.
Rubella	Birth defects in child of pregnant woman who acquires disease, especially during first 4 months of pregnancy.	Droplets or direct contact with nose or nasal secretions of infected person. Infection of fetus. Infants with congenital rubella also spread infection.	Mild, with a rash, slight fever, swollen lymph nodes possible. Up to 50% of cases inapparent.	None known. Acetaminophen to ease discomfort. Pregnant women should be isolated from known cases. Contact investigation.
Smallpox	Declared eradicated by WHO, October 1979. Cause of much suffering and death (40% of victims).	Most often through respiratory discharges. Also contact with lesions and fomites.	Chills, high fever, headache, backache, severe malaise, vomiting. Sometimes seizures, delirium, coma. Lesions around mouth and throat, rash, pus-filled blisters that break, sometimes leaving deep, pitted scars.	Worldwide vaccination program led to eradication.
Mumps	Extremely painful disease in adult males.	Airborne droplets and direct contact with saliva of infected person.	None, 30%. Vary widely, malaise, anorexia, myalgia, headache, low-grade fever. Earache, parotid gland swelling and tenderness. Complications may include orchitis, epididymitis, meningitis.	Vaccination. Exclusion from school for 9 days after onset. Contact investigation.

Treatment: No antibiotics are available to cure these viral diseases; treatment is symptomatic.

QUESTIONS FOR REVIEW

1. What are some complications that can occur with the common cold?
2. What is the most likely way by which a cold is acquired?
3. What symptoms indicate a secondary bacterial infection?
4. What is the best treatment for a cold?
5. What is the best way to avoid a cold?
6. What is the difference in meaning between influenza and the term *flu* as it is commonly used?
7. Why is influenza a dangerous disease?
8. Why has influenza been a difficult disease to prevent?
9. How is amantadine used in treating influenza?
10. What is the disease agent for infectious mononucleosis?
11. Why is mono called the college disease?
12. What complications may occur with infectious mononucleosis?
13. In what ways can chickenpox be a severe disease?
14. What is meant by the term "dewdrop on a petal"?
15. What complications may occur if a child scratches the lesions of chickenpox?
16. What is the goal of treatment in chickenpox?
17. When is VZIG used for chickenpox?
18. What is the cause of shingles?
19. How is shingles transmitted?
20. Where do the lesions for herpes zoster occur?
21. What may happen to an individual years after having an attack of shingles?
22. What are the unique characteristics among the symptoms of measles?
23. What danger is there to the fetus if a pregnant woman acquires rubella?
24. How can measles and rubella be prevented?
25. What is the historical significance of smallpox?
26. What characteristics of smallpox aided in its eradication?
27. What are the symptoms of smallpox?
28. What complications may occur with mumps?

FURTHER READING

Ackerman, S.J. "Flu Shots: Do You Need One?" *FDA Consumer,* Oct. '89, 23:8-11.

Adler, Stuart P. "Cytomegalovirus and Child Day Care: Evidence for an Increased Infection Rate Among Day-Care Workers." *New England Journal of Medicine,* Nov. 9, '89, 321:1290-1296.

Andiman, Ronald M. and Stuart S. Leicht. "Herpes Zoster on the Increase." *Patient Care,* Apr. 30, '88, 22:71-81.

"Another Way to Overtreat the Symptoms of a Cold." *Consumer Reports,* Feb. '91, 56:73.

Bagley, Janice L. "Colds & Flu: Transmission & Treatment." *American Druggist,* Sept. '89, 200:30-34.

Baum, Stephen G. and Carol F. Phillips. "Just Who Is at Risk for Mumps?" *Patient Care,* Feb. 28, '89, 23:48-54.

Bobo, J.K., et al. "Risk Factors for Delayed Immunization in a Random Sample of 1163 Children from Oregon and Washington." Feb. '93, (2):308-314.

Boldogh, Istran, Sazaly AbuBakar and Thomas Albrecht. "Activation of Proto-Oncogenes: An Immediate Early Event in Human Cytomegalovirus Infection." *Science,* Feb. 2, '90, 247:561-564.

Boyd, Robert F. *General Microbiology.* St. Louis: Mosby, 1988.

Bungay, Kathleen M. "Therapeutic Management of the Common Cold in Adults." *American Druggist,* Aug. '90, 202:99-105.

Cassidy, Jo. "Mononucleosis: What's in a Name?" *Current Health,* Sept. '90, 17:14-15.

Cohn, Jeffrey P. "Here Come the Bugs . . . Colds and Flu Season's Back. . . ." *FDA Consumer,* Nov. '88, 22:6-9.

Control of Communicable Disease in Man. Abram S. Benenson, ed. Fifteenth Edition, Washington, D.C.: American Public Health Association, 1990.

Cook, Lynn Crawford. "The Office Visitor Nobody Wants." *Health,* May '89, 21:78-81.

Devereaux, Kathryn. "Outwitting Winter Colds." *Women's Sports and Fitness,* Oct.-Nov. '88, 10:46-50.

Diamond, Jared. "A Pox upon Our Genes." *Natural History,* Feb. '90, 99:26-28.

Douglas, R. Gordon Jr. "Prophylaxis and Treatment of Influenza." *New England Journal of Medicine,* Feb. 15, '90, 322:433-450.

Edmonson, M. Bruce, et al. "Mild Measles and Secondary Vaccine Failure during a Sustained Outbreak in a Highly Vaccinated Population." *Journal of the American Medical Association,* May 9, '90, 263:2467-2471.

Feierman, Reuben and Paul Shea. "Cough and Cold Products that RPhs Recommend." *American Druggist,* Sept. '89, 200:39-42.

"From the Centers for Disease Control and Prevention. Influenza Activity—United States and Worldwide, the Composition of the 1993-94 Influenza Vaccine." *Journal of the American Medical Association,* Apr. 14, '93, 269(14):1778-1779.

Gannon, Kathi. "It's That Time Again: New Cold, Flu Remedies Hit Market." *Drug Topics,* Oct. 22, '90, 134:32-33.

Hopkins, Donald R. "Smallpox: Ten Years Gone." *American Journal of Public Health,* Dec. '88, 78:1589-1595.

Hopkins, Jack W. "The Eradication of Smallpox: Organizational Learning and Innovation in International Health Administration." *Journal of Developing Areas,* Apr. '88, 22:321-332.

"Hot Pepper and Herpes Pain." *Harvard Medical School Health Letter,* Sept. '89, 14:6-7.

Hussey, Gregory D. and Mary Klein. "A Randomized, Controlled Trial of Vitamin A in Children with Severe Measles." *New England Journal of Medicine,* July 19, '90, 323:160-164.

"Increase in Rubella and Congenital Rubella." *Journal of the American Medical Association,* Mar. 6, '91, 265:1076-1077.

Isaacs, David and Margaret Menser. "Measles, Mumps, Rubella, and Varicella." *Lancet,* June 9, '90, 335:1384-1387.

Jaret, Peter. "It All Starts with a Sneeze." *Health,* Nov. '88, 20:54-58.

Kamberg, Mary-Lane. "America's 10 Least Wanted: The Leading Causes of Death in the United States." *Current Health,* Sept. '90, 17:4-10.

Macknin, Michael L., Susan Mathew and Sharon VanderBrug Medendorp. "Effect of Inhaling Heated Vapor on Symptoms of the Common Cold." *Journal of the American Medical Association,* Aug. 22, '90, 264:989-991.

Margolis, Karen L., et al. "Frequency of Adverse Reactions to Influenza Vaccine in the Elderly." *Journal of the American Medical Association,* Sept. 5, '90, 264:1139-1141.

Marwick, Charles. "While Coping with This Season's Influenza, Experts Plan for Season Still to Come." *Journal of the American Medical Association,* Feb. 26, '88, 259:1131

Mast, Eric, et al. "Risk Factors for Measles in a Previously Vaccinated Population and Cost-Effectiveness of Revaccination Strategies." *Journal of the American Medical Association,* Nov. 21, '90, 264:2529-2533.

McCance, Kathryn L. and Sue E. Huether. *Pathophysiology: The Biologic Basis for Disease in Adults and Children*. St. Louis: Mosby, 1990.

McKinney, W. Paul and Gary P. Barnas. "Influenza Immunization in the Elderly." *American Journal of Public Health,* Oct. '89, 79:1422-1424.

Miller, E., et al. "Risk of Aseptic Meningitis after Measles, Mumps, and Rubella Vaccine in UK Children." *Lancet,* Apr. 17, '93, 341(8851):979-982.

Mostow, Steven R. "Closing in on the Common Cold?" *Patient Care,* Jan. 15, '90, 24:189-197.

Murph, Jody R., et al. "The Occupational Risk of Cytomegalovirus Infection Among Day-Care Providers." *Journal of the American Medical Association,* Feb. 6, '91, 265:603-608.

Murray, Patrick R., et al. *Medical Microbiology*. St. Louis: Mosby, 1990.

Radetsky, Peter. "Taming the Wily Rhinovirus." *Discover,* Apr. '89, 10:38-43.

Rados, Bill. ". . . And Here's Help; Modern Pharmacy's Answers to Chicken Soup." *FDA Consumer,* Nov. '88, 22:7-9.

Rossen, Anne E. "Comeback Diseases: They're No Joke . . . Don't Let Them Get the Last Laugh." *Current Health,* Jan. '91, 17:26-27.

Sixby, John W., et al. "Detection of a Second Widespread Strain of Epstein-Barr Virus." *Lancet,* Sept. 30, '89, 2:761-765.

Smith, M. B. and W. Feldman. "Over-the-Counter Cold Medications. A Critical Review of Clinical Trials Between 1950 and 1991." *Journal of the American Medical Association*. May 5, '93, 269(17):2258-2263.

Springer, Timothy. "Stalking the Cold Trail: The Shortcut to Medical Breakthroughs." *New Republic,* Oct. 29, '90, 203:17-20.

Sternberg, Ken. "At Start of Second Smallpox-Free Decade, Debate Continues about Keeping Virus." *Journal of the American Medical Association,* Oct. 21, '88, 260:2172.

Straus, Stephen E. "Clinical and Biological Differences between Recurrent Herpes Simplex Virus and Varicella-Zoster Virus Infections." *Journal of the American Medical Association,* Dec. 22, '89, 262:3455-3458.

Straus, Stephen E. "Shingles, Sorrows, Salves and Solutions." (Clinical), *Journal of the American Medical Association,* Apr. 14, '93, 269(14):1836-1839.

Sumaya, Ciro V. "Mononucleosis in Children: An Update." *Patient Care,* Nov. 15, '90, 24:139-148.

Thornton, James S. "Common Concerns about the Common Cold." *Physician and Sportsmedicine,* June '90, 18:120-124.

Thornton, Russell, Tim Miller and Jonathan Warren. "American Indian Population Recovery following Smallpox Epidemics." *American Anthropologist,* Mar. '91, 93:28-45.

Ukens, Carol. "Flu Season Starts Slowly, But Worst May Be Yet to Come." *Drug Topics,* Jan. 21, '91, 135:90-91.

Voelker, Rebecca. "Outbreaks Make Officials Consider Need for Better Measles Vaccine." *American Medical News,* Apr. 22, '91, 34:4-5.

Wacker, Bob. "Virus on Ice." *Health,* Dec. '89, 21:48-51.

Welch, Dawn. "The Cold War: When the Sniffles Start, Should You Ride or Rest?" *Bicycling,* Feb. '91, 32:64-67.

Willis, Judith Levine. "Mumps and Measles Make a Comeback." *Consumer's Research Magazine,* Sept. '89, 72:23-26.

Chapter 9

Viral Diseases Acquired through the Alimentary and Other Routes

O B J E C T I V E S

1 Explain the importance of the polio vaccine.

2 Distinguish between hepatitis A and hepatitis B.

3 State steps to take when someone is bitten by a wild or domestic animal.

4 Describe the effects of rabies without treatment.

5 Identify possible symptoms of encephalitis.

6 Distinguish between herpes simplex virus 1 and 2.

7 Indicate when warts need to be treated.

8 Discuss the history of AIDS.

9 Identify means of transmission, symptoms, treatment, prevention, and control for diseases in this chapter.

POLIOMYELITIS (INFANTILE PARALYSIS, POLIO)

One of the most dramatic medical events in the 1950s was the development of a vaccine for polio. Dr. Jonas E. Salk (Figure 9-1) devised the first vaccine for polio, and 6 years later, Dr. Albert Sabin (Figure 9-2) developed the second, which has almost entirely replaced Salk vaccine. Polio was first recognized in 1840 and became epidemic in Norway and Sweden in 1905. During the first half of this century, the disease became pandemic, and the word *polio* produced as much fear in the American people and peoples all over the world as the word *AIDS* does today. Paralysis and death were synonymous with polio, or infantile paralysis as it was called in the early days. Symbolic of the paralyzing form of the disease was the dreaded "iron lung," a monstrous armor of iron into which the victims were slid until only their heads were free (Figure 9-3). This machine was an artificial respirator, the forerunner of the much simpler apparatuses used in hospitals today. Polio can range from asymptomatic illness to paralysis and major illness, depending upon the course of the infection. It is caused by poliovirus, an *enterovirus*. Originally, polio was a disease

DID YOU KNOW?

Polio may be the next disease to be declared eradicated worldwide. The Pan American Health Organization (PAHO) is near to its goal of eradication in the Americas. Since January 1991, no cases have been reported in North, Central, or South America. If no cases are reported for the next 3 years, PAHO will be able to certify the eradication of the disease in the Western hemisphere. Meanwhile, WHO is conducting a campaign in Asia and Africa with a goal of eradication by 2000. If that goal is reached, then polio will be history and the second infectious disease to be eradicated in all parts of the world.

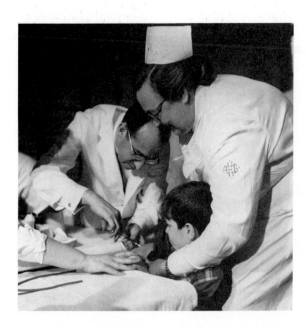

FIGURE 9-1   Dr. Jonas Salk, developer of the first vaccine for poliomyelitis.

FIGURE 9-2   Dr. Albert Sabin developed an oral polio vaccine that has almost entirely replaced Salk vaccine in the United States.

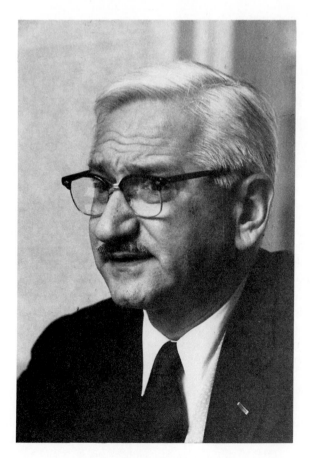

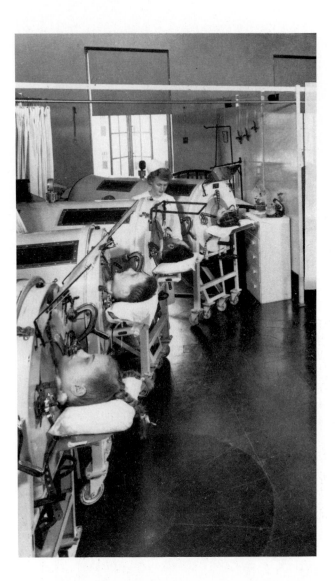

FIGURE 9-3 The so-called iron lung was used to assist people with paralytic polio in breathing.

of children, but in recent years it has occurred more often in people over age 15. Minor outbreaks still occur, usually among nonimmunized segments of the population, such as the Amish of Pennsylvania, where there was an outbreak in 1979. Figure 9-4 shows the decrease in cases following the development of the vaccines. Polio usually has an incubation period of 7 to 14 days, although it has been known to range from 3 to 35 days. The period of communicability is not accurately known, but the disease is most infectious during the first few days before and after the onset of symptoms. The virus exists in the feces for 3 to 6 weeks or longer. Most people are susceptible to the disease, but susceptibility to the paralytic form increases with age at time of infection. There are three types of the polio virus, and immunity following infection is type specific.

Transmission.   Direct contact through close association with someone who has the disease is necessary for infection with the poliomyelitis virus. The main means

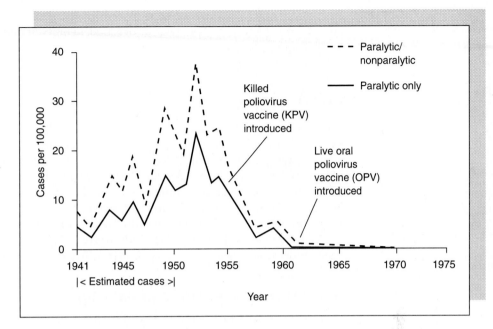

FIGURE 9-4 Polio incidence in the United States. Salk vaccine was introduced in 1955, and Sabin vaccine in 1961 to 1962. The solid line represents paralytic polio only; the dotted line represents both paralytic and nonparalytic polio.

of transmission is the fecal-oral route when there are poor methods of sanitation. Where sanitation is good, it is spread more by pharyngeal secretions. The organism is easier to detect and lasts longer in feces than in secretions from the throat.

Symptoms

The symptoms for poliomyelitis vary, depending upon the progression of the disease. Although the word "polio" brought fear to all at one time, it was only due to hearing about the worst cases. For most, polio is a comparatively mild disease. There are four possible outcomes of infection: (1) Asymptomatic illness occurs in at least 90% of poliovirus infections. (2) Minor illness with fever, headache, malaise, sore throat, and vomiting occurs in approximately 5% of patients. (3) Nonparalytic poliomyelitis with back pain and muscle spasms in addition to the symptoms of minor illness occurs in 1% to 2% of patients. (4) Paralytic polio with spinal and/or cranial paralysis occurs 3 to 4 days after minor illness has subsided. This form occurs in 0.1% to 2.0% of infected individuals. The extent of paralysis varies, depending upon how many nerves are affected. Only one leg may be involved, or the individual may have progressive paralysis that eventually affects vital organs and leads to death.

Treatment

Other than analgesics to relieve pain, there is no treatment for polio. Physical therapy is used to counteract muscle atrophy.

Prevention

Immunization for polio should begin at 2 months. Routine immunization of adults is not recommended except those at risk because of occupation or travel to high-risk areas.

Control   Since the greatest risk of infection is during the prodromal period, isolation is unnecessary. Identifying contacts in order to identify individuals who are ill and provide appropriate treatment is recommended.

VIRAL HEPATITIS

There are at least five different viruses that cause hepatitis (inflammation of the liver). The most common are hepatitis A and hepatitis B, which will be discussed in this chapter. Non-A, non-B hepatitis, now referred to as hepatitis C, is the form transmitted by unclean needles and found frequently among drug users. Figure 9-5 shows the comparative number of reported cases for the first three types of hepatitis. Figures 9-6 and 9-7 show the reported cases of hepatitis A and hepatitis B by state. Hepatitis D, or delta hepatitis, occurs only in someone who has hepatitis B, since it needs the B virus for its own survival. No outbreaks of hepatitis E have been reported in this country. It is similar to hepatitis A.

HEPATITIS A (INFECTIOUS HEPATITIS)

Hepatitis A, formerly called infectious hepatitis, occurs in all parts of the world. In developed countries, it occurs frequently in day-care centers where there are diapered children, among intravenous drug users, individuals who practice unprotected intercourse, and among travelers to countries where it is endemic. Epidemic cycles have not occurred in the United States since 1971, but in 1983, the number of reported cases started to increase, as shown in Figure 9-5. The primary reservoir of infection is people, although it has been found in chimpanzees and other non-human primates. The average incubation period is 28 to 30 days. Hepatitis A is communicable during the last part of the incubation period to a few days after the

FIGURE 9-5   Hepatitis by year, United States, 1952 to 1990.

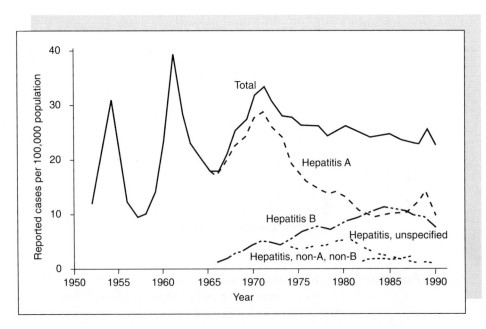

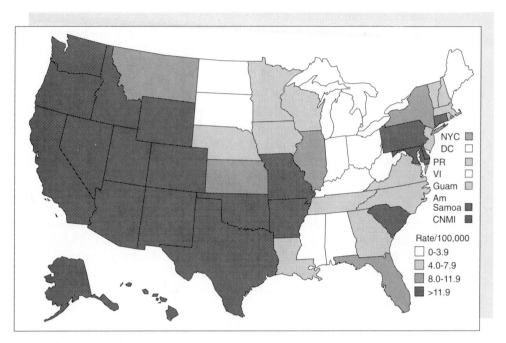

FIGURE 9-6   Hepatitis A—reported cases, per 100,000 population, United States, 1989.

FIGURE 9-7   Hepatitis B—reported cases, per 100,000 population, United States, 1989.

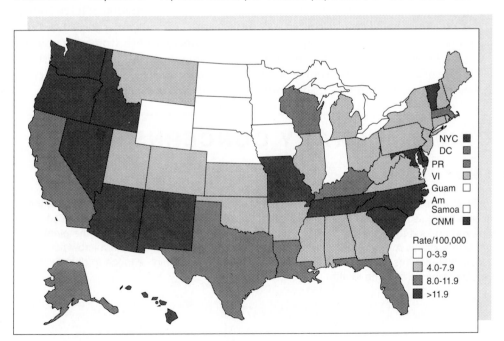

onset of jaundice. (Jaundice does not occur in some cases, particularly children—see Symptoms.) Susceptibility is general, and the low incidence of reported cases among children suggests that some infections are asymptomatic.

Transmission   The virus is present in the feces of infected persons and transmitted person to person by the fecal-oral route. Most often this occurs when the infected person handles food and contaminated food is eaten by others. The virus may also be present in shellfish from contaminated water and, if not cooked at a high enough temperature, transmitted to humans. Transmission of hepatitis A by blood is rare, but individuals who have had it should not donate blood.

Symptoms   There is usually a sudden onset with fever, malaise, anorexia, nausea, and abdominal discomfort, followed within a few days by jaundice (in some cases). The illness is usually mild, lasting 1 to 2 weeks. The severity of the illness generally increases with age. Children are often asymptomatic or have flulike symptoms but no jaundice. A diagnosis can only be made with liver function tests. The few fatalities that occur are in older patients.

Treatment   There is no specific treatment.

Prevention/Control   The public needs to be educated about good sanitation and personal hygiene. There should be particular emphasis on proper handwashing and sanitary disposal of feces. Individuals working in day-care centers need to use proper methods to minimize the possibility of fecal-oral transmission. Thorough handwashing after changing diapers and before meals is mandatory. Immunoglobulin (IgM) should be given to staff and attendees at any center where a case occurs. Administration of IG to families of attendees should also be considered. Travelers to high-risk areas should be given prophylactic doses of IgM. Oysters, clams, and other shellfish from contaminated areas should be heated at a high temperature for 4 minutes or steamed for 90 seconds. In case of an epidemic, the source of the infection needs to be identified by epidemiologic studies. Any common source of infection should be eliminated.

CONTEMPORARY CONCERNS

Better Safe than Sick

Microwaving food bought at a fast-food place can reduce the risk of catching hepatitis A. When a worker who routinely picked up food for his fellow employees came down with hepatitis A that was traced to a cook at a local fast-food restaurant, scientists could not understand why he became ill with the infection while the other 12 workers who ate the same food did not. Further investigation showed that he ate his food on the way back to the plant, but the others reheated theirs in the microwave, evidently at a temperature high enough to destroy the organism.

In case of an epidemic, the source of the infection needs to be identified by epidemiologic studies. Any common source of infection should be eliminated.

HEPATITIS B (SERUM HEPATITIS)

This viral hepatitis has a slower onset than infectious hepatitis. The average incubation period is 60 to 90 days, and blood from the victim is thought to be infective weeks before the symptoms appear and to remain infective through the carrier stage, which may be for life. The disease is milder and sometimes asymptomatic in children.

Transmission

Blood, saliva, semen, and vaginal fluids have shown to be infectious. Contaminated needles, syringes, and other intravenous equipment are important vehicles for spreading the disease. The infection may also be spread by contamination of sores or exposure of mucous membranes to contaminated blood or blood transfusion. Donated blood that has been screened is considered relatively safe. Since the advent of AIDS, screening of blood for hepatitis (and other) antibodies has become routine. The chance of receiving contaminated blood through transfusion is 1 "in a million" today. The infection can also be acquired through homosexual or heterosexual intercourse.

Symptoms

The symptoms of hepatitis B include insidious onset of anorexia, vague abdominal discomfort, nausea, vomiting, and sometimes rash and jaundice. Type B has a higher mortality rate than type A, particularly in people over 40.

Treatment

None available.

Prevention/Control

Vaccines are available, but their high cost prohibits general use. Vaccination is recommended for those at increased and continuing risk of infection and for all newborns. Blood must be continually screened, and all needles and syringes sterilized, or if they are disposable, proper methods of disposal must be used.

RABIES (HYDROPHOBIA)

Rabies is a disease of animals, especially bats, skunks, foxes, raccoons, dogs, cats, and cattle (Figure 9-8). The disease is communicated to humans by the bite of a rabid animal. Without treatment, it is almost always fatal. Figure 9-9 shows the number of cases in the United States and Puerto Rico by year. It is estimated that 30,000 deaths occur worldwide each year, mostly in developing countries. In the 10 years from 1980 to 1989, 12 deaths occurred in the United States.

The incubation period is usually 2 to 8 weeks, depending on a number of factors. Incubation periods have been known to be as little as 5 days to a year or more. The period of communicability varies, depending on the mammal involved. Dogs and cats are communicable for 3 to 10 days before the onset of symptoms and for as

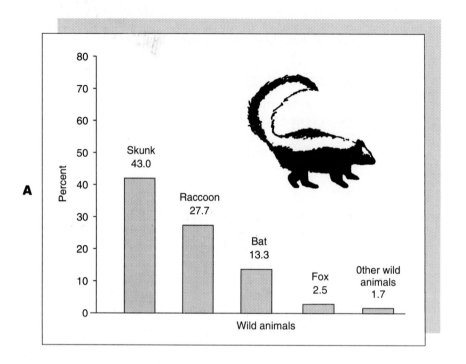

A

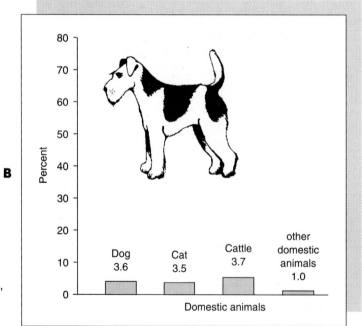

B

FIGURE 9-8 Distribution of animal rabies among **A,** wild animals, **B,** domestic animals in the United States, 1987.

long as the disease lasts. All warm-blooded mammals are susceptible, and there is no known natural immunity in humans.

Transmission Transmission is most often by introduction of the saliva of an infected animal by a bite or scratch into the muscle tissue. A few cases have resulted from corneal

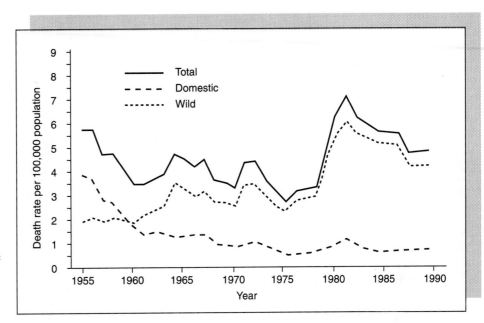

FIGURE 9-9 Rabies from wild and domestic animals, by year, United States and Puerto Rico, 1955 to 1990.

transplants when the organs were removed from individuals with undiagnosed CNS disease. No other person-to-person transmission has ever been documented. Transmission by air has been demonstrated in caves, and in Latin America transmission from bats to domestic animals is common. Insectivorous bats (the common kind in the United States) rarely transmit the disease.

Symptoms   The severity of the wound site in relation to nerve supply, distance from the brain, the amount of virus introduced, and layers of clothing are all factors in determining how quickly symptoms appear. The initial symptoms are local or radiating pain or burning and a sensation of cold, itching, and tingling at the bite site. There are also typical symptoms of fever, malaise, headache, anorexia, nausea, sore throat, and persistent loose cough. Then the patient will begin to show nervousness, anxiety, irritability, hyperesthesia (increased sensitivity to sensory stimuli), pupillary dilation, tachycardia, shallow respirations, and excessive salivation, tears, and perspiration. About 2 to 10 days after onset of these symptoms, the victim experiences restlessness, hyperactivity, disorientation, and in some cases, seizures. There is often an intense thirst, but attempts to drink induce violent, painful spasms in the throat (the reason for the name hydrophobia). Eye and facial muscles may become paralyzed. Coma and death follow 3 to 20 days after the onset of symptoms. Figure 9-10 shows the sequence of events following inoculation of rabies virus.

Treatment   Rabies is generally fatal if not treated promptly. Wound treatment and immunization must be given as soon as possible after the bite occurs. Any animal bite should be washed thoroughly (cleaned and flushed with water). The wound should not be sutured or closed. Although a person's own defenses may keep them from developing rabies even after being bitten by an infected animal, wound treatment must be given as soon as possible after the bite occurs. Vaccines that are used in the United States at this time are rabies vaccine, human diploid cell (HDCV), rabies vaccine

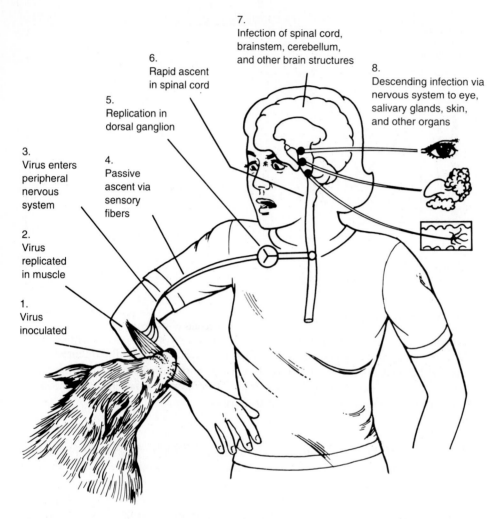

7.
Infection of spinal cord,
brainstem, cerebellum,
and other brain structures

6.
Rapid ascent
in spinal cord

8.
Descending infection via
nervous system to eye,
salivary glands, skin,
and other organs

5.
Replication in
dorsal ganglion

3.
Virus enters
peripheral
nervous
system

4.
Passive
ascent via
sensory
fibers

2.
Virus
replicated
in muscle

1.
Virus
inoculated

FIGURE 9-10 Progression of rabies virus infection. Numbered steps describe sequence of events.

adsorbed (RVA), and rabies immune globulin, human (HRIG). When or if these vaccines are administered depends upon the circumstances of the case involved as shown in Tables 9-1 and 9-2.

Prevention For prevention of rabies, registration, licensing, and vaccination of all dogs and cats is recommended. Stray, ownerless animals should be impounded and vaccinated or destroyed as necessary. An animal of any species that is acting strange or sick should not be picked up or handled. These animals should be reported to the police and/ or local health department. Any pet animal that has bitten a person with no provocation should be caged and observed for 10 days for signs of rabies. If a wild animal bites a person, it should be destroyed immediately and the head kept (on ice) and turned in for testing. Individuals at high risk (those who work with animals) should receive vaccinations.

TABLE 9-1 Rabies postexposure prophylaxis guide, United States, 1991

Animal Type	Evaluation and Disposition of Animal	Postexposure Prophylaxis Recommendations
Dogs and cats	Healthy and available for 10 days observation	Should not begin prophylaxis unless animal develops symptoms of rabies*
	Rabid or suspected rabid	Immediate vaccination
	Unknown (escaped)	Consult public health officials
Skunks, raccoons, bats, foxes, and most other carnivores; woodchucks	Regarded as rabid unless geographic area is known to be free of rabies or until animal proven negative by laboratory tests†	Immediate vaccination
Livestock, rodents, and lagomorphs (rabbits and hares)	Consider individually	Consult public health officials. Bites of squirrels, hamsters, guinea pigs, gerbils, chipmunks, rats, mice, other rodents, rabbits, and hares almost never require antirabies treatment

*During the 10-day holding period, begin treatment with HRIG and HDCV or RVA at first sign of rabies in a dog or cat that has bitten someone. The symptomatic animal should be killed immediately and tested.

†The animal should be killed and tested as soon as possible. Holding for observation is not recommended. Discontinue vaccine if immunofluorescence test results of the animal are negative.

TABLE 9-2 Rabies postexposure prophylaxis schedule, United States, 1991

Vaccination status	Treatment*	Regimen*
Not previously vaccinated	Local wound cleansing	All postexposure treatment should begin with immediate thorough cleansing of all wounds with soap and water.
	HRIG	20 IU/kg body weight. If anatomically feasible, up to one half the dose should be infiltrated around the wound(s) and the rest should be administered in the same syringe or into the same anatomic site as vaccine. Because HRIG may partially suppress active production of antibody, no more than the recommended dose should be given.
	Vaccine	HDCV or RVA, 1.0 ml, IM (deltoid area†), one each on days 0, 3, 7, 14, and 28.
Previously vaccinated‡	Local wound cleansing	All postexposure treatment should begin with immediate thorough cleansing of all wounds with soap and water.
	HRIG	HRIG should not be administered.
	Vaccine	HDCV or RVA, 1.0 ml, IM (deltoid area†), one each on days 0 and 3.

*These regimens are applicable for all age groups, including children.

†The deltoid area is the only acceptable site of vaccination for adults and older children. For younger children, the outer aspect of the thigh may be used. Vaccine should never be administered in the gluteal area.

‡Any person with a history of preexposure vaccination with HDCV or RVA; prior postexposure prophylaxis with HDCV or RVA; or previous vaccination with any other type of rabies vaccine and a documented history of antibody response to the prior vaccination.

Control   Respiratory secretions of someone bitten by a rabid animal may contain the virus, and contacts must be protected from them until it is determined that the victim does not have the disease. Any animal known to have bitten someone needs to be held for observation for 10 days. Valuable dogs and cats should not be killed unless it is established that they do have the disease. Unwanted dogs and cats and wild animals should be killed immediately and the brain checked for rabies.

ENCEPHALITIS

Encephalitis is a severe inflammation of the brain usually caused by mosquito-borne or tick-borne virus. In addition, encephalitis may be a sequella of another viral infection, such as polio, rabies, or mumps. This discussion will confine itself to arthropod-borne viral encephalitides (plural of encephalitis). Different strains of the virus occur in different parts of the country. Eastern equine encephalitis (EEE) is recognized in the eastern and north-central sections of the United States; western equine encephalitis (WEE) in the western and central states; St. Louis and Lacrosse encephalitis in most of the states; California encephalitis in forested areas of the country (Figure 9-11). These and other kinds of viral encephalitis occur in other parts of the world also.

Encephalitis occurs more in summer and early fall, particularly when conditions have been right for breeding many mosquitoes. The winter reservoir for most of these viruses is unknown. The incubation period is usually 5 to 15 days. There is no person-to-person transmission. People are more susceptible in infancy and old age.

FIGURE 9-11   Distribution of California encephalitis, 1966 to 1981.

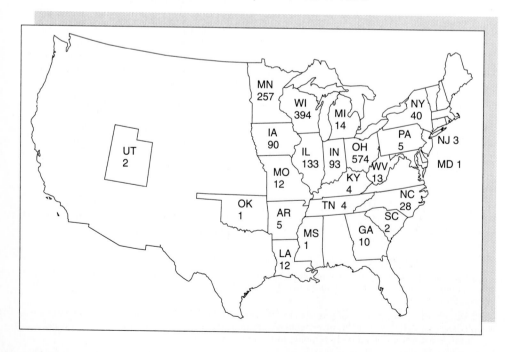

Transmission   These viral encephalitides are transmitted by the bite of an infected mosquito.

Symptoms   Viral encephalitis usually begins with sudden onset of fever, headache, and vomiting and progresses to include stiff neck and back, drowsiness, coma, paralysis, convulsions, muscular incoordination, and psychoses.

Treatment   There is no specific treatment for viral encephalitis. Analgesics for pain and other supportive therapy are used.

Prevention/Control   The following are ways to prevent and control viral encephalitis: control of mosquitoes by spraying and destruction of breeding places; use of screened living quarters and mosquito bed nets if necessary; avoidance of exposure to mosquitoes during times when they are known to bite; and use of repellants.

HERPES SIMPLEX

Herpes simplex is a recurrent, localized viral infection. Herpes simplex virus type I generally infects the upper part of the body, usually the lips and face. Herpes simplex virus type 2 generally infects the lower part of the body, most often the genital area. Infections from both types can occur in any part of the body depending on sexual practices and area exposed. (The incubation period for both types is 2 to 12 days. The viruses are found worldwide, and everyone is susceptible.) Both viruses can enter through a break in the skin or through the mucous membrane. Reactivation, which may or may not occur, can be due to a number of traumatic events, including stress or anything else that impairs the effectiveness of the immune system. Individuals with acquired immune deficiency syndrome (AIDS) are especially vulnerable to reactivation, which can lead to a generalized infection and death. Once a person is infected with either type, they are infected for life.

Most adults (70% to 90%) have been exposed to HSV type I (worldwide). Visible symptoms occur in only about 10% of the cases. Once the virus enters the body it is there for life. In about 60% of those infected, the disease is reactivated in later life and may occur as sores around the mouth during periods of stress or lowered resistance. The virus has been found in saliva for as long as 7 weeks after the lesion is healed.

Genital herpes, most often caused by herpes virus type II, is infective for about 7 to 12 days. Asymptomatic shedding of virus is probably common for both types.

Transmission   Transmission is by contact with saliva of infected individuals or by sexual activities. Both kinds can be transmitted by oral-genital or oral-anal contact.

Symptoms   Herpes may be asymptomatic or there may be varying degrees of typical prodromal symptoms. Itching and tingling precede the development of vesicular lesions around the mouth or in the genital or anal regions. The lesions are usually painful. There may also be fever, swollen glands, and painful urination. If lesions are internal, the

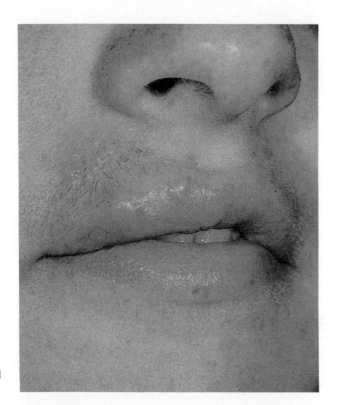

FIGURE 9-12 Herpes simplex on the lips and face.

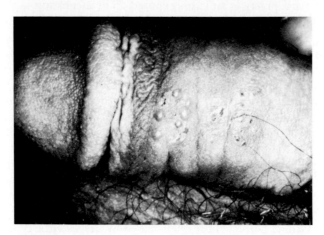

FIGURE 9-13 Genital herpes.

symptoms may not be noticed. Figure 9-12 is an example of oral herpes. The fluid-filled vesicles break open and heal in 1 to 3 weeks during the primary infection; the interval is shorter in reactivated disease. Figure 9-13 is an example of genital herpes.

The virus can also cause conjunctivitis or a corneal ulcer, encephalitis, meningitis, or herpetic whitlow, an infection of the fingers that sometimes occurs in nurses, dentists, and others working with infected people.

Treatment   An analgesic-antipyretic (pain and fever reducer) may be prescribed for a primary infection. If the mouth is affected, a mouthwash with a numbing agent may be used. Calamine or another drying lotion may be used to make the lesions on the lips and face less painful. Acyclovir, which comes in tablets or ointment form, has been found to reduce viral shedding, diminish pain, and speed up the healing for primary infections. It is also used prophylactically. As stated before, *there is no cure* for herpes infections at this time. Once a person is infected with the virus, it is with them for life.

Prevention/Control   Although personal hygiene is always a good practice to follow, the high rate of infection among adults makes it unlikely that oral herpes infection can be avoided. The use of condoms in sexual practices may reduce the risk of acquiring herpes in the genital or anal area. Close contact with anyone having apparent infection should be avoided. Individuals with herpetic lesions should be isolated from newborns, children, and immunosuppressed individuals. For pregnant women, a cesarean section is recommended before the membranes rupture, since a herpes infection can be fatal for the newborn child.

WARTS

Warts are caused by the human papilloma virus (HPV). There are a number of different kinds, including common warts, which usually appear on sites subject to injury, such as the hands, face, knees, or scalp, particularly in young children (Figure 9-14). They are firm, sharply defined, round or irregular, flesh-colored to brown growths. They may grow up to about one-quarter inch in diameter and often have a rough surface. Flat warts occur mainly on the wrists, the backs of hands, and the face. They are flesh colored and flat topped and may itch. Filiform warts appear more often in overweight, middle-aged people. They are long and slender and occur

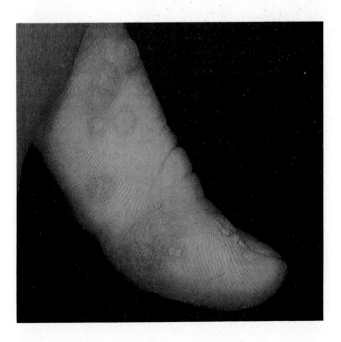

FIGURE 9-14 Common warts.

on the eyelids, armpits, or neck. Plantar warts appear as a hard, horny, rough-surfaced area on the sole of the foot. They may occur singly or in a cluster. Genital warts are pink and cauliflowerlike (Figure 9-15).

The incubation period for warts is usually 2 to 3 months but may be as short as 1 or as long as 20 months. Warts wherever they occur are communicable, probably as long as the lesions are present. Young children generally have more common or flat warts, but genital warts are more prevalent in sexually active young adults. Plantar warts occur more often in school-age children and adolescents. Individuals whose immune system is depressed, such as those with human immunodeficiency virus (HIV), are more susceptible to warts.

Transmission   Warts are usually transmitted by direct contact. Autoinoculation is also possible. Plantar warts may be acquired by walking barefoot on contaminated floors. Genital warts are usually transmitted by sexual contact.

Symptoms   Warts by themselves cause no pain or discomfort. If they become infected or if they are in a location such as plantar warts, where weight is placed upon them, or under a nail, they can be uncomfortable and painful.

FIGURE 9-15 Genital warts.

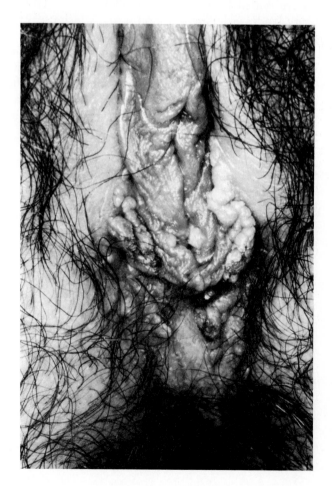

Treatment When the body builds up enough resistance, warts will disappear spontaneously. However, this can take months or years. If they are in a location that causes problems, such as plantar warts, there are procedures to help get rid of them. These may or may not be effective, and many times the warts return.

Prevention/Control In order to reduce the risk of getting warts, bath sandals should be worn on shower room floors or pool decks. Individuals should avoid direct contact with lesions on self or others. The chance of acquiring genital warts may be reduced by using condoms.

ACQUIRED IMMUNE DEFICIENCY SYNDROME (AIDS, HIV INFECTION)
RISE IN OPPORTUNISTIC DISEASE

It wasn't a new group of symptoms that warned the Centers for Disease Control (CDC) in 1981 that a strange, death-dealing virus was invading human bodies; it was an increase in reported cases of two rare diseases. *Pneumocystis carinii,* a type of pneumonia that had previously affected only those with suppressed immune systems, was infecting healthy homosexual men in Los Angeles; later on, cases of Kaposi's sarcoma, a rare skin tumor that previously affected only elderly men in the United States, was reported among young homosexual men. Soon it was evident that there was an increasing epidemic of opportunistic diseases, those that affect people with inefficient immune defenses. Opportunistic infections were also increasing in intravenous drug users and hemophiliacs, suggesting that the cause of the epidemic had something to do with transmission of blood as well as homosexual activity.

IDENTIFYING THE VIRUS

In 1984, scientists in France and America identified the virus responsible for the new epidemic. The French named it lymphadenopathy-associated virus (LAV), while the Americans named it human T-cell lymphotropic virus, strain III (HTLV III). In 1986, it was renamed human immunodeficiency virus (HIV).

The virus infects a cell known as a T-helper cell that is crucial in the immune system's defense of the body (see Chapter 2). Figure 9-16 is a highly magnified

CONTEMPORARY CONCERNS

The first 100,000 cases of AIDS took 8 years to accumulate while the second 100,000 were reported during a 2-year period (September 1989 through November 1991). Unless a vaccine is found or the pleading from victims and the warnings from health personnel are heeded by couples everywhere, this geometric progression will continue.

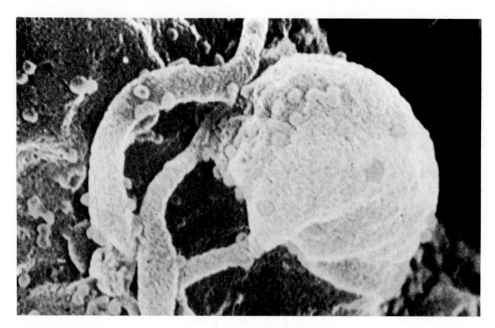

FIGURE 9-16 Human immunodeficiency virus released from infected T-helper cells (spherical particles) spread over adjacent T-helper cells, infecting them in turn. The individual AIDS particles are very tiny; over 200 million would fit on the period at the end of this sentence.

picture of AIDS virus infecting T-helper cells. Figure 9-17 is a comparison of the reaction of the immune system to an invading organism under normal conditions and when AIDS is present.

EPIDEMIOLOGY

As of May 31, 1991, more than 179,000 cases of AIDS had been reported to the CDC. Over 100,000 of these persons have died. AIDS has infected people of every race, age, sex, and sexual persuasion (Tables 9-3 and 9-4). In less than 10 years, it has become the second leading cause of death in males 25 to 44 years of age in the United States and has risen to number 5 on the list of leading causes of death among women in this group (Figure 9-18, *A* and *B*). Figure 9-19 shows the cases reported among various groups by year of diagnosis. AIDS cases have also been reported in every state (Figure 9-20).

AIDS has now been reported in countries all over the world, but the United States has reported the most cases. The incubation period is variable. It takes 1 to 3 months for antibodies to build up in the blood, and 2 to 10 years or longer from the time of HIV infection to a diagnosis of AIDS. The period of communicability is uncertain, but is thought to start soon after infection with HIV and to last throughout life.

Transmission In order for a person to acquire AIDS, semen, vaginal secretions, or blood of an individual infected with HIV must be introduced into their bloodstream. This has occurred through sexual intercourse, sharing HIV-contaminated needles and syringes, and through transfusions of infected blood or its components. The AIDS virus has been detected in saliva, tears, urine, and bronchial secretions, but no cases have been reported because of contact with these secretions. There has also been no evidence that AIDS has ever been transmitted by a mosquito or other biting

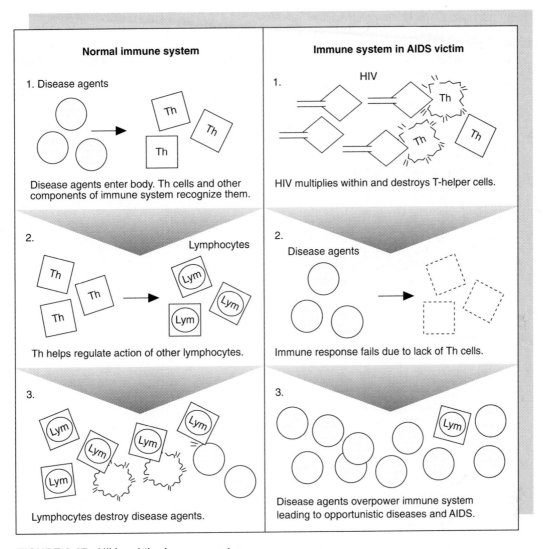

FIGURE 9-17   HIV and the immune system.

insect. One of the greatest tragedies of the AIDS epidemic is the number of infants who are infected by HIV–infected mothers before, during, or shortly after birth (see Figure 9-19, C).

Symptoms   A person may be infected with HIV and be asymptomatic (have no symptoms). This is now referred to as "HIV + without symptoms", and the individual is infectious. Within 3 months of the invasion of the virus, most people have non-specific signs and symptoms including fatigue, fever, night sweats, weight loss, diarrhea, lymphadenopathy, or cough. If a person with these symptoms tests positive for HIV, they are considered to have ARC, or AIDS-related complex. If the individual then develops one of the opportunistic diseases listed for AIDS such as Kaposi's sarcoma (Figure 9-21), then they are diagnosed as having AIDS. Both

TABLE 9-3 Characteristics of persons who have died from AIDS—United States, 1981–1990

Characteristic	No.	(%)
Total	*100,777*	*(100.0)*
HIV exposure group		
Homosexual/bisexual men	59,586	(59.1)
Intravenous-drug users		
Women and heterosexual men	21,126	(21.0)
Homosexual/bisexual men	6,894	(6.8)
Persons with hemophilia		
Adult/adolescent	945	(0.9)
Child	74	(0.1)
Transfusion recipient		
Adult/adolescent	2,793	(2.8)
Child	150	(0.1)
Heterosexual contact	3,587	(3.6)
Persons born in countries where HIV infection occurs primarily through heterosexual contact	1,160	(1.2)
Perinatal	1,186	(1.2)
No identified risk	3,276	(3.3)
Race/ethnicity		
White, non-Hispanic	55,494	(55.1)
Black, non-Hispanic	28,575	(28.4)
Hispanic	15,805	(15.7)
Asian/Pacific Islander	608	(0.6)
American Indian/Alaskan Native	138	(0.1)
Unspecified	157	(0.2)
Age at death (yrs)		
<5	1,141	(1.1)
5-14	308	(0.3)
15-24	3,266	(3.2)
25-34	36,418	(36.1)
35-44	37,634	(37.3)
45-54	14,256	(14.1)
≥55	7,405	(7.3)
Unspecified	349	(0.3)
Sex		
Male	90,715	(90.0)
Female	10,056	(10.0)
Unspecified	6	(<0.1)

Source: National AIDS surveillance.

ARC and AIDS are now referred to as "HIV + with symptoms." Some victims are asymptomatic until signs of Kaposi's sarcoma (Figure 9-21) or another opportunistic infection suddenly appear. At the present time, it is not known how many people infected with HIV will develop ARC, nor how many with ARC will develop AIDS. With new methods of treatment, development of ARC or AIDS has been delayed 5 to 10 years. *Text continued on p. 238.*

TABLE 9-4 Characteristics of reported persons with AIDS and percent change in cases, by year of report and year of diagnosis—United States, 1989 and 1990

Category	1990 Reported Cases			1989 Reported Cases	% change 1989–1990	
	No.	(%)	Rate*		Reported	Diagnosed†
Sex						
Male	38,082	(87.9)	30.9	31,282	21.7	5.9
Female	5,257	(12.1)	4.1	3,948	33.2	17.4
Age (yrs)						
0-4	622	(1.4)	3.3	533	16.7	2.3
5-9	120	(0.3)	0.6	89	34.8	33.0
10-19	208	(0.5)	0.6	149	39.6	17.0
20-29	8,338	(19.2)	19.7	6,992	19.3	5.9
30-39	19,722	(45.5)	46.8	16,260	21.3	4.7
40-49	10,026	(23.1)	33.5	7,640	31.2	13.6
50-59	3,013	(7.0)	13.4	2,518	19.7	4.1
≥60	1,290	(3.0)	3.1	1,049	23.0	13.5
Race/ethnicity‡						
White	22,342	(51.6)	11.8	18,661	19.7	2.5
Black	13,186	(30.4)	42.5	10,336	27.6	12.0
Hispanic	7,322	(16.9)	31.9	5,829	25.6	13.3
Asian/Pacific Islander	260	(0.6)	3.8	239	8.8	−8.8
American Indian/Alaskan native	71	(0.2)	4.0	63	12.7	23.1
Region						
Northeast	13,572	(31.3)	26.7	10,710	26.7	−2.2
Midwest	4,068	(9.4)	6.8	3,491	16.5	12.7
South	14,331	(33.1)	16.8	11,010	30.2	14.9
West	9,624	(22.2)	18.2	8,511	13.1	3.3
U.S. territories	1,744	(4.0)	46.2	1,508	15.6	31.0
HIV exposure category						
Male homosexual/bisexual contact	23,738	(54.8)	—	19,891	19.3	5.2
History of intravenous drug use						
Women and heterosexual men	10,018	(23.1)	—	8,089	23.8	7.9
Male homosexual/bisexual contact	2,295	(5.3)	—	2,214	3.7	−2.7
Persons with hemophilia						
Adult/adolescent	340	(0.8)	—	289	17.6	−2.9
Child	31	(0.1)	—	25	24.0	16.7
Transfusion recipients						
Adult/adolescent	866	(2.0)	—	777	11.5	−1.0
Child	39	(0.1)	—	40	−2.5	−2.6
Heterosexual contacts	2,289	(5.3)	—	1,631	40.3	40.9
Born pattern II country§	422	(1.0)	—	379	11.3	−10.1
Perinatal	681	(1.6)	—	565	20.5	7.8
No identified risk	2,620	(6.0)	—	1,330	—	—
Total	*43,339*	*(100.0)*	*17.2*	*35,230*	*23.0*	*7.2*

*Per 100,000 population.

†Diagnosed cases adjusted for estimated delays in reporting.

‡Excludes persons with unspecified race/ethnicity.

§Persons born in countries where heterosexual transmission predominates.

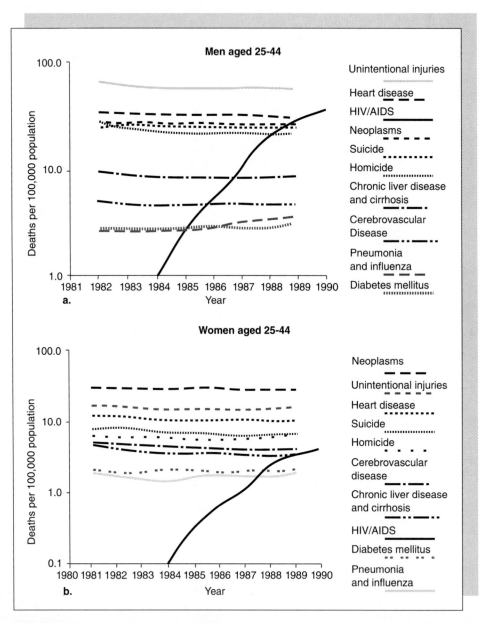

FIGURE 9-18   A, Leading causes of death among men 25-44 years of age—United States, 1981 to 1989. **B,** Leading cause of death among women 25-44 years of age—United States, 1980 to 1989.

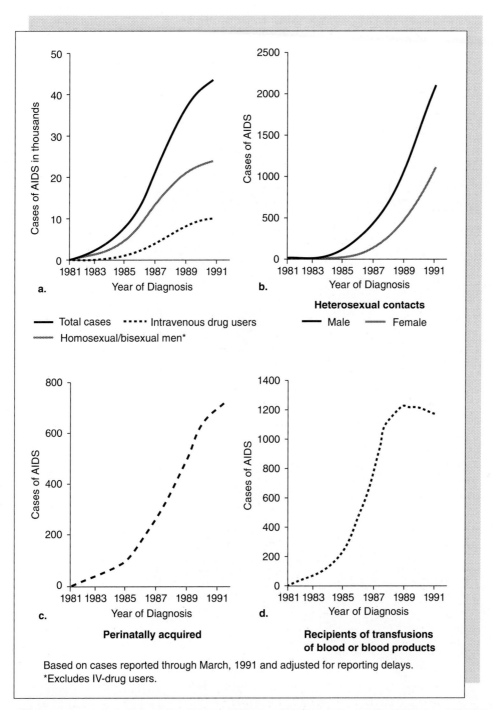

FIGURE 9-19   AIDS cases, by year of diagnosis—United States, 1981 to 1991. **A,** Total cases, cases among homosexual/bisexual men, and cases among women and heterosexual men reporting intravenous drug use. **B,** Cases among persons reporting heterosexual contact with persons with, or at high risk for, HIV infection. **C,** Perinatally acquired pediatric AIDS cases. **D,** Cases among recipients of transfusions of blood or blood products.

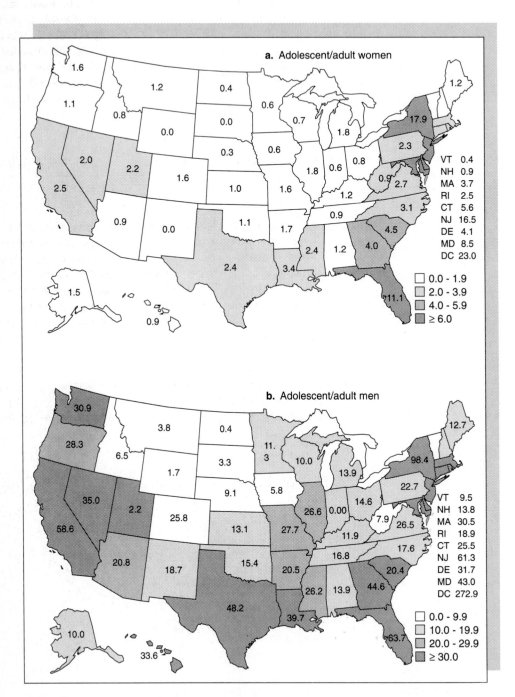

FIGURE 9-20 Rate of reported AIDS cases, per 100,000 population, among adolescents and adults, by sex and state of residence—United States, 1990.

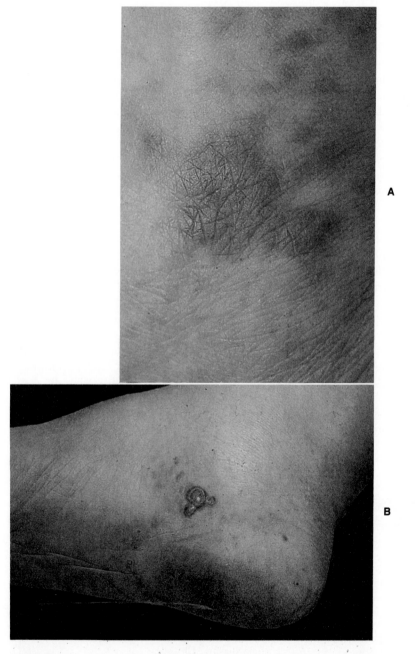

FIGURE 9-21   Symptoms of Kaposi's sarcoma. **A,** Early lesion consisting of purplish macules and plaques. **B,** Purple nodules are most commonly seen on the lower legs.

Treatment   A cure for AIDS has not been found. So far, zidovudine (formerly called azido-thymidine [AZT]) and other drugs have only slowed down the course of the disease. Treatment for the opportunistic infections is given when available. Researchers are working all the time to develop better treatment.

Prevention   The only sure means of prevention is sexual relations with uninfected individuals only, use of only sterilized needles for injections, and use of sterile gloves and equipment by all health care personnel. These seem like viable rules to follow, but unfortunately there are too many factors involved. Persons who use illicit drugs often do not care how they get their shots. People who drink too much may not care who their sex partners are. Even health care personnel are sometimes careless or, particularly in emergency situations, too rushed to take proper precautions. And many individuals will not take the time to find out the sexual history of their sex partners. The use of condoms will decrease the risk of infection and is probably the best means of prevention at present.

Control   Since prevention of AIDS transmission is not a realistic expectation at present, the best hope for stopping the epidemic is a vaccine. At first it was thought that no vaccine was possible, but now researchers are more hopeful. However, a vaccine is probably many years away. In the meantime, people need to realize that the only way this disease can be controlled is for everyone who is sexually active to have the facts. Sexual relations with someone who is not known well enough to rule out any possibility of having the virus (including a negative blood test if necessary) is an open invitation to infection with HIV. Communication between partners and with public health personnel to help with contact investigation, and developing monogamous long-term relationships will also help control this devastating disease.

SUMMARY

The table summarizes relevant data on viral diseases acquired through the alimentary and other routes.

SUMMARY TABLE	Viral diseases acquired through the alimentary and other routes			
Diseases	**Special Characteristics**	**Transmission**	**Common Symptoms**	**Prevention/ Control**
Poliomyelitis	Once a dreaded disease, now rare because of vaccine.	Direct contact with respiratory secretions or oral-fecal route in areas of poor sanitation.	Asymptomatic, 90%; typical prodromal symptoms, 5%; prodromal plus back pain and muscle spasms, 1%-2%; paralysis, 0.1% to 2%.	Immunization in early childhood. Contact investigation for possible treatment.

Treatment: At present, immunization is the main defense against viral diseases. A few drugs and antibiotics have been developed that relieve symptoms or extend lives, but there are no cures.

SUMMARY TABLE	Viral diseases acquired through the alimentary and other routes—cont'd			
Diseases	**Special Characteristics**	**Transmission**	**Common Symptoms**	**Prevention/ Control**
Hepatitis A	Rare in United States; reported cases began to rise. Also called infectious hepatitis.	Oral-fecal.	Sudden onset of fever, malaise, anorexia, nausea, abdominal discomfort; jaundice.	Good sanitation and personal hygiene. IgM prophylactic for at-risk individuals.
Hepatitis B	Also called serum hepatitis. Higher mortality rate than A.	Blood-to-blood or blood-to-mucus contact.	Insidious onset of anorexia, abdominal discomfort, nausea, and vomiting.	Vaccination for those at high risk. Proper disposal and sterilization of all needles and syringes.
Rabies	Animal disease communicated to humans by a bite. Almost always fatal without treatment.	Introduction of saliva of infected animal into bloodstream. No case of person-to-person transmission.	Local or radiating pain or burning, sensation of cold, itching, and tingling at bite site. Typical prodromal symptoms plus persistent loose cough. Nervousness, anxiety, irritability, hyperesthesia, pupillary dilation, tachycardia, shallow respiration, excessive saliva, tears, perspiration; 2 to 10 days later, other CNS disorders, intense thirst, and hydrophobia.	Registration, licensing, and vaccination of all dogs and cats. Wild and stray animal control. Vaccinations for high-risk individuals.
Encephalitis	Inflammation of the brain. Sequela of other viral illness. Occurs more in summer and early fall.	By bite of an infected mosquito.	Sudden onset of fever, headache, and vomiting. Progresses to stiff neck, and back, drowsiness, coma, paralysis, convulsions, muscular incoordination, and psychoses.	Mosquito control and elimination of breeding places. Avoidance of mosquitoes during times when they are known to bite. Use of repellants.
Herpes simplex 1	Generally infects the lips and face. Once the virus enters the body it is there for life. Reactivated in 60% of those infected. Occurs mostly in children.	By contact with saliva of infected individuals.	May be asymptomatic or may have typical prodromal symptoms. Vesicular lesions.	Avoid close contact with infected individuals. Isolate persons with lesions from newborns, children, and immunosuppressed individuals.

Continued.

SUMMARY TABLE Viral diseases acquired through the alimentary and other routes—cont'd				
Disease	**Special Characteristics**	**Transmission**	**Common Symptoms**	**Prevention/ Control**
Herpes simplex 2	Usually located in the genital area or on the cervix in women. Occurs mostly in adults.	By sexual contact.	Lesions in first attack typically painful and vesicular. Possible fever, swollen glands, painful urination.	Cesarean section to protect newborn. Condoms in sexual practices reduce risk.
Warts	Various kinds: common, flat, filiform, plantar, genital. Usually disappear without treatment in time.	Direct contact or autoinoculation.	None unless infected or in weight-bearing area.	Avoid direct contact with lesions. Use condoms to reduce risk of genital warts.
Acquired immune deficiency syndrome (AIDS)	First reported in 1981 among homosexual males in United States. Now found in all kinds of people, male and female, young and old, heterosexual and homosexual. First leading cause of death among 25- to 44-year-old males. No recovered cases have been documented. Over 179,000 cases reported; over 100,000 of these have died.	Introduction of blood, semen, or vaginal secretions of infected person into bloodstream. Usually by sexual intercourse, anal sex, unclean needles, or mother-to-fetus transmission.	Typical prodromal symptoms. Opportunistic diseases.	Sexual relations with uninfected individuals only, use of sterilized needles only, use of sterile gloves and equipment by health care personnel at all times. Use of condoms to decrease risk of infection. Education of the public.

QUESTIONS FOR REVIEW

1. What was the "iron lung?"
2. Among what people do outbreaks of polio still occur?
3. What are the four possible outcomes of poliomyelitis?
4. What five viruses are known to cause hepatitis?
5. Compare the means and results of infection with viral hepatitis A and viral hepatitis B.
6. Why is infection with hepatitis A a particular concern in day-care centers?
7. What determines the time from the bite of a rabid animal to symptoms in the victim?
8. Why is it necessary to determine whether an animal that has bitten someone without provocation is rabid?
9. What are the initial symptoms of rabies?

10. What is the treatment for a bite from an animal with rabies?
11. What is the cause of viral encephalitis?
12. What symptoms are specific for encephalitis?
13. What is the difference between infections caused by herpes simplex virus I and those caused by herpes simplex virus II?
14. For how long after the sores have healed can the herpes virus I still be found in saliva?
15. Who is susceptible to herpetic whitlow?
16. How does acyclovir help a herpes infection?
17. What five kinds of wart were discussed in the text?
18. How are warts transmitted?
19. When might warts cause symptoms?
20. What opportunistic infections are most often connected with AIDS?
21. What is the difference between LAV, HTLV III, and HIV?
22. How does AIDS cause damage to the immune system?
23. How is AIDS transmitted?
24. What are the symptoms of AIDS?
25. How may AIDS be prevented/controlled?

FURTHER READING

Alter, Miriam J., et al. "The Changing Epidemiology of Hepatitis B in the United States: Need for Alternative Vaccination Strategies." *Journal of the American Medical Association,* Mar. 2, '90, 263:1218–1222.

Bayer, Ronald. "Public Health Policy and the AIDS Epidemic." *New England Journal of Medicine,* May 23, '91, 324:1500–1504.

Beale, A.J. "Polio Vaccines: Time for a Change in Immunization Policy?" *Lancet,* Apr. 7, '90, 335:839–842.

Boyd, Robert F. *General Microbiology.* St. Louis: Mosby, 1988.

Brennan, Troyen A. "Transmission of the Human Immunodeficiency Virus in the Health Care Setting—Time for Action." *New England Journal of Medicine,* May 23, '91, 324:1504–1509.

Brown, Phyllida. "Amphetamines and the HIV Connection." *New Scientist,* May 11, '91, 130:13.

Brown, Phyllida. "Could Herpes Speed Up AIDS?" *New Scientist,* Feb. 9, '91, 129:28.

Bryson, Y., et al. "Risk of Acquisition of Genital Herpes Simplex Virus, Type 2 in Sex Partners of Persons with Genital Herpes: A Prospective Couple Study." *Journal of Infectious Disease,* Apr. '93, 167 (4):942–946.

Collison, Michele N-K. "Dramatic Increase in Genital-Warts Disease among Students Worries College Health Officials." *Chronicle of Higher Education,* May 31, '89, 35:A23.

Control of Communicable Disease in Man. Abram S. Benenson, ed. Fifteenth Edition, Washington, D.C.: American Public Health Association, 1990.

Cowen, Ron. "Herpes May Disarm Immune System." *Science News,* May 26, '90, 137:326.

Cuzzell, Janice Z. "Clues: Pain, Burning, and Itching." *American Journal of Nursing,* July '90, 90:15–16.

Daniels, Norman. "Duty to Treat or Right to Refuse?" *Hastings Center Report,* Mar. '91, 21:36–46.

Drastura, Jenny. "Rabies: From Superstition to Science." *Dog World,* Jan. '91, 76:19.

Flieger, Ken. "Mad Dogs and Friendly Skunks: Controlling Rabies." *FDA Consumer,* June '90, 24:22–27.

Gellin, Bruce G., David E. Rogers. "Ask the Right Question about HIV." *Medical World News,* Apr. '91, 32:53.

Goldsmith, Marsha F. "AIDS Vaccines Inch Closer to Useful Existence." *Journal of the American Medical Association,* Mar. 20, '91, 265:1356–1357.

Gutman, L. T., M. E. Herman-Giddens and W. C. Phelps. "Transmission of Human Genital Papillomavirus Disease: Comparison of Data from Adults and Children." *Pediatrics.* Jan. '93, 91(1):31–38.

Hein, Karen. "Fighting AIDS in Adolescents." *Issues in Science and Technology,* Spring '91, 7:67–72.

Henderson, Donald A. "How Smallpox Showed the Way." *World Health,* Dec. '89, pp. 19–21.

Ho, Mei-Shang, et al. "Viral Gastroenteritis Aboard a Cruise Ship." *Lancet,* Oct. 21, '89, 8669:961–964.

Holland, Lisa. "The ABCs of Hepatitis." *Good Housekeeping,* Apr. '91, 212:239.

Kaplowitz, Lisa G., David Baker, et al. "Prolonged Continuous Acyclovir Treatment of Normal Adults with Frequently Recurring Genital Herpes Simplex Virus Infection." *Journal of the American Medical Association,* Feb. 13, '91, 265:747–751.

Levi, Sassoon, et al. "*Campylobacter pylori* and Duodenal Ulcers: The Gastrin Link." *Lancet,* May 27, '89, 8648:1167–1168.

Marcus, R., et al. "Risk of Human Immunodeficiency Virus Infection Among Emergency Department Workers." *American Journal of Medicine,* Apr. '93, 94 (4):363–370.

McCance, Kathryn L. and Sue E. Huether. *Pathophysiology: The Biologic Basis for Disease in Adults and Children.* St. Louis: Mosby, 1990.

McKillip, Jack. "The Effect of Mandatory Premarital HIV Testing on Marriage: The Case of Illinois." *American Journal of Public Health,* May '91, 81:650–653.

Munsat, Theodore L. "Poliomyelitis—New Problems with an Old Disease." *New England Journal of Medicine,* Apr. 25, '91, 324:1206–1207.

Murray, et al. *Medical Microbiology.* St. Louis: Mosby, 1990.

Myers, T. "Factors Affecting Gay and Bisexual Men's Decisions and Intentions to Seek HIV Testing." *American Journal of Public Health.* May, '93, 83 (5):701–704.

Nicholson, Karl G. "Rabies." *Lancet,* May 19, '90, 335:1201–1205.

Nuovo, Gerard J., Bader M. Pedemonte. "Human Papillomavirus Types and Recurrent Cervical Warts." *Journal of the American Medical Association,* Mar. 2, '90, 263:1223–1226.

Orr, D. P. "Factors Associated with Condom Use by Sexually Active Male Adolescents at Risk for Sexually Transmitted Disease." *Pediatrics,* May, '93, 91 (5):873–879.

Palca, Joseph. "The True Source of HIV?" *Science,* May 10, '91, 252:771.

Power, C., et al. "Cytomegalovirus and Rasmussen's Encephalitis." *Lancet,* Nov. 24, '90, 336:1282–1284.

Randall, Teri. "Rest of World Ready to Follow This Hemisphere's Approach to Eliminating Polio in Near Future." *Journal of the American Medical Association,* Feb. 20, '91, 265:839–840.

Raub, William. "From the National Institutes of Health." *Journal of the American Medical Association,* Mar. 6, '91, 265:1075.

Rooney, J. F., et al. "Oral Acyclovir to Suppress Frequently Recurrent Herpes Labialis. A Double-Blind, Placebo-Controlled Trial." *Annals of Internal Medicine,* Feb. 15, '93, 118 (4):268–272.

Spence, Annette. "Herpes Update." *Self,* Sept. '90, 12:262–264.

Tiollais, Pierre, Maria-Annick Buendia. "Hepatitis B Virus." *Scientific American,* Apr. '91, 264:116–123.

"Treatment of Herpes Simplex Labialis." *Lancet,* June 23, '90, 335:1501–1502.

Voeller, Bruce. "AIDS and Heterosexual Anal Intercourse." *Archives of Sexual Behavior,* June '91, 20:233–276.

Whitley, Richard J. "Viral Encephalitis." *New England Journal of Medicine,* July 26, '90, 323:242–250.

Whitley, Richard, Ann Arvin, et al. "Predictors of Morbidity and Mortality in Neonates with Herpes Simplex Virus Infections." *New England Journal of Medicine,* Feb. 14, '91, 324: 450–454.

Zoler, Mitchel L. "Advances on All Hepatitis Fronts." *Medical World News,* Nov. '90, 31:20.

Chapter 10

Diseases Caused by Fungi

O B J E C T I V E S

1 Compare coccidioidomycosis and histoplasmosis.

2 Identify factors that predispose an individual to candidiasis.

3 State the location for the various forms of tinea.

4 State symptoms, treatment, prevention, and control for the diseases in this chapter.

COCCIDIOIDOMYCOSIS (VALLEY FEVER)

This fungal disease is found mainly in the southwestern United States and Central and South America (Figure 10-1). It is found in two forms, primary coccidioidomycosis, which is an acute respiratory disease, and progressive coccidioidomycosis, a progressive, chronic, frequently fatal disease. The progressive form occurs more frequently in dark-skinned men, pregnant women, and individuals whose immune

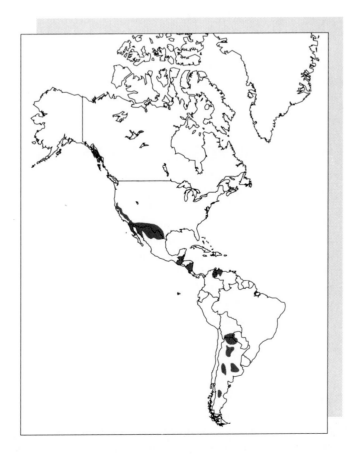

FIGURE 10-1 Geographic distribution of coccidioidomycosis in North, Central, and South America.

245

systems are suppressed. The fungus, *Coccidioides immitis,* is reservoired in the soil. In the United States it is found from California to southern Texas. Incubation is 1 to 4 weeks for primary infection and variable for progressive coccidioidomycosis. The disease is not communicable. Susceptibility is general, but one attack confers lifelong immunity.

Transmission

Transmission is generally by inhalation of the spores found in the soil in endemic areas.

Symptoms

The primary illness may be asymptomatic or resemble a flulike illness with cough, fever, sore throat, chills, malaise, headache, and in some cases an itchy rash. About 5% of infected individuals develop tender red nodules on their legs, especially the shins, with joint pain in the knees and ankles. The primary disease generally heals spontaneously within a few weeks. In rare cases (1 in 1000) the disease disseminates throughout the body, causing fever and abscesses. Disseminated coccidioidomycosis is frequently fatal (up to 60% of cases).

Treatment

The primary form usually requires only bed rest and relief of symptoms. Various antifungal agents are effective in treating more severe primary cases and the disseminated form.

Prevention/Control

Dust control measures should be used in endemic areas. Individuals from nonendemic areas need to be careful about selecting occupations where they will be exposed to dust. Skin testing can be done to determine exposure. Individuals who have to work in risky locations should wear dust masks.

HISTOPLASMOSIS (SPELUNKER'S DISEASE)

Raising chickens would not seem to be a very dangerous occupation, but in certain parts of the United States, chickens can provide the source of an infection that in its most severe form can be fatal. The organism that causes this fungal infection, *Histoplasma capsulatum,* is found in the feces of bats and birds, particularly chickens and starlings. It grows in soil with a high nitrogen content and has been endemic in the Midwest for many years but is now spreading to other parts of the country (Figure 10-2). Areas of infection are also found in South and Central America, Africa, Europe, eastern Asia, and Australia. When the soil of chicken houses or bat caves is stirred up by raking, windy conditions, or some other means, the spores rise into the air and may be inhaled by anyone in the area. The incubation period is 5 to 18 days. Susceptibility is general, and inapparent infections are common, leading to increased resistance.

Transmission

There is no person-to-person transmission. Inhalation of spores from the soil that have become airborne is the main means of transmission. A person can also become infected if the spores are rubbed into an open sore, but this type of transmission is rare. Figure 10-3 shows the common sources of infection with histoplasmosis.

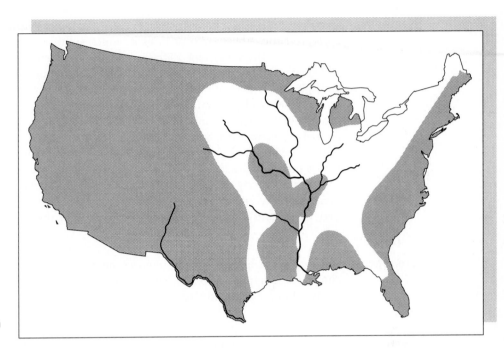

FIGURE 10-2   Endemic areas (white) of histoplasmosis in North America.

FIGURE 10-3   Possible sources of histoplasmosis.

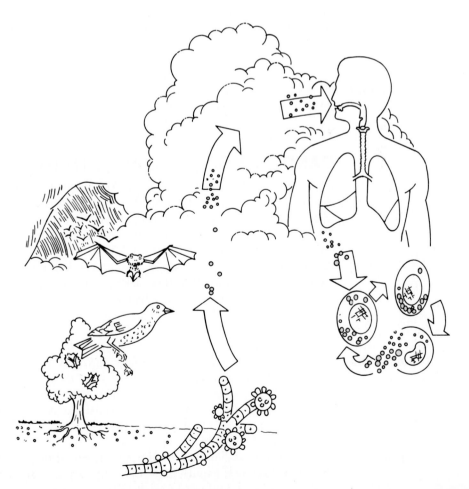

Symptoms   The primary lesion for histoplasmosis is in the lungs. Most often, the individual is asymptomatic. There are four cases in which symptoms appear: (1) primary acute, with flulike symptoms such as fever, malaise, headache, myalgia, anorexia, cough, and chest pain; there may also be small scattered nodules in the lung, lymph nodes, and spleen; (2) acute disseminated, with enlarged liver and spleen, swollen lymph nodes, fever, and prostration; can be fatal without treatment; (3) chronic disseminated, with variable symptoms, which may include fever, anemia, hepatitis, endocarditis, meningitis, ulcers of mouth, larynx, stomach, or bowel, and infection of the adrenal glands; this too is usually fatal unless treated; (4) chronic pulmonary, which mimics tuberculosis and causes a productive cough, difficult breathing, and sometimes bloody sputum. Eventually there is weight loss, extreme weakness, breathlessness, and cyanosis (dark bluish or purplish skin). Periods of remission may occur, and often there is spontaneous cure of this type.

Treatment   Primary acute histoplasmosis requires no treatment. For the other three kinds, antifungal therapy is effective, either amphotericin B or ketoconazole. This is generally a long-term treatment of about 10 weeks.

Prevention   Protective masks should be used when working in areas that may be contaminated, such as chicken coops and their surrounding soil, bat-infested caves, and starling nesting places. Dusty, contaminated areas should be sprayed with water or oil to reduce dust.

Control   In case of an outbreak, there should be investigation of contacts to determine whether there is an environmental source of infection that can be eliminated.

CANDIDIASIS (MONILIASIS, THRUSH)

Candidiasis is an opportunistic yeastlike fungal infection of the skin or mucous membranes. It is generally caused by *Candida albicans*. It often occurs in babies (diaper rash), in the mouth (thrush), or in the vulvovaginal area (moniliasis). The infection occurs worldwide, and the fungus is a natural inhabitant of the human body. The incubation period for candidiasis is variable. Thrush, in infants, has an incubation period of 2 to 5 days. Candidiasis is communicable as long as the lesions are present. A number of factors make people susceptible to the fungus, including diabetes mellitus, use of broad-spectrum antibiotics, cancer chemotherapy, and AIDS.

Transmission   Candidiasis can be transmitted by secretions or excretions of infected individuals or carriers. A baby can get thrush while passing through the birth canal of a mother with the infection; candidiasis can be transmitted through sexual intercourse, and endogenous infections occur whenever resistance is lowered.

Symptoms   Symptoms for candidiasis depend upon the site of the infection. When on the skin, there is a scaly, red, papular rash, often appearing in creases of skin, such as under

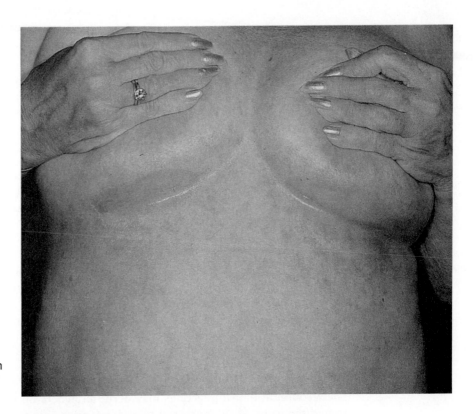

FIGURE 10-4 Rash in breast area caused by candidiasis.

FIGURE 10-5 Rash in vaginal area caused by candidiasis.

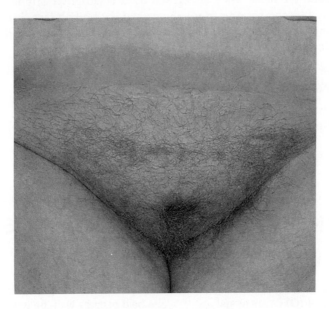

the breasts (Figure 10-4) or in the vaginal area (Figure 10-5). In diaper rash, there are papules at the edges of the rash.

Candidiasis in the mouth is called thrush and causes cream-colored or bluish white patches on the tongue, mouth, or pharynx. They may cause only a burning sensation in the mouths and throats of adults, but in infants they can swell and cause difficulty in breathing.

When candidiasis occurs in the vagina, there is a white or yellow "cheesy" discharge that is extremely itchy. There are white or gray raised patches on the vaginal wall, and intercourse may be painful. Different symptoms occur when the infection is in the kidneys, lungs, brain, endocardium, esophagus, nails, or eye, all of which are susceptible to infection by the fungus. The infection may also be systemic and cause chills, high fever, low blood pressure, prostration, and sometimes a rash.

Treatment

The first aim of treatment is to control the underlying condition that allowed this opportunistic infection to occur. There are many antifungal drugs that are effective in treating candidiasis, and some, particularly effective for vaginal infection, are now sold over the counter.

Prevention-Control

Treatment of vaginal candidiasis in pregnant women can prevent thrush in the newborn. Partner treatment is necessary, since the infection can be transmitted through sexual intercourse. The effectiveness of the immune system can be improved by maintaining a healthful lifestyle.

DERMATOPHYTOSES (TINEA)

These common fungal infections may occur anywhere on the skin and under and around the nails. They are caused by dermatophytes (fungi). The word *tinea,* followed by the Latin term for the part of the body infected, is often used. The most common infections are tinea capitis (head), tinea corporis (body), tinea cruris (inguinal), tinea pedis (foot), and tinea unguium (nail).

TINEA CAPITIS

This occurs mainly in children and is commonly referred to as ringworm of the scalp. It is more common in large cities and overcrowded conditions. The reservoir

CONTEMPORARY CONCERNS

Fungal infections can be easily recognized and often treated by over-the-counter (OTC) antifungal cream, lotions, or powder depending on the location. But if you still have the infection after 4 weeks, you should check with your doctor about using an oral antibiotic, griseofulvin, which should clear up the problem. Don't forget to check your pets for telltale bald patches with the typical red ringworm appearance as they can be a source of the infection.

Tinea capitis and tinea unguium are most likely to need the prescription drug before they disappear.

for most of the organisms is people, although some have animal hosts. Incubation is 10 to 14 days, and the fungus is communicable through contaminated materials as long as the lesions are present.

Transmission

The infection is transmitted by direct or indirect contact. The backs of theater seats, barber clippers, toilet articles, combs, hairbrushes, or clothing and hats that have been contaminated with hair from an infected person are common fomites. Animals also can transmit the infection and sometimes are carriers.

Symptoms

Tinea capitis begins as a small papule and spreads across the head or bearded areas. Figure 10-6 shows a patch of scaly baldness left on the back of a boy's head by the fungal infection. The hairs that are in the area of infection become brittle and break off easily. One variety of tinea capitis is characterized by a mousy odor. In this kind, there are small, yellowish, cuplike crusts that appear stuck on the scalp. The hair does not break off but becomes gray and lusterless and eventually falls out. The baldness caused by this infection may be permanent.

Treatment

The treatment of choice is an antifungal drug, griseofulvin, which is taken by mouth for at least 4 weeks. There are also over-the-counter remedies that may be effective if the infection is mild. If there is a secondary bacterial infection, antibiotics may be used.

Prevention

Parents and children should be educated to the danger of acquiring the infection from infected children and animals. If there is an epidemic, for most species involved, ultraviolet light (Wood's lamp) can detect lesions on the head; this can be used before children enter school. Children with unkempt hair should be examined for lesions.

FIGURE 10-6 Tinea capitis.

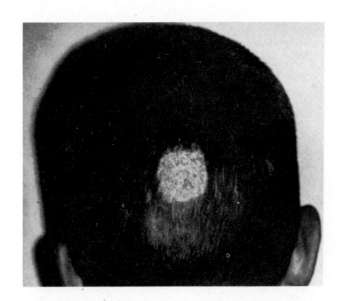

Control   If the cases are mild, daily washing of the hair will remove loose hairs. In severe cases, hair should be washed daily and covered with a cap. Household contacts, pets, and farm animals should be examined and treated if infected.

TINEA CORPORIS AND TINEA CRURIS

These fungal infections occur worldwide, and males are more often infected than females. Tinea cruris infects the skin in the pubic area and almost always in males. It is commonly called jock itch. The reservoir for the organisms that cause tinea corporis is in humans, animals, and soil. For tinea cruris, it is usually in men. The incubation period is 4 to 10 days, and the infection is communicable as long as lesions are present or as long as infective fungus is on contaminated materials. Friction and excessive perspiration in the armpits or inguinal area will predispose to fungal infection.

Transmission   Fungal infections are transmitted by direct or indirect contact with skin of an infected person or lesions of infected animals. Floors, shower stalls, benches, and similar locations can also be a source of infection.

Symptoms   This fungus disease of the body begins with red, slightly elevated scaly patches that contain minute vesicles or papules. The lesions are ring shaped, and new patches arise on the periphery while the central area clears up, leading to the "ringworm" appearance (Figure 10-7). The periphery may be dry and scaly or moist and crusted. Often there is considerable itching.

Treatment   The individual must bathe thoroughly and frequently with soap and water. Scabs and crusts are removed, and a fungicide ointment applied. An oral fungicide is also effective.

Prevention   Towels and clothing used for workouts should be laundered with hot water and/ or a fungicidal agent; showers and gymnasiums should be kept antiseptic with

FIGURE 10-7   Tinea corporis.

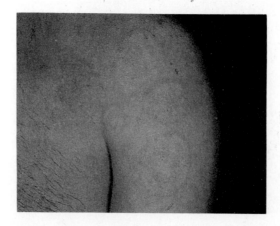

frequent washing of benches and floors with a fungicidal agent. Showers and dressing rooms should be hosed, with allowance for rapid draining, at regular intervals.

Control   Individuals who are being treated for a tinea infection should be excluded from swimming pools and activities likely to lead to exposure of others. Clothing of infected individuals should be laundered frequently with a fungicidal agent. School and household contacts and pets should be examined for identification and treatment of a possible source.

TINEA PEDIS

This fungus infection of the foot, especially between the toes, is commonly called athlete's foot. It is the most common of all the fungal skin diseases. The fungus infects adults more often than children, males more than females. The infections occur more often and are more severe in hot weather. Warm, moist conditions (such as exist between sweaty toes) predispose to the infection. The reservoir of infection is people. The incubation period is unknown, but the infection is communicable as long as lesions are present or infective spores are on contaminated materials. Some people seem more susceptible than others, and inapparent infections occur. Those who are susceptible may have repeated attacks.

Transmission   Same as for tinea corporis.

Symptoms   There is scaling or cracking between the toes and watery blisters (Figure 10-8). In severe cases, lesions may appear on other parts of the body, particularly the hands, but this is an allergic reaction to the fungus products and not infective. Itching can be severe, and cracking can become extremely painful.

Treatment   Fungicide in salve or powder form should be applied after every bath or shower. Feet should be kept dry and exposed to the air as much as possible.

FIGURE 10-8   Tinea pedis.

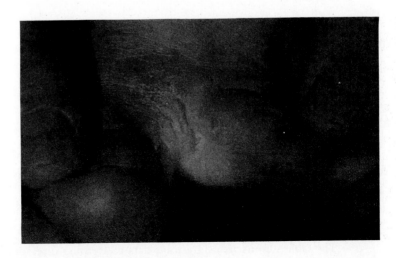

Prevention   Same as for tinea corporis, except that special attention to drying between toes after bathing and regular use of a fungicidal powder will reduce chances of infection.

Public and private pools used to have a foot bath for swimmers to walk through as they went from the dressing rooms to the pool. It is now known that unless someone changes these foot baths every 10 to 15 minutes, the solution no longer is effective and will eventually support the growth of tinea, thus spreading the infection.

Open (from the top) dressing facilities that can be kept comparatively dry by the sun and scrubbed nightly with disinfectant (fungicide) are best. A fungicide should be applied to the pool decks and dressing rooms / office area at night to reduce the risk of spreading tinea pedis. These measures should also be applied to locker / shower rooms in schools and sports facilities.

Control   In some cases, tinea pedis is very difficult to eradicate. If this is the case, socks and shoes of infected individuals need to be boiled if possible or replaced if not. Inspection of individuals before entering locker rooms or shower facilities should be done regularly, and those who have lesions on their feet should be restricted from usage of public areas.

TINEA UNGUIUM

Tinea can also infect the fingernails or toenails. It more commonly affects the toenails. It may infect one or more nails and is a fairly common occurrence. The reservoir of infection is people, sometimes animals or soil. The incubation period is unknown; infection is communicable as long as the lesion is present. If a nail is injured, it is more susceptible to infection, and reinfection often occurs.

Transmission   There is a low rate of transmission, and it is thought to spread mainly by direct contact with infected skin or nails.

Symptoms   The infected nail gradually thickens and becomes discolored, and cheesy-looking material collects under the nail. In some cases, the nail becomes chalky and disintegrates.

Treatment   The treatment of choice is griseofulvin by mouth. It is given until the nails grow out. There are other topical applications that can be purchased over the counter, but they are not generally effective.

Prevention   Same as for tinea pedis.

Control   There are no specific control measures, since the infection is not often transmitted, even to family members.

SUMMARY

The table summarizes significant data concerning diseases caused by fungi.

| | **SUMMARY TABLE**   Diseases caused by fungi | | | |
Diseases	**Special Characteristics**	**Transmission**	**Common Symptoms**	**Prevention/ Control**
Coccidioidomy-cosis	Mainly in south-western United States. Common name: valley fever. May be acute or chronic. Fungus spores found in soil from California to southern Texas.	Inhalation of spores from soil. Most favorable conditions—summer dust and windstorms.	May be asymptomatic or may have flulike symptoms and an itchy rash. Rarely disseminates but if so, may be fatal. May have lesions in lung similar to TB. May also be systemic abscesses.	Dust control measures. Masks for working in high-risk areas. Tests for susceptibility. Strong immunity after recovery.
Histoplasmosis	Endemic in Midwest and East, spreading to other parts of country. Bats and birds carry organism in feces. Spore form of fungus found in soil around bat-infested caves, chicken houses, etc.	Inhalation of spores from soil. No person-to-person transmission.	Primary lesion in lungs. May be asymptomatic or may be flulike illness, acute disseminated, chronic disseminated, or chronic pulmonary. Last three may be fatal if untreated, but spontaneous remissions occur also.	Protective masks in high-risk areas. Dusty contaminated areas sprayed with water or oil. In outbreak, contact investigation for environmental source.
Candidiasis	Opportunistic yeastlike fungus. Natural inhabitant of human body. Different locations, different forms, e.g., thrush, moniliasis, diaper rash. Resistance lowered by chemotherapy, antibiotics, AIDS, diabetes, and other diseases.	Endogenous infection or contact with excretions or secretions of infected individuals.	Depend on site of infection, e.g., scaly, red, papular rash in creases of skin. Cream-colored or bluish white patches in mouth or pharynx can cause breathing difficulty. Cheesy discharge from vaginal area, extreme pruritis. Systemic infection causes chills, high fever, low blood pressure, prostration, rash.	Treat infected pregnant women; treat sexual partners; improve immune system.
Dermatophy-toses Tinea capitis	Mainly in children (ringworm of the scalp).	Contact, direct or indirect, with hair or articles used by infected person, or sometimes with animals.	Begins as a small papule and spreads across head or bearded areas. Hairs become brittle and break easily.	Education of parents and children. Daily washing of hair and wearing of cap in severe cases. Examination and treatment of contacts and pets.

Continued.

SUMMARY TABLE	Diseases caused by fungi—cont'd			
Diseases	**Special Characteristics**	**Transmission**	**Common Symptoms**	**Prevention/ Control**
Tinea corporis and tinea cruris	Ringworm of the body and pubic area (jock itch). More common in men. Friction and excessive perspiration are factors.	Same as tinea capitis.	Red, slightly elevated scaly patches that contain tiny vesicles or papules. Periphery may be dry and scaly or moist and crusted. Considerable itching.	Launder towels and clothing used for workouts in hot water. Antiseptic measures used in gymnasiums, showers, dressing rooms. Exclude infected persons from swimming pools and other activities at high risk for exposing others. Examine school and household contacts and pets for possible source.
Tinea pedis	"Athlete's foot," most common fungal infection. Fungus thrives in warm, moist conditions. Interdigital.	Same as tinea corporis.	Scaling or cracking between toes, watery blisters. Severe itching and pain possible.	Feet kept dry, fungicidal salve or powder application after bath or shower. Contaminated socks and shoes disinfected.
Tinea unguium	Infection of toenails and sometimes fingernails.	Direct contact with infected skin or nails.	Nail thickens, becomes discolored; cheesy-looking material collects under nails.	Same as for tinea corporis.

QUESTIONS FOR REVIEW

1. In what part(s) of the country is coccidioidomycosis found?
2. How is coccidioidomycosis transmitted?
3. When is coccidioidomycosis fatal?
4. In what part of the country is histoplasmosis found?
5. What are the common sources of infection for histoplasmosis?
6. In what five ways may infection with histoplasmosis affect the individual?
7. How can coccidioidomycosis and histoplasmosis be avoided?
8. What are the common sites for infection with candida?
9. What symptoms occur at each site of candidiasis?
10. What factors predispose an individual to candidiasis?
11. Why is treatment of pregnant women with candidiasis important?
12. What are the most common sites of tinea infections?
13. What treatments are effective for tinea infections?

14. How are the symptoms for the various kinds of tinea infection alike and how do they differ?
15. How can each kind of tinea discussed in the chapter be prevented and controlled?

FURTHER READING

Ampel, N. M., C. O. Dols and J. N. Galgiani. "Coccidioidomycosis During Human Immunodeficiency Virus Infection: Results of a Prospective Study in a Coccidioidal Endemic Area." *American Journal of Medicine,* Mar. '93, 94 (3):235-240.

Banov, Charles H., John H. Epstein and Leonard B. Grayson. "Treating the Itch That Persists." *Patient Care,* Oct. 15, '89, 23:79-90.

Boyd, Robert F. *General Microbiology.* St. Louis: Mosby, 1988.

"Cave-Associated Histoplasmosis in Costa Rica." *Journal of the American Medical Association,* June 24, '88, 250:3535-3536.

Chessin, Lawrence N. "Targeting Systemic Mycoses." *Patient Care,* Aug. 15, '88, 22:121-137.

Cinque, Chris. "Tennis Shoe Dermatitis: Making a Surefire Diagnosis." *Physician and Sportsmedicine,* Dec. '89, 17:123-137.

Control of Communicable Disease in Man. Abram S. Benenson, ed, Fifteenth Edition, Washington, D.C.: American Public Health Association, 1990.

Dismukes, William E. et al. "A Randomized, Double-Blind Trial of Nystatin Therapy for the Candidiasis Hypersensitivity Syndrome." *New England Journal of Medicine,* Dec. 20, '90, 323:1717-1723.

Foxman, Betsy. "The Epidemiology of Vulvovaginal Candidiasis: Risk Factors." *American Journal of Public Health,* Mar. '90, 80:320-322.

"From the Centers for Disease Control and Prevention. Coccidioidomycosis—United States, 1991-1992." *Journal of the American Medical Association,* Mar. '93, 269 (9):1098-1099.

Matthews, Ruth, et al. "Candida and AIDS: Evidence for Protective Antibody." *Lancet,* July 30, '88, 2:203-205.

McBride, A. and B. A. Cohen. "Tinea Pedis in Children." *American Journal of Diseases of Children,* '92, 146 (7), 844-847.

McCance, Kathryn L. and Sue E. Huether. *Pathophysiology: The Biologic Basis for Disease in Adults and Children.* St. Louis: Mosby, 1990.

Murray, Patrick, et al. *Medical Microbiology.* St. Louis: Mosby, 1990.

Odom, R. "Pathophysiology of Dermatophyte Infections." *Journal of the American Academy of Dermatology,* May, '93, 28 (5 Pt 1): S2-S7.

Rajah, V. and A. Essa. "Histoplasmosis of the Oral Cavity, Oropharynx and Larynx." *Journal of Laryngology and Otology,* Jan. '93, 107 (1): 58-61.

Ramsey, Michael L. "Athlete's Foot: Clinical Update." *Physician and Sportsmedicine,* Oct. '89, 29:29-36.

Reed, B. D. and A. Eyler. "Vaginal Infections: Diagnosis and Management." *American Family Physician,* June '93, 47 (8):1805-1818.

Rezabek, G. H. and A. D. Friedman. "Superficial Fungal Infections of the Skin. Diagnosis and Current Treatment Recommendations." *Drugs,* May, '92, 43 (5): 674-682.

Rosen, Ted. "Dermatophytosis: Practical Tips for Avoiding Common Mistakes." *Consultant,* Aug. '89, 29:29–36.

Rosen, Ted. "Tinea Versicolor and Candidiasis: Practical Tips for Avoiding Common Mistakes." *Consultant,* Aug. '89, 29:40–43.

Scully, Robert E. et al. "A 40-Year-Old Man with Dysphagia, Chest Pain, Fever, and a Subcarinal Mass." *New England Journal of Medicine,* Apr. 11, '91, 324:1040–1047.

Chapter *11*

Diseases Caused by Protozoa and Metazoa

O B J E C T I V E S

1 State means of avoiding giardiasis and amebiasis.

2 Describe precautions that should be taken to prevent toxoplasmosis.

3 Explain why malaria is still a problem in the world.

4 Describe the sequence that produces the periodic chills and other symptoms in malaria.

5 Distinguish among pinworm, roundworm, hookworm, and tapeworm.

6 Discuss the source of trichinosis.

7 Distinguish among the three kinds of parasitic lice that cause pediculosis.

8 Identify symptoms, treatment, prevention, and control for the diseases discussed in this chapter.

GIARDIASIS

Giardiasis is an infection of the small intestine caused by a protozoan, *Giardia lamblia*. The disease occurs worldwide but is most common in developing countries and other areas where sanitation and hygiene are poor. In the United States, it is found more often in children. It is more common in people who have returned from countries where it is endemic and in campers who drink water from contaminated streams without purifying it. The incubation period is 5 to 25 days or longer. The disease is communicable as long as the person has the infection. Many people are asymptomatic carriers.

Transmission Giardiasis is acquired by ingesting the cysts in fecally contaminated water or by the fecal-oral transfer of cysts, person to person. Figure 11-1 shows how giardiasis is spread. Many victims are asymptomatic and transmission is more likely to be by

---

DID YOU KNOW?

Waterborne giardiasis has been increasing in the United States with 95 outbreaks reported over the last 25 years. *Giardia* is also the most frequently isolated intestinal protozoan from populations worldwide and the most common pathogenic parasite in the United States.

It has been estimated that 60% of all *Giardia* infections are acquired through water and that water could have gone through a city's purification system. Studies have strongly suggested that *Giardia* can be transmitted through the city water supplies if they have not used filtration technology capable of removing *Giardia* cysts. Giardiasis has been diagnosed among residents of areas where only mechanical filtration and chlorination were used to purify the water. Evidently, mechanical filtration and chlorination are not enough to guarantee a pure water supply.

Fraser, G. Graham, and Kenneth R. Cooke: "Endemic Giardiasis and Municipal Water Supply." *American Journal of Public Health,* 1992; 81:760-762.

those without symptoms. Individuals who are symptomatic would be restricted in socialization and activities, to a greater or lesser extent, depending on the severity of the symptoms. Chlorine used in water treatment does not destroy the cysts.

Symptoms   When there are symptoms from giardiasis, they are gastrointestinal. They include abdominal cramps, pale, loose, greasy stools, and nausea. With chronic giardiasis, there may be fatigue and weight loss.

Treatment   The drug of choice for giardiasis is metronidazole. There are other drugs that can be used alternatively, and flurazolidone is used in suspension for very young children. Severe diarrhea may necessitate fluid replacement.

Prevention   The best means of prevention is education of the public in personal hygiene and the need for handwashing before eating and after toilet use. Protection of public water supplies from contamination with human or animal feces and sanitary disposal of

FIGURE 11-1   Cycle of giardiasis.

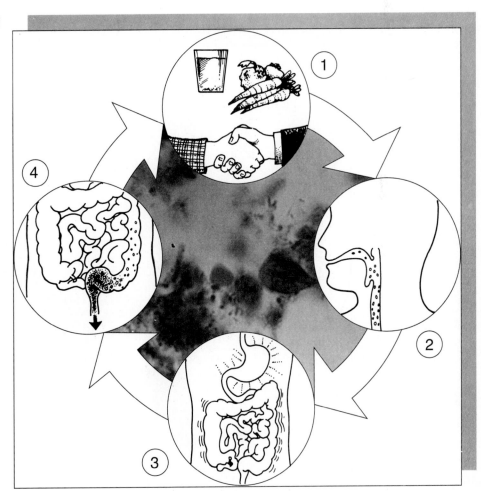

feces are also mandatory. Campers need to boil or filter any water not connected to a city purification system.

Control   If there is an outbreak, contacts should be examined for signs of infection, and there should be a search for environmental sources that can be eliminated.

AMEBIASIS (AMEBIC DYSENTERY)

This acute or chronic disease is caused by a tiny parasitic protozoan named *Entamoeba histolytica*. The infection may or may not be symptomatic. Amebiasis occurs world-wide but is found more often in areas where sanitation is poor. Incidence in the United States averages from 1% to 3% but is higher in mental institutions and among homosexual males who have many sexual partners. The incubation period is commonly 2 to 4 weeks, and the disease is communicable as long as an infected individual is passing cysts. Most persons who harbor the organism do not develop disease.

FIGURE 11-2 Cycle of amebiasis.

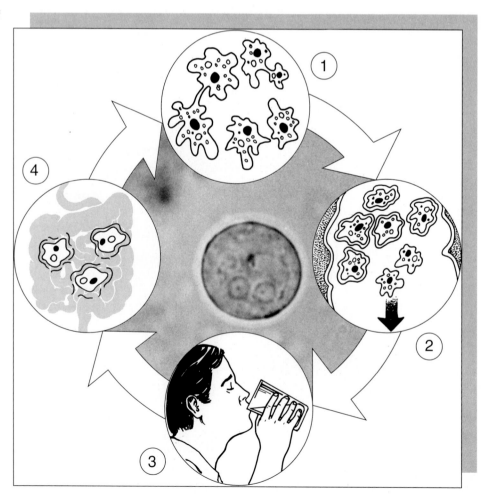

Transmission   Transmission occurs principally through ingesting feces-contaminated food and water. It may also occur sexually through oral-anal contact. The cycle by which amebiasis is spread is shown in Figure 11-2.

Symptoms   Symptoms of the acute form of amebic dysentery include sudden high fever, chills, abdominal cramping, profuse, bloody diarrhea with **tenesmus,** and abdominal pain. Chronic amebic dysentery lasts 1 to 4 years, with periods of bloody, mucoid diarrhea, mild fever, and abdominal cramps. Complications may lead to more serious illness including abscess of the liver.

Treatment   A number of different drugs are used in treatment, depending upon the severity and nature of the disease.

Prevention   As with any disease that is passed through feces, the emphasis in prevention is on education of the public in sanitary disposal of feces and thorough handwashing after defecation. Any fruits and vegetables need to be cleaned and cooked correctly, and water that may be contaminated needs to be boiled if other purification methods are not available. High-risk individuals need to be warned of the dangers of oral-fecal transmission.

Control   Infected individuals should be excluded from food handling and working with patients in health care institutions. Contacts should be investigated for infection and a search conducted for a possible source.

TOXOPLASMOSIS

One of the most common infectious diseases, toxoplasmosis usually produces no ill effects except when transmitted by a woman to her unborn child or in people with immunodeficiency. The protozoan *Toxoplasma gondii* causes the infection. The most common method for people to get it is through eating undercooked lamb or pork. About 25% of the pork and 10% of the lamb eaten by humans contains the *Toxoplasma* organisms. These organisms also multiply in the intestines of cats, and about 1% of cats excrete cysts containing *Toxoplasma* eggs in their feces. The infection occurs worldwide in mammals and birds. Cats acquire the infection from eating infected birds and mammals (particularly rodents) and are the main host, although other animals act as intermediate hosts.

Transmission   Toxoplasmosis is transmitted from the host to humans in the cysts, that can live outside the host. As has been stated, the most common means of infection is through eating undercooked meat. Since the cysts are in the feces of the host, cat boxes and unprotected sandboxes may also contain them. Children who play in these areas may become infected. One of the most serious forms of infection occurs when a pregnant woman has a primary infection and it is transmitted through the placenta to the unborn child. Figure 11-3 shows the different means by which toxoplasmosis may be transmitted.

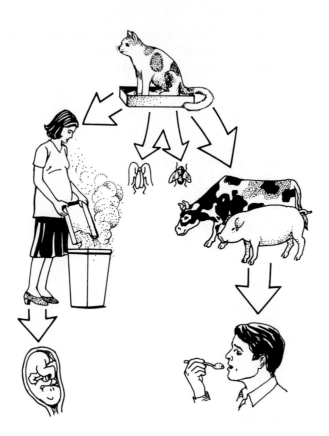

FIGURE 11-3 Transmission of toxoplasmosis.

Symptoms If toxoplasmosis is acquired in the first trimester of pregnancy, it often results in stillbirth. Infants who survive have congenital toxoplasmosis. Many problems may arise because of this infection, such as hydrocephalus and **hepatosplenomegaly.** Some defects do not become evident for months or years. The symptoms for the acute form of histoplasmosis are similar to those for mononucleosis. Immunodeficient patients may have a generalized infection with encephalitis, fever, headache, vomiting, delirium, convulsions, and a rash. Complications of the generalized infection include myocarditis, pneumonitis, and hepatitis.

Treatment Treatment is not necessary unless the infection is during early pregnancy or there are complications. Immunocompromised individuals including AIDS patients need to have prophylactic treatment throughout life. Several drugs are effective and used for these cases.

Prevention All meats should be cooked thoroughly. If cats are kept inside and fed only commercially prepared cat food, then they should not become infected. Litter boxes should be cleaned frequently and children not allowed near them. Pregnant women should not be involved with cleaning litter boxes or have contact with strange cats. Sandboxes should be protected from stray cats. The public and, especially, pregnant women should be educated as to the dangers and means of acquiring toxoplasmosis.

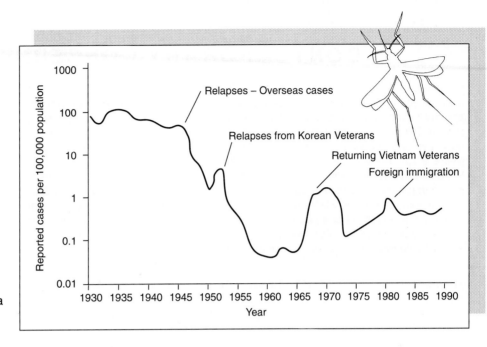

FIGURE 11-4   Reported cases of malaria by year—United States, 1930 to 1990.

Control   If infection with toxoplasmosis occurs, contacts should be examined and the source of the infection identified.

MALARIA

Malaria is the single most important disease hazard for people traveling to foreign countries. Malaria is no longer endemic in most Western countries but is brought into the United States by travelers who have been in Asia, Africa, or Latin America, where it is most prevalent. Figure 11-4 shows reported cases and some of the reasons for the variation in number of cases from 1930 to 1990 in the United States. Malaria is a disease caused by four species of plasmodium, *Plasmodium vivax, P. malariae, P. falciparum,* and *P. ovale.* The incubation period varies from 12 days to 10 months or longer, depending on the infecting strain. Untreated or insufficiently treated patients may be a source of mosquito infection for 1 to more than 3 years. There is a fatality rate of 10% for untreated cases. Individuals with certain genetic traits seem to have some natural immunity, and adults in endemic areas have built up tolerance to the infection. Otherwise, susceptibility is universal. The World Health Organization has been trying to eliminate malaria in the developing nations, but little progress has been made in the last 20 years, since the mosquitoes have developed resistance to insecticides, and the plasmodia have developed resistance to drugs.

Transmission   Malaria is most often transmitted by the bite of an infected female *Anopheles* mosquito. It can also be transmitted by injection or transfusion of the blood of infected persons or by contaminated needles. Congenital infection is rare. When an infected mosquito bites, it injects the plasmodia into the bloodstream of the victim. The infective microorganisms move through the circulation to the liver, where they

CONTEMPORARY CONCERNS

Malaria causes disease in 270 million and kills 2 million a year. To date, there has been no widely approved vaccine for malaria, but Manuel Patarroyo, a Colombian scientist, has developed one and used it in 20,000 people in Latin America. He claims a 70% success rate, but Britain's Medical Research Council has refused human trials twice, saying that there were not enough data.

Those in the United States at greatest risk are armed forces members and people who travel to endemic areas. Army medical researchers have asked for permission to test the vaccine on volunteers. Although there are reports of failure to get the same results (70% effectiveness) in attempts to replicate the experiment, scientists at Walter Reed Medical Center believe that the earlier researchers failed to follow Patarroyo's specifications precisely. To correct this, vaccine for the test was produced in an FDA certified lab, and Patarroyo has collaborated closely with the Walter Reed group. Stephen Hoffman, chief Navy malaria researcher, believes that, considering the enormity of the problem, all possibilities for a vaccine should be explored.

Marshal, Eliot. "Malaria Vaccine on Trial at Last?" *Science,* 255:1063–1064, February 28, 1992.

---

form cystlike cells. When the cysts rupture, they invade **erythrocytes** (red blood cells) and feed on the **hemoglobin** (iron-containing pigment). Eventually, the erythrocytes rupture, releasing the contents into the bloodstream to infect other erythrocytes. At this point, the person becomes a reservoir for malaria and infects any mosquito that feeds on him or her. When the infected mosquito bites a person, the cycle continues as shown in Figure 11-5.

Symptoms   The classic symptoms of malaria are chills, fever, myalgia, and headache, interspersed with periods of well-being. Acute attacks occur when the erythrocytes rupture, releasing their contents into the bloodstream. These attacks have three stages: (1) cold stage—chills and shaking that last 1 to 2 hours; (2) hot stage—high fever up to 107° F, which lasts 3 to 4 hours; (3) wet stage—profuse sweating that lasts 2 to 4 hours. Other more serious symptoms may occur and vary with the form of the disease. The cycles of wellness and malarial attacks may continue for as long as 50 years.

Treatment   For all but *P. falciparum,* treatment with chloroquine is effective, and the victim usually recovers in 3 to 4 days. Quinine and other drugs, used together, are effective against *P. falciparum,* which has become resistant to chloroquine, but 10 days of treatment is necessary.

Prevention   Since a mosquito is the means by which malaria is transmitted, one of the most important preventive measures is elimination of any breeding places. In endemic areas, screens need to be used in living and sleeping areas, and bed nets impregnated with an insecticide can also reduce the risk of acquiring the disease. Insecticides are also helpful when applied to the skin of people who may be exposed to the *Anopheles*

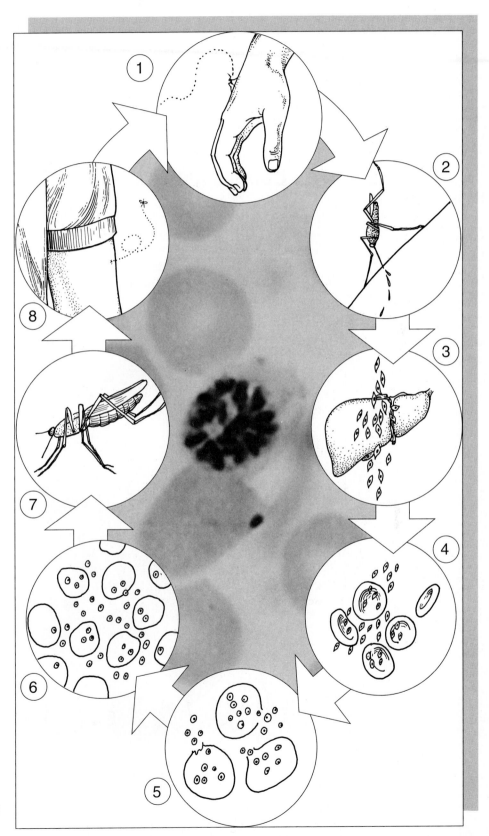

FIGURE 11-5 Cycle of malaria.

mosquito. Blood donors need to be questioned about possible infection with malaria. Finally, drugs should be used prophylactically for those traveling to an endemic area.

Control   If someone is diagnosed with malaria, an investigation should be made to determine the source. If it is a case of needle sharing, all participants must be treated.

ENTEROBIASIS (PINWORM INFECTION)

This is the most prevalent infection with worms in the United States. Children are the main victims, with as many as one fifth of all children in the United States infected at one time. The infection occurs worldwide and among all socioeconomic classes. Humans are the reservoir of infection. There is no evidence of an animal reservoir for these helminths. The life cycle (incubation period) of the worm is 2 to 6 weeks. The disease is communicable as long as the eggs are being discharged, usually about 2 weeks. Everyone is susceptible to pinworm infestation.

FIGURE 11-6   Cycle of enterobiasis.

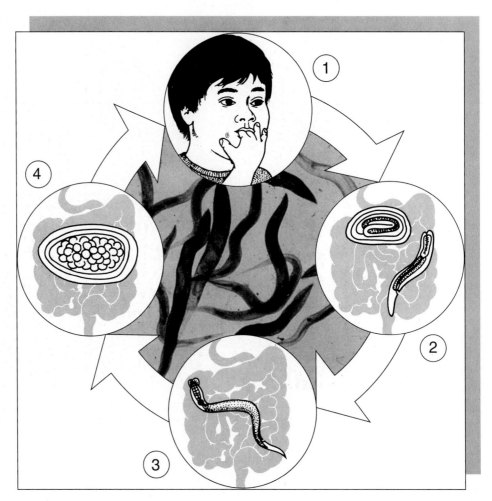

Transmission   The pinworms live in the human intestine. Female worms are white and usually about a third of an inch long. They migrate to the **perianal** (around the anus) area at night to lay their eggs. Direct transmission occurs when a person's hands transfer the eggs from the anus to the mouth. Indirect transmission occurs by contact with clothing, bedding, food, or other articles that have been contaminated with the eggs. In households where there is heavy contamination, dustborne infection may occur. Figure 11-6 shows how pinworm infestation may occur.

Symptoms   In some cases, there are no symptoms, but for most, tickling and intense itching at night are present. The itching disturbs sleep, and scratching may lead to a secondary infection. Rarely, complications may occur, such as appendicitis and vaginitis.

Treatment   When pinworm infestation is suspected, a physician will apply cellophane tape to the anal area and examine it under the microscope for signs of the eggs. Drugs can destroy the worms, but everyone in the family needs to be treated to avoid reinfection.

Prevention   Education of children in personal hygiene is the best means of prevention. Emphasis should be placed on keeping the hands away from the mouth (discourage fingernail biting), daily bathing (preferably showers), the need for handwashing after defecation and before handling food, and changing underwear daily.

Control   All members of the family should be examined, and the source of the infection identified. Families should adhere to cleanliness as far as bed linens, underclothing, and other articles that might be contaminated.

ASCARIASIS (ROUNDWORM INFECTION)

Infection with roundworms occurs worldwide in approximately 1 billion people. In the U.S., about 4 million are infected. It is more prevalent in the South, particularly among children 4 to 12 years old. Up to 90% of the population may be infected in poorer countries, while only about 1% have a light infestation in the United States and other developed countries. Although the disease is largely asymptomatic, the worms compete for food with the host and in children can retard growth because of malnutrition. It takes approximately 60 days for eggs to appear in the feces after their ingestion (incubation period). The reservoir is in humans or the soil. The disease is communicable as long as female worms live in the intestine. Infective eggs can also live in the soil for years. Everyone is susceptible to infestation with these worms.

Transmission   Ascariasis is acquired by humans through ingestion of soil contaminated with human feces that harbor the eggs. This process can occur directly by eating contaminated soil or indirectly by eating raw vegetables grown in contaminated soil and not well washed. After the eggs are eaten, they hatch and release larvae, which penetrate the intestinal wall and reach the lungs through the bloodstream. The larvae grow in the lungs, pass into the alveoli, ascend the trachea, and are then swallowed, thus entering the gastrointestinal tract. Here they grow to maturity, mate, and the female lays her eggs, which pass out with the feces, beginning the cycle anew. Figure 11-7 shows the cycle for ascariasis.

FIGURE 11-7 Cycle of ascariasis.

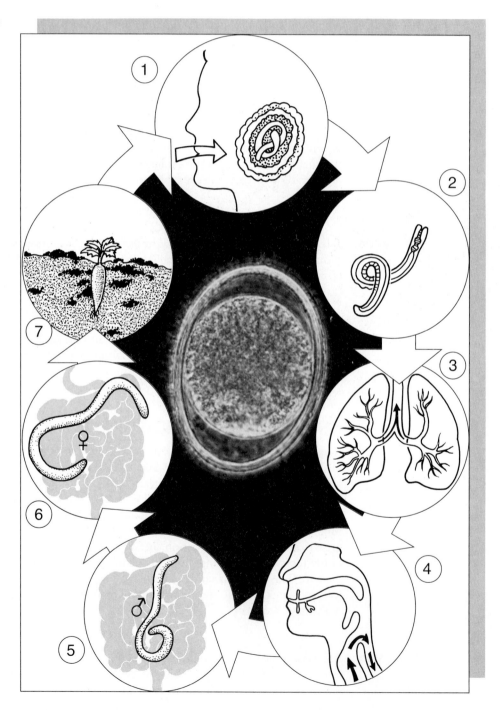

Symptoms Often, the first sign of a roundworm infection may be a live worm noticed in the stools or one that passes out of the mouth or nose. There may be mild stomach discomfort, and if the infection is severe, stomach pain, vomiting, restlessness, disturbed sleep, and, in extreme cases, intestinal obstruction.

Treatment Antiworm medications are effective in temporarily paralyzing the worms so that they can be expelled by peristaltic movements of the intestines.

Prevention Proper sanitation methods to keep soil from being polluted with feces, and training children to wash hands before eating and handling food, are the best methods of prevention.

Control The source of infection should be identified and any environmental sources eliminated. Family members should be checked and treated if necessary.

TRICHINOSIS

Infection with the worm responsible for trichinosis occurs when meat containing the cyst is ingested. These cysts are found primarily in pork and are infective when the pork is not cooked thoroughly. The reservoir for the organism is in swine, dogs, cats, rats, and many wild animals, including fox, wolf, and bear. Gastrointestinal symptoms may appear within a few days of eating the meat; systemic symptoms usually appear in 8 to 15 days, but this varies from 5 to 45 days, depending upon the number of worms ingested. There is no person-to-person communicability, but animal hosts remain infective for months. Figure 11-8 shows reported

FIGURE 11-8 Reported trichinosis cases—United States, 1947 to 1990.

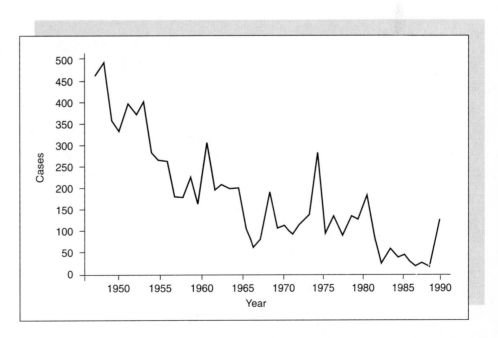

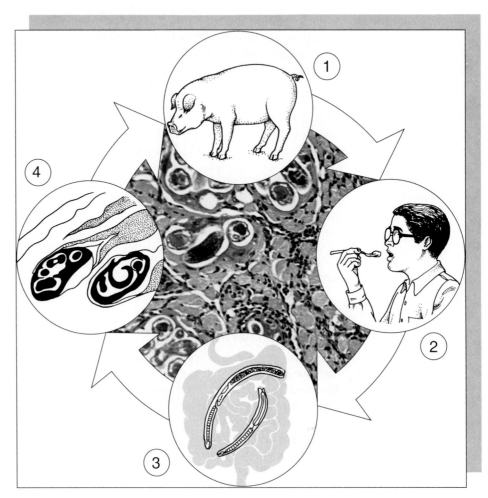

FIGURE 11-9 Cycle of trichinosis.

cases in the United States for 1947 to 1990. Although there has been a steady decline, outbreaks still occur. Everyone is susceptible to trichinosis, and an initial infection results in partial immunity.

Transmission　Humans acquire the disease by eating raw or insufficiently cooked meat containing the encysted larvae. Although beef is not a source, hamburger is sometimes purposely or inadvertently mixed with pork and, if undercooked, can also contain infective cysts. Figure 11-9 shows how infection with trichinosis may occur.

Symptoms　Ingesting just a few worms usually causes no symptoms. A heavy amount of worms may cause diarrhea and vomiting within a day or two of eating the meat. A week later, more symptoms may occur as the larvae spread through the body. These symptoms include fever, swelling around the eyelids, and severe muscle pains. In most people, the symptoms gradually disappear, but in rare cases, the person may become seriously ill and die.

Treatment Different drugs are used during the intestinal stage and the muscular stage. Corticosteroids may be used in severe cases.

Prevention The disease can be prevented by thorough cooking of all pork, pork products, and any meats that may be mixed with pork or contain the worms, such as bear meat.

Control The source of infection should be identified, and any remaining infected meat confiscated. Other family members and persons who have eaten suspected meat should be examined for infection.

HOOKWORM DISEASE

Sandy soil, high humidity, a warm climate, and failure to wear shoes provide the conditions for acquiring hookworm disease. It occurs mostly in tropical and subtropical countries where poor sanitation allows human feces to get into the soil. In the United States, the disease is most common in the Southeast. Incubation may be from a few weeks to several months, depending upon degree of infection and condition of the host. The disease is not communicated from person to person, but infected individuals can contaminate the soil for several years. If conditions are favorable, the larvae will remain infective in the soil for several weeks. Everyone is susceptible to the hookworm. Some immunity is thought to develop after the first infection.

Transmission Humans are infected when infective larvae penetrate the skin, usually the foot. The larvae pass through the circulatory system to the lungs, enter the alveoli, migrate up the windpipe, and are swallowed, entering the gastrointestinal tract. Here they mature, mate, and the female deposits eggs, which are excreted in the feces to begin the cycle again. Figure 11-10 shows the cycle of hookworm disease.

Symptoms A red, intensely itchy rash may develop at the point of entry, usually on the feet. This is called ground itch and may last several days. If the infestation is light, there may be no symptoms. In heavier infestations, after the ground itch, the migration of the larvae through the lungs may produce a cough and pneumonia. When the adult worms form in the intestines, there may be abdominal discomfort. The most serious result of hookworm disease is the loss of blood, which can lead to anemia, enlarged heart (from increased oxygen demand), and heart failure.

Treatment Administration of drugs to destroy the worms and correction of any iron deficiency through diet or iron supplements are the usual treatment.

Prevention Hookworm disease can be prevented by the sanitary disposal of human feces and the wearing of shoes in endemic areas.

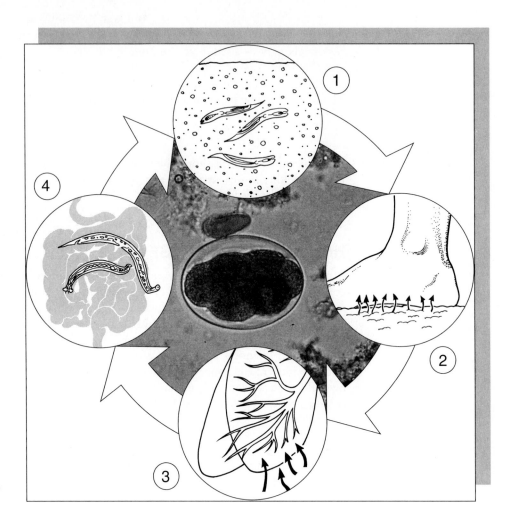

FIGURE 11-10 Cycle of hookworm disease.

Control The source of the infection should be identified and eliminated.

TAENIASIS (TAPEWORM DISEASE)

People may become infected with various species of tapeworm that are sometimes present in beef, pork, or fish. These worms can grow to be 20 or 30 feet long and lodge in the intestines. The occurrence of tapeworm disease is worldwide, particularly where beef and pork are eaten raw and where sanitary conditions allow swine and cattle to have access to human feces. It is rare in the United States but is frequently found in immigrants from other countries. From the time of ingestion, it takes 8 to 14 weeks for the eggs to appear in the stools. Pork tapeworm is communicable person to person, but the others are not. The eggs of beef and pork tapeworm may be released into the environment for as long as they are in the intestines, sometimes as long as 30 years. The eggs may remain infective in the environment for months. Everyone is susceptible to tapeworm infection.

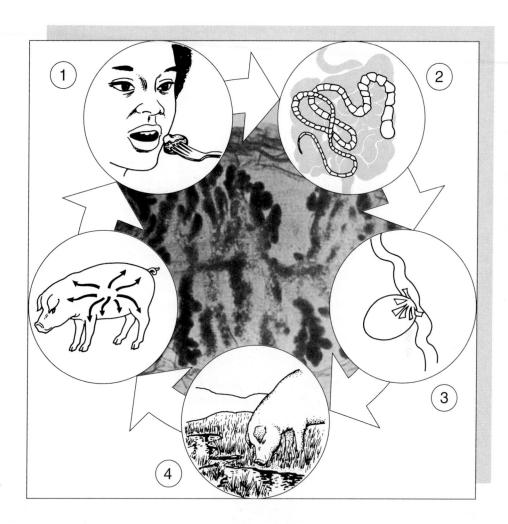

FIGURE 11-11 Cycle of tapeworm disease.

Transmission   Humans acquire tapeworms by ingesting undercooked or raw meat or fish or by hand-to-mouth contact in some cases. Figure 11-11 shows the life cycle of a tapeworm.

Symptoms   Even though these worms become very large, there may be no symptoms besides mild abdominal discomfort and diarrhea. In the case of the tapeworm found in pork, a more serious effect occurs when the embryos escape from the egg shells, penetrate the intestinal wall, move into the circulation, and are carried to various tissues where they develop into cysts that may lead to dangerous systemic and central nervous system symptoms.

Treatment   Drugs are available that are effective in the treatment of tapeworm.

Prevention   Means of prevention include education of the public regarding proper cooking of meats and sanitary disposal of human feces. If beef or pork are frozen to $-5°$

centigrade (23° Fahrenheit) for more than 4 days, the infecting organism will be destroyed.

Control Rigid sanitation measures should be taken and the source of the infection identified and eliminated.

SCABIES

Scabies results from infestation with mites that burrow under the skin and lay eggs. Figure 11-12 is an enlarged view of *Sarcoptes scabiei,* the scabies mite. Scabies infestation can occur anywhere, and although it was once thought to be a sign of poverty or poor sanitation, recent outbreaks in the United States and Europe have developed in all socioeconomic groups. The incubation period is 2 to 6 weeks before itching begins in persons who are newly infected. For those who have been exposed before, it is 1 to 4 days after reexposure. Scabies is highly communicable until mites and eggs are destroyed. Some individuals seem to be more resistant than others to the infection, and those who have had one infestation are not infected as easily as before.

Transmission The scabies mite is usually acquired by skin-to-skin contact. Sexual relations are often a means of transmission.

Symptoms The major symptom is itching that is greater at night. Evidence of the presence of the mites is visible as papules, vesicles, or tiny burrow lines. They generally appear

FIGURE 11-12 Scabies mite.

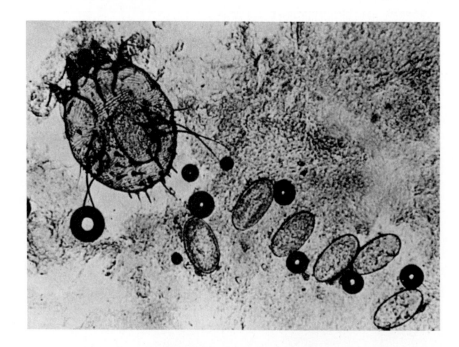

between fingers, anterior surfaces of wrists and elbows, in the armpit, at the waistline, on nipples in females, and genitalia in males. In infants, the burrows may appear on the head and neck. Scratching of the lesions can lead to secondary bacterial infections.

Treatment   Topical application of an insecticide, lindane, is the treatment for scabies, immediately preceded and followed the next day by a soap-and-water bath. Itching often persists for 1 to 2 weeks, even after the treatment has eliminated the mites.

Prevention   The best prevention for scabies is education of the public on the means of transmission and the need for early diagnosis and treatment of infested individuals and their contacts.

Control   Contacts need to be examined to determine the source of infection and administer treatment.

PEDICULOSIS

Three kinds of parasitic lice feed on human blood and cause pediculosis: *Pediculus capitis,* the head louse; *P. humanus,* the body louse (Figure 11-13); and *Phthirus pubis,*

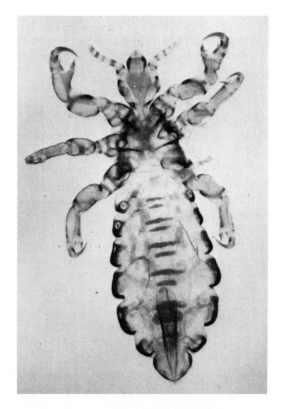

FIGURE 11-13   Body louse.

the crab louse. *P. capitis* is the most common species and feeds on the scalp and, rarely, in the eyebrows, eyelashes, and beard. It occurs where there are overcrowded conditions and poor personal hygiene and generally affects children. *P. corporis* stays in the seams of clothing, close to the skin, and lives only to feed on blood. Prolonged wearing of the same clothing, overcrowding, and poor personal hygiene are factors in this infestation. (This is the body louse mentioned in Chapter 7 as the means by which typhus fever is spread.) *P. pubis* is usually found in the pubic area but may also be in other hairy parts of the body. Infestation with lice may occur in any part of the world, and outbreaks of head lice are common among schoolchildren and in institutions. The eggs of the lice hatch in about a week, and the lice reach sexual maturity in 8 to 10 days, when mating takes place and more eggs are laid. Everyone is susceptible to louse infestation if suitable conditions are present.

Transmission
The means of transmission for head and body lice is direct contact with an infested person or indirect contact with their belongings. Pubic or crab lice are acquired through sexual intercourse or use of infested bedding. When an individual develops a fever, lice leave them, and thus crowding and illness with fever increase transmission from person to person.

Symptoms
For head lice, there is severe itching; matted, foul-smelling, lusterless hair (severe cases); swollen lymph nodes; and a rash on the body. The adult lice crawl down the hair shafts and deposit oval, gray-white nits (eggs) on the hair shafts. When body lice are present, there are usually small red papules on the shoulders, trunk, or buttocks, which change to hives from scratching. If the infestation is not treated, the skin becomes dry, discolored, thickly encrusted, and scaly, and there may be a bacterial infection and scarring. Pubic lice cause skin irritation from scratching, which is usually more obvious than the bites. Small gray-blue spots may appear on the thighs and upper body.

Treatment
Treatment for head lice is a lindane cream rubbed into the scalp at night, then rinsed out in the morning with lindane shampoo. This treatment is repeated the following night. A fine-tooth comb dipped in vinegar is used to remove nits from the hair. Washing the hair with ordinary shampoo will remove crustations. Body lice may be removed by bathing with soap and water. In severe cases, lindane may have to be used. The lice can be removed from clothes by washing, ironing, or dry cleaning. Pubic lice are treated with lindane cream or lotion that is left on for 24 hours, or by shampooing with lindane shampoo. Treatment is repeated in 1 week, and clothes and bed sheets must be laundered to prevent reinfestation. There are other preparations that can be used in treating pediculosis if lindane is not effective.

Prevention
All primary schoolchildren should be inspected regularly for head lice. If conditions are present that favor body lice, then children should be inspected for these also. The public should be educated on the value of laundering clothing and bedding in hot water or dry cleaning to destroy the nits and lice. Children should be cautioned against borrowing combs or other cosmetic supplies or clothing capable of trans-

mitting the lice. Contact with infested individuals and their belongings should be avoided.

Control   Infested individuals should be isolated from contact with others until 24 hours after treatment with lindane or other effective insecticide. Along with treatment of infested individuals, clothing, bedding, and other possible vehicles of transmission must be disinfected. Household and other close contacts should be examined and treated when necessary.

SUMMARY

The table summarizes relevant data on diseases caused by protozoa and metazoa.

SUMMARY TABLE	Diseases caused by protozoa and metazoa			
Diseases	**Special Characteristics**	**Transmission**	**Common Symptoms**	**Prevention/ Control**
Giardiasis	Found more in children in the United States. Common in travelers from endemic areas and campers drinking impure water.	Ingestion of cysts in contaminated water or by fecal-oral route, person to person.	Often none. When present, abdominal cramps; pale, loose, greasy stools; nausea.	Sanitary disposal of feces, thorough handwashing after defecation, well-cleaned raw fruits and vegetables. Exclusion of infected individuals from food preparation.
Toxoplasmosis	Dangerous for unborn child if mother is infected and for immunodeficient individuals.	Most common: ingestion of undercooked lamb or pork. Also by contact with feces of cats and some other animals.	Acute form similar to mononucleosis. Generalized form in immunodeficient patients: encephalitis, fever, headache, vomiting, delirium, convulsions, rash.	Thorough cooking of lamb and pork. Keep cats inside and feed only commercially prepared cat food. Clean litter boxes frequently; do not allow children to play in them or pregnant women to clean them. Cover sandboxes when not in use to keep cats out.

Continued.

SUMMARY TABLE   Diseases caused by protozoa and metazoa—cont'd

Diseases	Special Characteristics	Transmission	Common Symptoms	Prevention/ Control
Malaria	Single most important disease hazard for travelers to Asia, Africa, Latin America. WHO efforts to eliminate malaria hampered by insecticide-resistant mosquitoes and drug-resistant plasmodia.	By the bite of an infected female *Anopheles* mosquito. Also by injection or transfusion of blood from an infected person or with contaminated needles.	Chills, fever, myalgia, headache.	Elimination of breeding places for mosquitoes; screened living and sleeping areas; insecticides.
Enterobiasis (pinworm)	Most prevalent infection with worms in the United States. Mostly in children.	Direct from anal area to mouth. Indirect on contaminated articles. Rarely by inhalation of dust.	Tickling and intense itching at night in anal area.	Emphasis on good personal hygiene for children, particularly handwashing after defecation. Daily change of underwear and cleanliness of bed linens.
Ascariasis (roundworm)	More prevalent in southern United States and among children 4-12.	Ingestion of contaminated soil or unwashed contaminated raw vegetables or fruit.	Mild cases: stomach discomfort. Severe cases: stomach pain, vomiting, restlessness, disturbed sleep. Extreme cases: intestinal obstruction.	Good sanitation and training of children in personal hygiene.
Trichinosis	Cysts found primarily in pork.	Ingestion of raw or insufficiently cooked meat containing encysted larvae.	At first, diarrhea, vomiting. Later, fever, swelling around eyelids, severe muscle pains.	Thorough cooking of pork, pork products.
Hookworm	Most common in southeastern United States. Worm usually enters through foot.	Penetration of skin, usually the foot, by infective larvae. Eggs are produced in intestines, excreted in feces.	Red, intensely itchy rash at point of entry. Abdominal discomfort. Cough, pneumonia, anemia, and complications possible.	Sanitary disposal of human feces, wearing of shoes.
Taeniasis (tapeworm)	Can grow to be 20 to 30 feet long in intestines.	Usually by ingesting undercooked or raw meat or fish.	Mild abdominal discomfort, diarrhea. Pork tapeworm may produce serious systemic effects.	Thorough cooking of all meats and sanitary disposal of human feces.
Scabies (mites)	Mites burrow under the skin.	Skin-to-skin contact.	Itching that increases at night. Papules, vesicles, or tiny burrow lines.	Education of the public on means of transmission; early diagnosis and treatment.

		SUMMARY TABLE Diseases caused by protozoa and metazoa—cont'd		
Diseases	**Special Characteristics**	**Transmission**	**Common Symptoms**	**Prevention/ Control**
Pediculosis (lice)	Head louse, body louse, and pubic louse (crabs).	Direct contact with an infested person, their bedding, or other articles they have used or worn.	Head lice: severe itching, foul-smelling, lusterless hair, swollen lymph nodes, rash. Body lice: small red papules on shoulders, trunk, or buttocks; hives. Skin becomes dry, discolored, encrusted and scaly without treatment. Pubic lice: itching, skin irritation from scratching; small gray-blue spots on thighs and upper body.	Inspection of all primary schoolchildren for head lice. Inspection for body lice when infestation likely. Avoidance of physical contact with infested individuals. Public education on laundering and cleaning procedures to destroy nits and lice. Infested individuals should be isolated until 24 hours after treatment.

QUESTIONS FOR REVIEW

1. What groups of people are more likely to acquire giardiasis?
2. What precautions can be taken to prevent giardiasis?
3. What similarities are there between amebiasis and giardiasis?
4. For what people is toxoplasmosis most dangerous? Why?
5. What is the most common method for acquiring toxoplasmosis?
6. What precautions can be taken to prevent transmission of toxoplasmosis by cats?
7. Why have efforts by WHO to control and eliminate malaria failed in recent years?
8. How is malaria transmitted?
9. When persons with malaria have an acute attack of chills and other symptoms, what has taken place in their bodies?
10. Describe the three stages of an acute attack of malaria.
11. What means of prevention are recommended for malaria?
12. Why are children more likely to have pinworms?
13. What causes the nocturnal itching of pinworms?
14. What methods are recommended for prevention of pinworms?
15. Where in the United States is roundworm most prevalent?
16. How are roundworms transmitted?
17. What method is used to expel roundworms?
18. What meat is usually the source of trichinosis?
19. How can trichinosis be prevented?
20. How do humans become infected with hookworm?
21. What is the most serious result of hookworm disease?
22. In which meats can tapeworms be found?

23. To what dangerous results can infection with pork tapeworm lead? How?
24. How is scabies transmitted?
25. Describe the infestation and results caused by the three kinds of parasitic lice discussed in the text.
26. What means of treatment, prevention, and control are used for lice?

FURTHER READING

Addiss, D. G., et al. "Epidemiology of Giardiasis in Wisconsin: Increasing Incidence of Reported Cases and Unexplained Seasonal Trends." *American Journal of Tropical Medicine and Hygiene,* July '92, 47(1):13-19.

"Ascariasis." *Lancet,* May 6, '89, 1:887-889.

Boyd, Robert F. *General Microbiology.* St. Louis: Mosby, 1988.

Casemore, David P. "Foodborne Illness: Foodborne Protozoal Infection." *Lancet,* Dec. 8, '90, 336:1427-1432.

Cherfas, Jeremy. "Malaria Vaccines: The Failed Promise." *Science,* Jan. 26, '90, 247:402-403.

Clore, Ellen Rudy and Leah Ann Longyear. "Comprehensive Pediculosis Screening Programs for Elementary Schools." *Journal of School Health,* May '90, 60:212-214.

Cohn, M. S. "Superficial Fungal Infections. Topical and Oral Treatment of Common Types." *Postgraduate Medicine.* Feb. 1, '92, 91(2):239-244, 249-52.

Control of Communicable Disease in Man. Abram S. Benenson, ed. Fifteenth Edition, Washington, D. C.: American Public Health Association, 1990.

Cook, C. C. "Prevention and Treatment of Malaria." *Lancet,* Jan. 2, '88, 1:32-37.

DiNapoli, Joan B., et al. "Eradication of Head Lice with a Single Treatment." *American Journal of Public Health,* Aug. '88, 78:878-880.

Doglioni, C., et al. "Gastric Giardiasis." *Journal of Clinical Pathology.* Nov. '92 (11):964-967.

Dvorak, A. M. "Giardia Lamblia." *New England Journal of Medicine,* Apr. 8, '93, 328(14):1010.

"From the Centers for Disease Control: International Task Force for Disease Eradication." *Journal of the American Medical Association,* Oct. 14, '92, 268(14):1841.

Gilman, Robert H., et al. "Rapid Reinfection by *Giardia lamblia* after Treatment in a Hyperendemic Third World Community." *Lancet,* Feb. 13, '88, 1:343-345.

Graham, Barbara. "A New Bug In Town: Why City Dwellers Are Coming Down with 'Backpacker's Disease.'" *Health,* Oct. '90, 22:30-32.

Hoffman, S. L. "Diagnosis, Treatment, and Prevention of Malaria." *Medical Clinics of North America,* Nov. '92, 76(6):1327-1355.

Hoffman, Stephen L. "Prevention of Malaria." *Journal of the American Medical Association,* Jan. 10, '91, 205:308-309.

Hunter, Beatrice Trum. "Giardiasis: The Most Common Parasitic Infection." *Consumers' Research Magazine.* Apr. '93, 76:8-9.

Jackson, George J. "Parasitic Protozoa and Worms Relevant to the U.S." *Food Technology,* May '90, 44:106-110.

Jeannel, D., et al. "What Is Known about the Prevention of Congenital Toxoplasmosis?" *Lancet,* Aug. 11, '90, 330:350-352.

Kent, George P., et al. "Epidemic Giardiasis Caused by a Contaminated Public Water Supply." *American Journal of Public Health,* Feb. '88, 78:139-143.

Khuroo, Mohammad Sultan, Showkat Ali Zargar and Rakesh Mahajan. "Hepatobiliary and Pancreatic Ascariasis in India." *Lancet,* June 23, '90, 335:1503-1506.

Lauerman, John F. "Mosquito with a Mission: Why the World Is No Longer Safe from Malaria." *Health,* Mar. '91, 23:58-60.

Marshall, Eliot. "Malaria Research What Next?" *Science,* Jan. 26, '90, 247:388-391.

McCabe, Robert and Jack S. Remington. "Toxoplasmosis: The Time Has Come." *New England Journal of Medicine,* Feb. 4, '88, 318:313-315.

McCance, Kathryn L. and Sue E. Huether. *Pathophysiology: The Biologic Basis for Disease in Adults and Children.* St. Louis: Mosby, 1990.

McComber, Diane R., Rebecca Clark and D.F. Cox. "Consumer Preference for Pork Loin Roasts Cooked to 100 degrees F and 185 degrees F." *Journal of the American Dietetic Association,* Dec. '90, 90:1718-1719.

Mintz, E. D., et al. "Foodborne Giardiasis in a Corporate Office Setting." *Journal of Infectious Disease,* Jan. '93, 167(1):250-253.

"Mosquito Transmitted Malaria California and Florida." *Journal of the American Medical Association,* Mar. 13, '91, 285:1230-1231.

Murray, Patrick, et al. *Medical Microbiology.* St. Louis: Mosby, 1990.

Novotny, Thomas E., et al. "Prevalence of *Giardia Lamblia* and Risk Factors for Infection Among Children Attending Day Care Facilities in Denver." *Public Health Reports,* Jan. Feb. '90, 105:72-75.

Ongarth, Jerry C., et al. "Backcountry Water Treatment to Prevent Giardiasis." *American Journal of Public Health,* Dec. '89, 70:1633-1637.

Playfair, J.H.L., J.M. Blackwell and H.R.P. Miller. "Parasitic Diseases." *Lancet,* May 26, '90, 335:1263-1266.

Porter, D. H., et al. "Food Borne Outbreak of *Giardia lamblia.*" *American Journal of Public Health,* Oct. '90, 80:1258-1259.

Porter, John D., et al. "*Giardia* Transmission in a Swimming Pool." *American Journal of Public Health,* June '88, 70:650-653.

Pruksachatkunakorn, C. A. M. Duarte, and L. Schachner. "Scabies: How to Find and Stop the Itch." *Postgraduate Medicine,* May 1, '92, 91(6):263-266, 269.

Quick, R., et al. "Restaurant-Associated Outbreak of Giardiasis." *Journal of Infectious Disease,* Sept. '92, 166(3):673-676.

Schantz, Peter M. "The Dangers of Eating Raw Fish." *New England Journal of Medicine,* Apr. 27, '89, 320:1143-1145.

Sorvillo, Frank J., et al. "Declining Rates of Amebiasis in Los Angeles County." *American Journal of Public Health,* Nov. '88, 78:1503-1504.

Steketee, Richard W., et al. "Recurrent Outbreaks of Giardiasis in a Child Day Care Center, Wisconsin." *American Journal of Public Health,* Apr. '88, 78:485-490.

Taplin, David., et al. "Community Control of Scabies." *Lancet,* Apr. 27, '91, 337:1016-1018.

Wallace, M. R., R. J. Rossetti, and P. E. Olson. "Cats and Toxoplasmosis Risk in HIV-Infected Adults." *Journal of the American Medical Association.* 269(1):76-77.

"Walrus without Tears." *Lancet,* Jan. 27, '90, 335:202-203.

Warren, Kenneth S., "Hookworm Control." *Lancet,* Oct. 15, '88, 2:887-888.

Young, Theresa A. and Judith Levine Wilis. "Of Lice and Children: Going to the Head of Class." *FDA Consumer,* Nov. '88, 23:28-31.

Chapter 12

Cardiovascular and Cerebrovascular Disease

O B J E C T I V E S

1 Describe the disease process in atherosclerosis.

2 Distinguish among major risk factors for atherosclerosis that can be and *cannot* be altered.

3 Identify five risk factors that *may* be related to the development of atherosclerosis.

4 Distinguish among essential, secondary, and malignant hypertension.

5 Explain the significance of angina pectoris.

6 Explain possible causes of congenital heart defects.

7 Describe the cardiovascular diseases in this chapter, including predisposing factors, symptoms, prevention, and treatment.

8 Identify the signs of a cerebrovascular accident (stroke).

PHYSIOLOGY OF THE CARDIOVASCULAR SYSTEM

The cardiovascular system is composed of the heart (Figure 12-1), blood vessels (Figure 12-2), and lymphatics (Figure 12-3). The heart is a muscular pump that consists of four chambers: two atria or upper chambers and two ventricles or lower

FIGURE 12-1 The human heart.

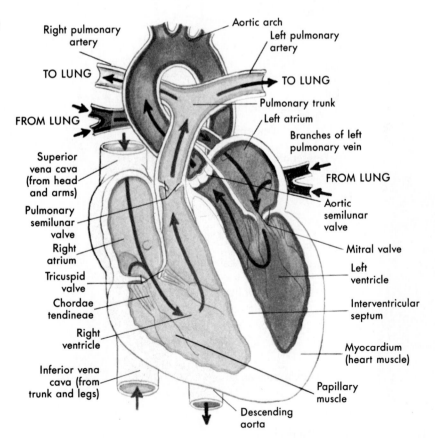

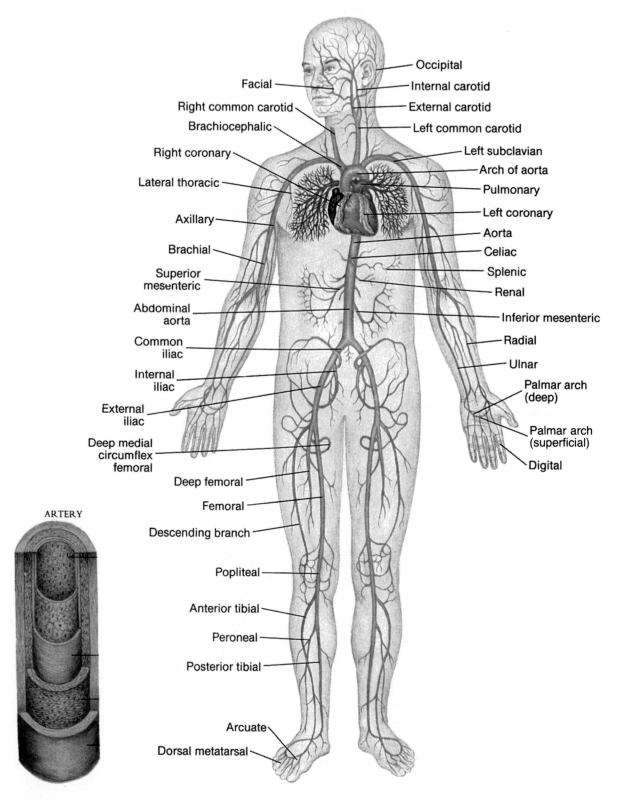

FIGURE 12-2 The arteries of the body.

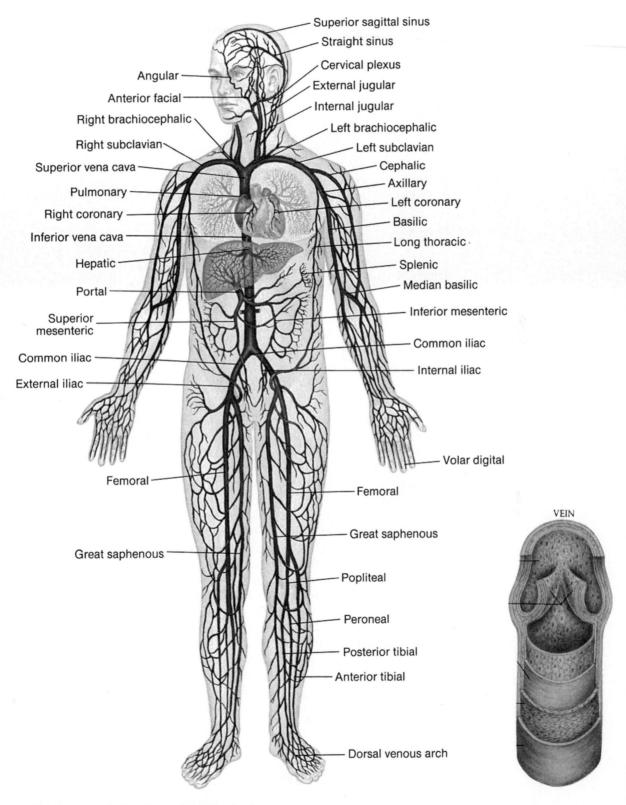

FIGURE 12-2, cont'd.   The veins of the body.

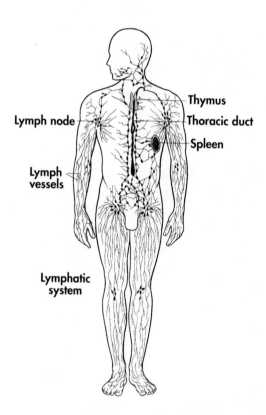

Thymus

Lymph node

Thoracic duct

Spleen

Lymph vessels

Lymphatic system

FIGURE 12-3 The lymphatic system.

chambers. Figure 12-4 shows the direction of blood flow through the chambers, valves, and blood vessels. Although the following description of blood flow discusses one side at a time, it is important to remember that both atria contract at the same time and both ventricles contract at the same time.

Blood returns to the heart from the upper and lower body by the superior (upper) and inferior (lower) venae cavae, into the right atrium (Figure 12-4). The blood passes from the atrium through the tricuspid valve into the right ventricle. Approximately 80% of the blood flows from the atrium to the ventricle by gravity. When the right atrium contracts, the rest of the blood is pushed into the ventricle. When the right ventricle contracts, the tricuspid valve is closed by the pressure of the blood, and the pulmonary semilunar valve opens, allowing blood to pass into the pulmonary arteries, which carry the blood to the lungs for oxygenation.

The oxygenated blood returns to the left atrium through the pulmonary veins and passes into the left ventricle, which is completely filled after left atrial contraction. Contraction of the ventricle then pushes the blood against the bicuspid valve, closing it, and against the aortic semilunar valve, causing it to open. The blood flows through the aorta and is distributed to the rest of the body, including the heart muscle itself, which has its own supply of veins and arteries. These are the coronary (from the Latin for *crown*) arteries and veins and are shown in Figure 12-9.

CONDUCTION SYSTEM

The heart has specialized conducting tissue that allows electrical impulses to regulate the heart beat. These structures are cardiac muscle like the rest of the heart but

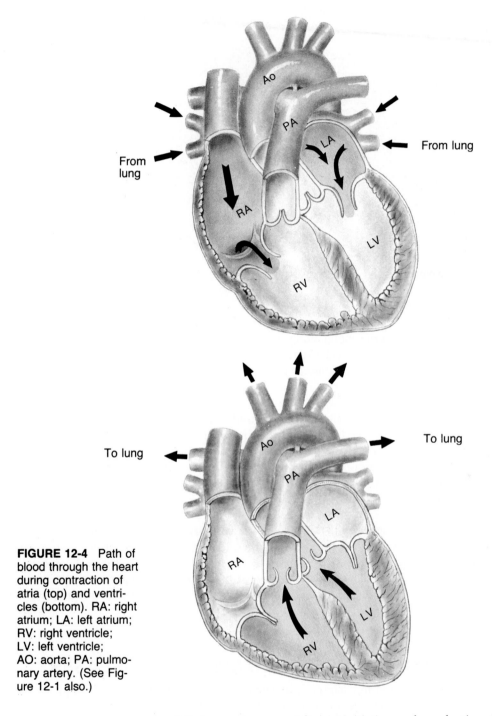

FIGURE 12-4 Path of blood through the heart during contraction of atria (top) and ventricles (bottom). RA: right atrium; LA: left atrium; RV: right ventricle; LV: left ventricle; AO: aorta; PA: pulmonary artery. (See Figure 12-1 also.)

modified enough to specialize in initiating and conducting the heart beat. The sinoatrial node, atrioventricular node, atrioventricular bundle, or bundle of His, and Purkinje fibers can be seen in Figure 12-5.

The *sinoatrial node* is the part of the heart called the pacemaker and initiates electrical contraction in the heart. The impulse generated at the sinoatrial node travels quickly through the muscle fibers of both atria to the atrioventricular node (AV node).

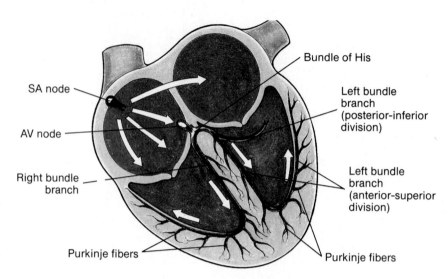

FIGURE 12-5 The conduction system of the heart.

At this point the conduction pauses to allow for contraction of the atrium. When the impulse passes from the atrioventricular node, it picks up speed and is relayed through the *atrioventricular bundle* and to the *Purkinje fibers,* which together stimulate the ventricles to contract.

This conduction system of the heart works with no noticeable flaws for many years for most people. But abnormal rhythms, referred to as *cardiac arrhythmias* or *cardiac dysrhythmias* can be caused by a number of disorders. These arrhythmias vary in severity from those that are mild, occur infrequently, and are accompanied by no other symptoms, to those that are life threatening, such as ventricular fibrillation. In any case, cardiac arrhythmias involve a disturbance of the heart's electrical conduction and the amount of blood being pumped from the heart. If the ability of the heart to pump blood to the body is impaired enough, it can lead to sudden death. It should be understood that an occasional irregular beat may happen to anyone and is not indicative of any problem. However, if irregular beats occur in a pattern over a period of time, a physician should be consulted. When the electrical conduction from the atria to the ventricles is slowed or blocked, a temporary or permanent pacemaker can be placed into or on the heart to maintain the contraction of the ventricles.

PREVENTION OF CARDIOVASCULAR DISEASES

As was discussed in Chapter 2, heredity, environment, and lifestyle all play a part in determining whether or not an individual will develop a chronic disease. Although research is going on today that may make it possible to alter genes and thus affect the heredity factor, it will be years before this can be done. There are also some elements in our environment that are difficult to control, but there are many we can change. Certainly we can make changes in the way we eat, sleep, work, and play. For those who make the effort, it can mean not only added years of life but added quality of life for the years they live.

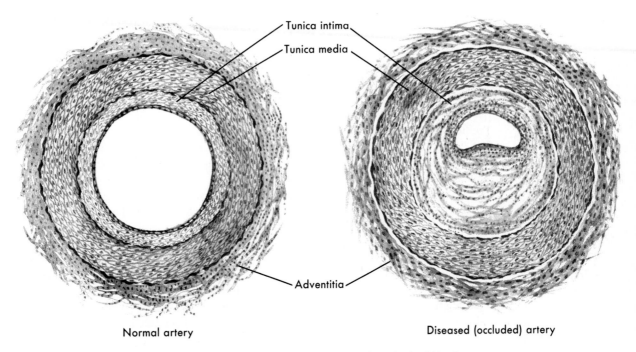

Tunica intima
Tunica media
Adventitia

Normal artery   Diseased (occluded) artery

FIGURE 12-6   Buildup of atheromatous plaque reduces the lumen (opening) within the artery.

Often cardiovascular disease is far advanced when diagnosed. According to studies and research, the onset of the disease can be as early as childhood. Educational and preventive measures need to begin in childhood and continue throughout life. Proper nutritional habits, abstention from smoking, regular activity, weight control, and stress management can greatly reduce the risk for atherosclerosis and hypertension. Atherosclerosis and hypertension are present in many cardiovascular diseases.

TYPES OF CARDIOVASCULAR DISEASE
ATHEROSCLEROSIS

Atherosclerosis is discussed first because of its involvement in many forms of cardiovascular disease. Information in this section will be referred to as other diseases of the heart and blood vessels are discussed.

The term *atherosclerosis* (AS) is from the Greek *athero* (gruel) plus *sclerosis* (hardening). Figure 12-6 shows the deposits of plaque on the endothelium (inner lining) of an artery. These fatty deposits resemble the fat observed on a fresh chicken.

The terms *arteriosclerosis* and *atherosclerosis* are often used interchangeably although technically, atherosclerosis is a form of arteriosclerosis. Arteriosclerosis refers to hardening of the arteries and loss of elasticity of the vessel walls. There are several disease processes that cause this. Most of these are rare, but atherosclerosis has become epidemic in economically developed societies, and in the Western world it is now the disease that most often leads to illness and death.

Because all nations do not have the high incidence of atherosclerosis found in the Western world, it seems reasonable to believe that the disease is not inevitable.

Studies have shown that when natives of Japan, which has a relatively low rate of atherosclerosis, immigrate to the United States, they soon develop the same rates of illness and death from atherosclerosis as persons born in the United States. Some factor or factors in our society or in our lifestyles must contribute significantly to the incidence of death from this cardiovascular disease.

Although atheromas can develop in any artery, the most common sites are the aorta and the coronary and cerebral arteries. As a result, myocardial infarcts (MIs), or heart attack, and cerebrovascular accidents (CVAs), or stroke, are the major results of AS. AS also affects other parts of the body, including the legs, where it can result in peripheral vascular disease, and gangrene (death of tissue usually because of an inadequate supply of oxygen to the area).

A number of theories of atherogenesis (the formation of atheromas) have developed. Figure 12-7 shows successive stages in the formation of an atherosclerotic plaque according to the reaction to injury theory. This theory, which seems to be the most popular, states that (1) the endothelium is somehow injured, perhaps by bacteria, nicotine, hyperlipidemia (too much fat), or high blood pressure. When any injury occurs in the body, our natural defenses are activated (see Chapter 3), and blood cells are able to attach to the endothelium; (2) cholesterol, foamy (containing lipids) macrophages, smooth muscle cells (which multiply), and other cellular debris are added to the lesion; and (3) it eventually becomes a fibrous plaque; (4)

FIGURE 12-7   Progression of atherosclerosis from normal artery **A** to complicated lesion with thrombus **D.**

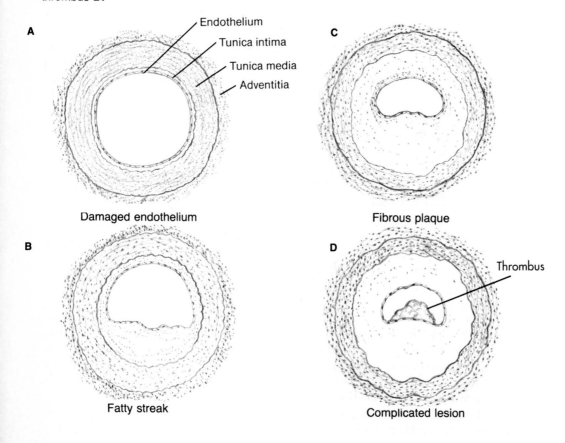

finally, a thrombus is formed, calcification may occur, and more lipids accumulate; it is then referred to as a "complicated lesion." Treatment for atherosclerosis in any of these stages may reverse the process.

The components of a plaque—cholesterol, foamy macrophages, smooth muscle cells, and cellular debris—are present in each plaque in varying amounts, resulting in differences between the lesions. It should also be remembered that this process occurs over many years of a person's lifetime (the beginning of atherosclerotic plaques has been found in young children), and there are no apparent signs until the disease is far advanced.

As the plaques increase in size, the lumen (opening) of the arteries becomes smaller (Figure 12-7). With progression of the disease, the flow of blood through the artery is restricted, leading to insufficient blood flow to tissue in the area. If the plaque is in a coronary artery or the aorta, and a thrombus (stationary clot) develops or an embolus (moving clot) occludes an artery, a myocardial infarct, or heart attack, may occur. If the plaque is in an artery supplying the brain and the above events occur, a cerebrovascular accident, or stroke, may be the result.

Predisposing Factors

It is known that atherosclerosis increases with *age*. As the passageways for blood through the arteries become narrower because of atheromas, ischemic heart disease (IHD), or insufficient blood supply to the heart, occurs. The formation of atheromas is probably not a natural result of age, but at present death from ischemic heart disease as a result of atherosclerosis increases as people get older.

Gender is another risk factor that cannot be changed. Before age 60, atherosclerosis is more prevalent in men than in women. After menopause, the difference decreases, and recent studies indicate that women are more at risk for cardiovascular disease than was expected by the scientific community. The problem is that almost all studies on heart disease in the past were done using men as the subjects and the results were applied to women as well.

Some families suffer a higher death rate from IHD than others. The term *familial hyperlipoproteinemias* is used to describe a group of inborn abnormalities in lipid metabolism. Individuals who have inherited one of these disorders tend to develop atherosclerosis, usually before the age of 50, if not treated. There might also be a tendency toward hypercholesterolemia in some families because of dietary and other habits supported by the social customs of the family.

It is not possible to choose not to age or to choose our sex or parents, or to choose to be born in a part of the world where the risk for atherosclerosis is low, but there are many ways by which all individuals can reduce their risk for atherosclerosis and IHD. The following risk factors for atherosclerosis can be reduced or eliminated.

HYPERLIPIDEMIA

Cholesterol is taken in the food we eat and is also manufactured in the liver. It is a major component of atheromatous plaques. There are a number of connections between cholesterol and atherosclerosis that have been verified by such studies as the well-publicized Framingham Study and the Multiple Risk Factor Intervention Trials (MRFIT), both of which have been ongoing for many years. Among those connections are the following:

1. Laboratory animals will develop atherosclerosis when fed diets that raise the level of cholesterol in their blood.
2. Genetic disorders that produce high levels of cholesterol in the blood lead to atherosclerosis and increased risk of IHD.
3. Most populations with relatively high levels of cholesterol in their blood have more deaths due to IHD.
4. Many different studies have shown that when patients with high cholesterol are treated by diet, regular exercise, and cholesterol-lowering drugs, cardiovascular mortality is reduced.

The damaging effects of a high cholesterol level received so much press when first recognized that the fact that other lipids (fats) in the blood also played a part in cardiovascular disease was largely ignored by advertisers eager to sell their products. Efforts to educate the public, as well as guidelines on advertising, are helping people make wiser choices when trying to reduce their risk of cardiovascular disease.

Lipoproteins. Lipids can be divided into five types according to their properties. All lipids in the plasma circulate attached to protein, thus the term *lipoprotein*. The lipids attached to the protein in varying amounts are phospholipids, cholesterol, and triglycerides. One type of lipoprotein, chylomicron, is composed primarily of triglycerides (80% to 95%) from dietary fats and is present only after a meal. The other four types are very-low-density lipoprotein (VLDL), intermediate-density lipoprotein (IDL), low-density lipoprotein (LDL), and high-density lipoprotein (HDL).

Of these five lipids, LDL is the lipid most strongly correlated with atherosclerosis and has the most cholesterol. It is sometimes referred to as the "bad" cholesterol. On the other hand, there is an inverse relationship between HDL and atherosclerosis. HDL removes cholesterol from the blood and sends it to the liver to be processed and excreted and may even remove it from atheromatous plaques. HDL has been called "good" cholesterol. Chylomicron and IDL are normally removed from the plasma very quickly or converted to LDL and do not accumulate. It is not yet known how atherogenic VLDL is. It is only certain that LDLs are atherogenic and HDLs are not. In fact, higher levels of HDLs lower the risk for heart disease.

Because HDLs lower the risk for heart disease, the level of LDL in the plasma does not always identify those at risk for atherosclerosis. It is possible to have low LDL and still be at risk because the HDL is also low. Conversely, LDL may be very high, but it is not considered a risk if the HDL is also high. The important measure for anyone is the ratio of total cholesterol to HDL. For men, a ratio of 4:1 is considered low risk, and for women a ratio of 3.8:1 is low risk (Table 12-1).

HYPERTENSION, OR HIGH BLOOD PRESSURE

There is no doubt that untreated hypertension accelerates atherogenesis and the incidence of heart disease. The Framingham Study has shown that there is a higher rate of IHD in individuals with diastolic pressures greater than 105 mm Hg (millimeters of mercury) than in individuals whose diastolic pressure is less than 85 mm Hg, and that after age 45 high blood pressure is a greater risk factor than high

TABLE 12-1 Ratio of total cholesterol to HDL cholesterol

Risk	Male	Female
Very low (½ average)	Under 3.4	Under 3.3
Low risk	4.0	3.8
Average risk	5.0	4.5
Moderate risk (2 × average)	9.5	7.0
High risk (3 × average)	Over 23	Over 11

cholesterol levels. Recent studies have found that, by age 55, women have the same incidence of hypertension as men. According to the data, hypertension is present in more than half of all women older than 55 and in two thirds of women over 65. Hypertension will be discussed in more detail later in the chapter.

SMOKING

The association between smoking and heart disease is well documented. Included in the findings are the following: when autopsies are performed, there is a greater degree of aortic and coronary atherosclerosis in smokers than in nonsmokers; when a smoker gives up smoking, his (most studies to date have been done on males) risk of dying of IHD decreases with each year that he is smoke-free; if a person smokes, there is a far greater risk of dying of a heart attack; since women have begun to smoke, their risk of coronary heart disease has been increasing; and finally, the death rate from IHD is 70% to 200% higher in men who smoke one or more packs of cigarettes a day than in those who don't smoke.

DIABETES MELLITUS

Diabetes seems to make people susceptible to atherosclerosis. It is estimated that about 75% of diabetics under the age of 40 have moderate to severe atherosclerosis in comparison to 5% of nondiabetics. Although research is still going on to find a definitive relationship, several factors are thought to increase the incidence of atherosclerosis in diabetics. *Hyperlipidemia* occurs in one third to one half of diabetics. Type II diabetics have *lower levels of HDL,* making them more susceptible to atherosclerosis. Diabetics also have *increased platelet adhesiveness,* which can affect atherogenesis. Finally, many type II diabetics are *obese* and have *hypertension,* both of which can contribute to the formation of atherosclerotic plaques.

MISCELLANEOUS FACTORS

There are other factors that may be related to the development of atherosclerosis. Although the relationship has not yet been verified by research, evidence of their connection is gradually accumulating. These include (1) competitive, stressful lifestyle with type A behavior; (2) hyperuricemia (excess uric acid in the blood); (3) obesity; (4) lack of regular exercise; (5) high intake of carbohydrates; and (6) use of oral contraceptives, particularly combined with smoking (this applies more to those who have used oral contraceptives in the past; oral contraceptives are thought to be safer today).

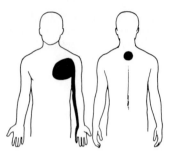

FIGURE 12-8 Some sites of pain and pressure for angina (left) and heart attack (right). Pain may occur elsewhere in the neck, shoulder, chest, or arms. Any severe pain in these areas should be reported to a physician.

Symptoms

Symptoms of atherosclerosis do not appear until the disease is far advanced. They occur when the lumen of the artery has become so small that the blood supply to a body part is restricted. If this happens to be in a coronary artery, then the decrease in oxygen to the heart causes angina pectoris, a severe pain and/or feeling of pressure in the region of the heart that usually radiates to the left shoulder and down the left arm. Other symptoms may occur, depending upon the severity of the attack. If the blood flow is restricted to the muscles of the legs, there is pain in the legs during walking that is relieved by rest. A decrease of blood flow in the arteries supplying the brain may cause transient ischemic attacks (TIAs), which produce symptoms and signs of a stroke (see Cerebrovascular Accident, page 311) but last less than 24 hours, and/or episodes of dizziness. Figure 12-8 shows possible sites for pain of angina and heart attack.

Prevention

Prevention depends upon controlling or eliminating risk factors (which are discussed under Predisposing Factors), as much as possible with medical care and a healthful lifestyle (see Chapter 2).

Treatment

The severity and location of the diseased arteries have to be considered in order to prescribe treatment. In studies conducted by the Stanford Center for Research in Disease Prevention, it has been shown that HDL levels are increased by the right diet and regular exercise alone. This beneficial effect has occurred in all groups tested (by the Stanford Center as well as other institutions), including people with coronary heart disease, the elderly, men, women, and children. And according to the National Institutes of Health (NIH), for most people, "quitting smoking and paying rigorous attention to diet, weight control, and exercise are all that's needed" to optimize lipid levels and reduce the risk of coronary heart disease (resulting from atherosclerosis). Drugs to decrease lipidemia are only used if dietary and lifestyle modifications do not succeed in lowering the LDL or increasing HDL or if lipid levels are dangerously high.

HYPERTENSION

Hypertension is another condition that is a strong risk factor for heart disease (see Atherosclerosis). Blood pressure is measured by use of a stethoscope and cuff called a sphygmomanometer. When a reading is taken, the systolic pressure is heard first, and the diastolic second. The systolic reading is the amount of pressure placed against the walls of the arteries when the ventricles are contracting. The diastolic reading is the amount of pressure placed against the walls of the arteries when the heart is at rest.

There is controversy among clinicians as to when to start treatment for hypertension. Normal blood pressure in most young adults is 120/80 (120 systolic and 80 diastolic). Highly trained athletes could be much lower. Borderline hypertension, according to the National Institutes of Health, is 140/90 to 160/95, with a diastolic pressure of 90 to 104 indicating a need for treatment.

Generally, readings need to be done more than once on individuals before they can be diagnosed as hypertensive, since there are fluctuations that occur naturally during the day. Since the diastolic reading indicates how much rest the heart is getting, there is more concern over a high diastolic reading than a high systolic reading. For some people, the trip to the doctor's office is enough to raise their blood pressure. Other factors, including emotional and physical stress, can cause the systolic pressure to rise temporarily. This is the reason that at least two readings are taken before a diagnosis of hypertension is given.

There are two types of hypertension, *essential* and *secondary*. Another term used when speaking of high blood pressure is malignant hypertension, a severe form in which the blood pressure rises rapidly, resulting in the possibility of injury to the arterioles. It may be present in either kind of hypertension.

ESSENTIAL HYPERTENSION

Also referred to as primary or idiopathic hypertension, essential hypertension is the most common form. It is estimated by the American Heart Association that 60,130,000 Americans (approximately one fourth) have high blood pressure. Although risk factors are known, an underlying cause has not been identified. The term *essential hypertension* may be confusing when the common meaning of *essential* is used; in referring to diseases, however, the words *essential, idiopathic,* and *primary* are used to indicate a condition that is present for which no cause has been identified.

Predisposing Factors

Risk factors for essential hypertension include family history, race, stress, obesity, high dietary intake of saturated fats or sodium, use of tobacco, use of oral contraceptives, and insufficient physical activity.

Some people are exposed to one or more of these factors and never develop hypertension. But people who do develop hypertension generally have one or more of these factors in their life. Family history, race, and aging cannot be controlled, but the rest can, and if they are, then essential hypertension can be reduced to normal and kept there.

Symptoms

Most people with hypertension have no symptoms until the disease causes changes in the blood vessels. Severely elevated blood pressure damages the inner walls of the arteries, causing fibrin accumulation, swelling, and, possibly, blood clots. The symptoms of advanced disease vary, depending on the location of the damaged vessels. If they are in the area of the brain, a cerebrovascular accident (CVA), or stroke, may occur; in the retina, blindness; in the heart, myocardial infarction; and in the kidneys, proteinuria, edema, and eventually, renal failure.

CONTEMPORARY CONCERNS

Heart Disease in Women

Studies on women and heart disease are beginning to get coverage in the medical journals. Because men tend to die younger than women, research on women was negligible until only a few years ago.

One of these studies dealt with employment status and heart disease risk factors in middle-aged women and was called the Rancho Bernardo Study.* Counter to what was commonly thought, middle-aged women employed in managerial positions are healthier than unemployed women.

*Kritz-Silverstein et al. "Employment Status and Heart Disease Risk Factors in Middle-Aged Women: The Rancho Bernardo Study." *American Journal of Public Health*, Feb. '92, 82:215-229.

Prevention   To prevent hypertension, any risk factors that can be changed should be. Persons with family histories of hypertension, stroke, or heart attack should have their blood pressure checked at least once a year. An annual checkup is wise for all young people and adults; anyone who has undergone a prolonged period of stress or who is obese should be checked more frequently.

Treatment   Exercise has proved to be just as effective as drugs in lowering blood pressure. A low-fat diet, salt restriction, and weight control can also help. If exercise, decreasing dietary fat and salt, and attaining the best body weight do not help, there are many drugs that can be used. The main categories are diuretics, beta blockers, calcium channel blockers, and ACE inhibitors that block a hormone known as angiotensin. Angiotensin has a strong influence on blood pressure. Some doctors will initiate drug therapy at a higher level of pressure than others, feeling that the side effects of the drugs may do more harm than a moderately raised pressure.

With proper treatment, most people are able to lower their pressure enough to avoid serious damage to the blood vessels. Unfortunately, it is difficult to get people to stay on a regular schedule of drugs and/or lifestyle changes, since symptoms are normally not present or are so mild as to be unnoticed.

SECONDARY HYPERTENSION

Secondary hypertension results from renal disease or other identifiable causes, including endocrine, vascular, and neurogenic disorders. Some of these will be discussed in Chapter 16.

CORONARY ARTERY DISEASE (CAD)

The heart has its own blood supply (Figure 12-9). When the supply of blood to the heart is insufficient, it is usually a result of coronary artery disease (CAD). This disease is more prevalent in white people, the middle-aged, and the elderly. Before

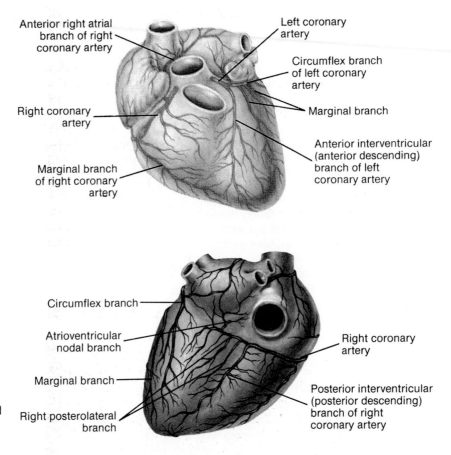

FIGURE 12-9 Blood vessels of anterior and posterior surface of heart.

menopause, women have less heart disease than men, but after menopause, their chances of a heart attack gradually increase. White males under the age of 45 in the United States have a six times greater risk than women of the same age. In males 45 to 54 there is a four- to fivefold difference, and by the eighth decade, there is only a twofold difference. The difference between men and women in susceptibility to CAD is not completely understood. It was thought that the female hormone estrogen had a protective effect, but when estrogen supplements were given to men in scientific studies, there was no difference in CAD mortality. It is possible that male hormones, including testosterone, are correlated with increased risk for CAD. As was stated earlier, researchers have just begun to use female subjects for cardiovascular research. This should result in more verifiable information.

Predisposing Factors

Atherosclerosis is the usual cause of CAD. When the atheromas, made of cholesterol, other fats, and cellular debris, build up on the walls of the coronary arteries, the blood flow to the heart muscle is reduced. This condition is referred to as cardiac ischemia. Narrowing of a vessel lumen results in slowing the movement of blood, and a thrombus may form. If the thrombus occludes the lumen or an embolus moves to the site, the blood flow may be shut off completely, leading to a myocardial infarction, to be discussed next. The predisposing factors for atherosclerosis were discussed earlier in the chapter.

DID YOU KNOW?

Two Hypertension Drugs Do Double Duty

Researchers at The University of Minnesota and the Mayo Clinic have found that two drugs commonly used to treat high blood pressure also prolong survival rate in heart attack patients and reduce the incidence of heart failures.

The reports are considered to be exceedingly important, since cardiovascular disease is the number one cause of death in the United States. Nearly twice as many people die of heart disease each year (nearly 600,000) in the United States as die of cancer and all other diseases combined.

The two drugs, captopril and enalapril, are effective in controlling blood pressure because they inactivate the process that causes blood vessels to constrict. Captopril was found to reduce overall death rate of patients (2200) who had suffered heart attack by 20% given 3 to 16 days after the attack. It also reduced the incidence of heart failure by 37% and repeat heart attacks by 25% in the same group.

Enalapril was used in another study of 4200 patients who were suffering from heart failure. Although there was only a small reduction in overall mortality rates, hospitalizations among the group dropped 36%, and deaths caused by progressive heart failure declined by 21%.

Symptoms Angina pectoris (generally shortened to angina) is the classic symptom of CAD. It is usually described as a squeezing or crushing tightness in the chest. The tightness may radiate to the left arm, neck, jaw, or shoulder blade, and sometimes is felt as a dull pain or burning (Figure 12-8). The pain or tightness may also be accompanied by nausea, vomiting, fainting, sweating, and cold hands and feet. These attacks often follow physical exertion, large meals, or stressful experiences.

Prevention Same as for atherosclerosis.

Treatment In addition to changes in lifestyle, drugs may be used to reduce oxygen consumption by the heart or to increase oxygen supply to the heart. Those now in use include nitrates, beta blockers, and calcium channel blockers, all of which (by different actions) increase oxygen supply to the heart and reduce myocardial demand for oxygen. Also, since excess platelets have been found to decrease the flow of blood to the heart, antiplatelet agents may be used.

Angioplasty, a procedure in which a balloon is inserted into the artery and then inflated, is sometimes used to treat CAD. This procedure helps to widen the lumen and establish an increased flow of blood to the heart (Figure 12-10).

Coronary artery bypass grafts are used to treat the condition surgically if the angina is severe, ventricular function is good, and the coronary arteries are in good condition. The techniques for this surgery have improved steadily, and one of the newest methods involves using an artery from the breast rather than a vein from the leg. These techniques are palliative rather than curative, since the atherosclerotic process will continue unless changes in diet, exercise, and other habits that are known to increase the risk of atherosclerosis occur.

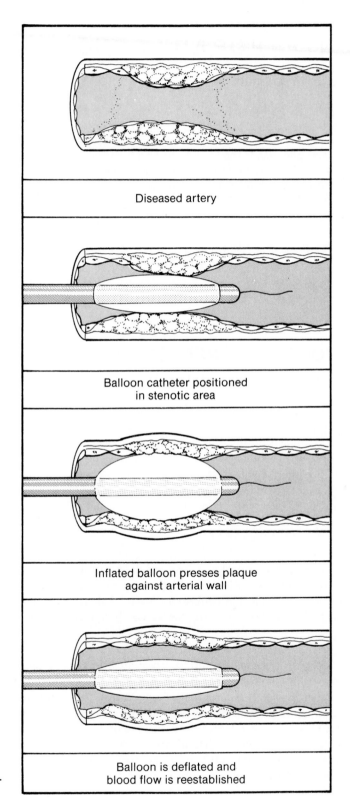

Diseased artery

Balloon catheter positioned
in stenotic area

Inflated balloon presses plaque
against arterial wall

Balloon is deflated and
blood flow is reestablished

FIGURE 12-10   Balloon angioplasty.

CONTEMPORARY CONCERNS

"Antisense" Angioplasty in Animals

A new DNA technique has been used on experimental animals at the Massachusetts Institute of Technology to prevent blood vessels from closing again after angioplasty has been performed. The procedure is called "antisense" and is used to block the action of a gene called c-myb, which makes the protein that causes muscle cells multiply and again narrow the arterial lumen.

The scientists developed a chemical message in the form of molecules called nucleotides that stopped the action of c-myb. The nucleotide was applied to the vessel walls of rats and rabbits that had had angioplasty, and the antisense message succeeded in preventing the build-up of muscle cells.

News Service Reports, Sept. 3, '92 (Duluth *News Tribune*).

MYOCARDIAL INFARCT (HEART ATTACK)

A heart attack, or myocardial infarct (MI), occurs when the blood flow is reduced, by atherosclerosis or a clot, through one or more of the coronary arteries, causing ischemia and necrosis (death of tissue, or infarct). Death often results from the cardiac damage or complications, particularly when treatment is delayed. Almost half of sudden deaths due to MI occur within 1 hour of the onset of symptoms, before the individual is hospitalized. Death occurs in 4 to 6 minutes if the heart stops beating, but if cardiopulmonary resuscitation (CPR) is begun immediately, the chances of survival are greatly increased. As was discussed earlier, females have lower mortality rates from CVD than males, especially before they reach menopause.

Predisposing Factors
The causes of myocardial infarct are the same as for coronary artery disease, since the latter leads to MI. A family history of MI, hypertension, smoking, elevated serum triglyceride and cholesterol levels, diabetes mellitus, obesity, sedentary lifestyle, and inability to control stress are all considered to be predisposing factors.

Symptoms
A persistent crushing pain in the chest area beneath the sternum (breastbone) is the most common symptom. This pain may radiate to the left arm, jaw, neck, or shoulder blades. It is often described as crushing, squeezing, or heavy and may be accompanied by vomiting, sweating, and difficulty in breathing. In some cases, the pain may not occur at all; indigestion is often the only sign. Angina of increasing frequency may indicate that an MI is imminent. Sometimes victims have a feeling of impending doom. They may also feel fatigued and experience vomiting and a feeling of suffocation.

Prevention
Same as for atherosclerosis.

Treatment   Immediate administration of CPR when the heart has stopped and emergency medical treatment can be lifesaving. Various drugs may be administered to relieve chest pain, stabilize heart rhythm, and reduce the load on the heart. Among these are antiarrhythmics, diuretics, nitroglycerin, and morphine.

RHEUMATIC HEART DISEASE

Rheumatic heart disease is a result of a systemic inflammatory disease of childhood (see Chapter 4, Rheumatic Fever) that generally follows a streptococcal infection. Inflammation of the heart (pancarditis, which includes endocarditis [Chapter 6], myocarditis, and pericarditis) can lead to heart damage, particularly to the valves. Eventually the valvular problem may lead to congestive heart failure. The incidence of rheumatic fever and its sequellae, including rheumatic heart disease, has decreased in the United States over the years since antibiotic treatment has become available. For the period from 1940 to 1982, the number of cases dropped from 20.6 per 100,000 population to 2.2. Periodically, however, there is a resurgence of the disease in the United States, and globally there are 15 to 20 million cases a year.

Predisposing Factors   The predisposing factor for rheumatic heart disease is rheumatic fever.

Symptoms   About 50% of those who develop rheumatic fever go on to develop pancarditis and/or damaged heart valves. The symptoms of acute rheumatic fever are very similar to those of other disorders (see Rheumatic Fever in Chapter 4), and because they do not occur for 1 to 5 weeks after the streptococcal infection, they may not be recognized as symptoms of rheumatic fever. The earliest sign of rheumatic heart disease may be a murmur, due to valve dysfunction, that has gone undetected for many years. There may also be other symptoms, including chest pain, extra heart sounds, heart block, and atrial fibrillation. However, once the acute stage of rheumatic fever is passed, there may be an undetected residual effect on the heart valves that is not diagnosed and only discovered years later when the individual is subjected to heart surgery (perhaps for another reason).

Prevention   Since rheumatic heart disease is always a result of rheumatic fever, which follows a streptococcal infection, prevention of rheumatic heart disease depends on early treatment of streptococcal infections and continued treatment and management of rheumatic fever should it develop.

Treatment   If there is severe valve dysfunction of the heart, then corrective valvular surgery can be performed. This seldom occurs before adolescence and, as was mentioned earlier, in the absence of apparent symptoms, may not be identified for many years.

CONGESTIVE HEART FAILURE

Although the heart is a single organ, heart failure may begin on the right or left side but will eventually affect the whole heart.

Congestive heart failure (CHF) occurs when the heart cannot keep up its work load of pumping blood to the lungs and the rest of the body. This inability generally occurs because the left ventricle has been damaged, but it may also result if the right ventricle is damaged. In either case, failure of one side of the heart will gradually affect the whole heart. It may be acute, as a direct result of MI, but it is generally a chronic disorder resulting in decreased pumping of blood from the heart and associated with retention of salt and water, which leads to swelling in the legs and ankles.

Right-sided heart failure is most often a result of right ventricular strain caused by disease of the lungs or pulmonary arteries and is referred to as *cor pulmonale*.

Predisposing Factors

CHF can be caused by a number of factors. Included in these are MI, hypertension, mitral stenosis (narrowing of the mitral valve opening) secondary to rheumatic heart disease, and aortic stenosis (Figure 12-11).

Symptoms

Fatigue, dyspnea (shortness of breath), enlarged neck veins when the victim is in an upright position, nocturia (excessive urination at night), and enlargement of the

FIGURE 12-11 Conditions leading to congestive heart failure.

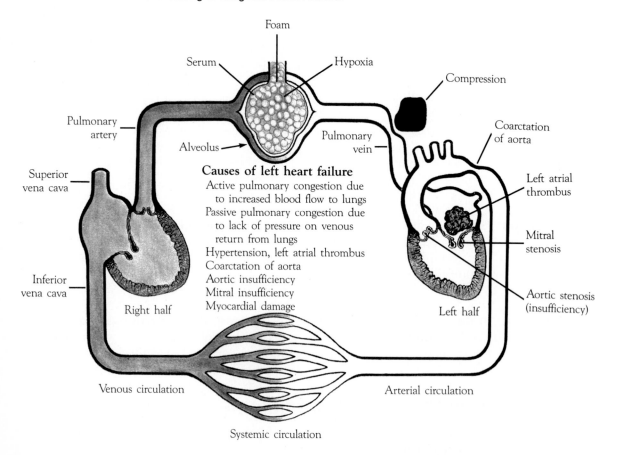

liver are among the signs of CHF. Patients sometimes have coldlike symptoms with a dry cough and confuse the condition with an allergic reaction.

Prevention   Same as for atherosclerosis.

Treatment   Bed rest with diuretics to reduce blood volume, digitalis to strengthen myocardial contractility, and vasodilators to increase cardiac output are among the therapies used to treat CHF.

THROMBOPHLEBITIS

Inflammation of a vein accompanied by formation of a thrombus is called thrombophlebitis. The disease usually occurs in an extremity, and most often a leg. If it is in a superficial vein, it is not as serious and is less likely to lead to an embolism. In the deep veins, the condition has to be monitored carefully, as the thrombus can become an embolus and travel to the lungs, resulting in pulmonary embolism, which can be fatal.

Predisposing Factors   There are a number of factors involved in the formation of thrombi. Anything that causes an alteration of the epithelial lining of the vein can lead to a thrombus. The process may occur as a result of surgery or trauma. Cardiovascular disorders, obesity, heredity, increasing age, an excess of platelets and overproduction of fibrinogen, use of oral contraceptives, and prolonged bed rest are also among the identified causes. Intravenous drug abuse and extensive use of the intravenous route for medication and diagnostic tests may cause superficial thrombophlebitis.

Symptoms   As the thrombus grows, chemicals are released, resulting in heat, pain, swelling, redness, tenderness, and hardness along the length of the affected vein in superficial thrombophlebitis. There may be no symptoms for deep-vein thrombophlebitis, or the patient may experience pain, fever, chills, malaise, and possibly swelling and cyanosis (blueness caused by reduced oxygen in the general circulation) of the affected arm or leg.

Prevention   Although some predisposing factors cannot be changed, reducing the risk factors for atherosclerosis, which have already been discussed, and making any other changes possible to reduce other risk factors will help to prevent thrombophlebitis.

Treatment   The main goal of treatment is to prevent the thrombus from becoming an embolus and traveling to the lungs. Pain relief is provided by administration of analgesics. Bed rest with elevation of the affected arm or leg, moist soaks, anticoagulants for deep-vein thrombophlebitis, and antiembolism stockings (after it is safe to walk) are used in treatment.

VARICOSE VEINS

Varicose veins are dilated and twisted veins, usually superficial, in which blood tends to accumulate and stagnate because of defective valves. Since they are near the surface, the pressure of the excess blood produces a bluish raised area along the line of the vein. Nodules can be seen pushing the skin in front of them (Figure 12-12). Most often varicose veins occur in the legs but may also appear in the rectal area as hemorrhoids.

Predisposing Factors
Factors that may contribute to the development of varicose veins are obesity, hormonal changes during pregnancy or at menopause, pressure on the pelvic veins during pregnancy, and standing for long periods.

Symptoms
There may be no symptoms or mild to severe symptoms, including cramps at night, dull aching, fatigability, and pain in feet and ankles.

Prevention
Avoiding obesity and long periods of standing can reduce the risk. If weight gain during pregnancy does not go beyond the optimal level, this may also reduce the risk for women.

Treatment
Surgery is possible but not advised unless the problem becomes severe. Antiembolism stockings, prescribed exercise (to improve blood flow), rest, and elevation of the extremity are the usual treatment.

FIGURE 12-12 Varicose veins.

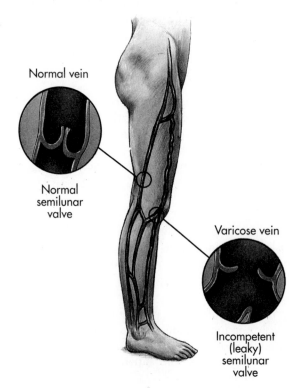

Normal vein

Normal semilunar valve

Varicose vein

Incompetent (leaky) semilunar valve

CONGENITAL HEART DEFECTS

An abnormality of the heart that is present from birth, congenital heart defect occurs in six to eight babies per 1000 born. Some defects are not apparent at birth may not become evident until adolescence or adulthood. The most common heart deformities are ventricular septal defect (VSD), patent ductus arteriosus (PDA), atrial septal defect (ASD), pulmonic stenosis, coarctation of the aorta, and tetralogy of Fallot (Figure 12-13).

Symptoms   Defects in the structures of the heart lead to insufficient or excessive circulation of the blood to the lungs or to the body. In some cases, deoxygenated blood might be pumped to the body instead of to the lungs. Or oxygenated blood might be pumped to the lungs instead of to the body. These conditions will cause cyanosis, difficulty in breathing, or both. Children with heart defects may tire rapidly with activity. As has been mentioned before, symptoms may not occur until adulthood.

Predisposing Factors   In most cases (over 90%) the cause is unknown. However, both environmental and genetic risk factors are thought to be involved. Environmental factors include conditions affecting the mother, such as rubella, smoking, and alcoholism and other

FIGURE 12-13 Three common congenital heart defects: **A,** ventricular septal defect; **B,** patent ductus arteriosus; **C,** atrial septal defect.

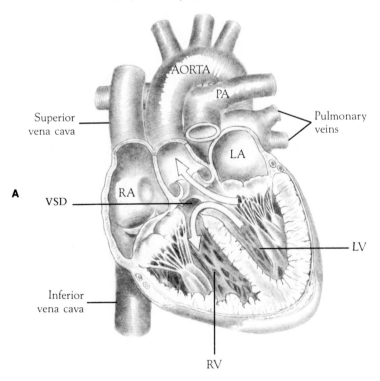

Superior vena cava

AORTA

PA

Pulmonary veins

LA

A

RA

VSD

LV

Inferior vena cava

RV

Continued.

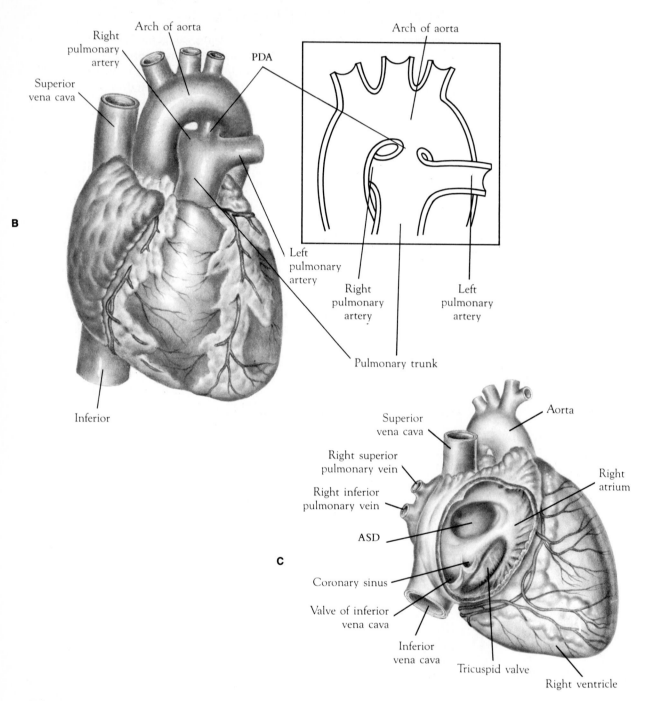

FIGURE 12-13, cont'd.

drug use. There is well documented evidence of the defects that can occur as a consequence of maternal rubella in the first trimester of pregnancy.

The age of the mother at time of pregnancy is a factor also because more defects tend to occur in babies as the mother's age increases, particularly over 40. Hereditary factors do not seem to play a significant role. Because a couple has one child with a birth defect does not mean that a second child will be affected.

Prevention Women need to abstain from alcohol if there is a chance that they could be pregnant, since some researchers believe that just one drink could cause a defect if it is taken early in the development of the fetus. If a woman is pregnant, she needs to stay away from anyone with rubella, and girls should not be vaccinated against rubella after puberty. Women over 40 should be aware of the possibility of congenital defects in the baby should they decide to have a child. During pregnancy, no drugs should be taken by the mother unless approved by the doctor.

Treatment Rest, oxygen, and various drugs may be used initially and offer temporary or indefinite relief. Some defects present at birth may get smaller or disappear as the child gets older. However, if the condition of the child (or adult in some cases) worsens, then surgery may be considered.

Surgical correction of heart disease caused by congenital defects is an area of medicine where there has been good progress, resulting in improved techniques. Corrective surgery is now available for most heart defects. Narrowed heart valves can be treated by balloon valvuloplasty, in which a catheter is introduced into the heart to widen the affected valve. In some cases, open heart surgery is necessary, and some conditions can be treated only by a heart transplant.

Children who have successful heart surgery gradually have a near-normal life span. However, they are more susceptible to endocarditis, and preventive antibiotics may be prescribed.

CEREBROVASCULAR DISEASE
CEREBROVASCULAR ACCIDENT (STROKE)

Although cerebrovascular accidents affect the brain, they are caused by disorders of or in the blood vessels.

A cerebrovascular accident (CVA), or stroke, is caused by a sudden impairment of cerebral circulation in one or more of the blood vessels supplying the brain. This impairment may be due to a thrombus, embolus, or hemorrhage. In older people, thrombosis is the most common cause. It tends to occur while the person is asleep or shortly after awakening. It can also occur during surgery or after a heart attack. An embolism, the second most common cause, may occur at any age but is more likely among people who have a history of some types of heart disease or after open-heart surgery. Hemorrhage may also occur at any age and results from chronic hypertension or aneurysms that cause sudden rupture of a cerebral artery.

The interruption or insufficiency of oxygen supply can lead to serious damage and death of cells in brain tissue. About half of the people who survive a CVA remain permanently disabled and experience another stroke within weeks, months, or years. CVA is the third most common cause of death in the United States today and the most common cause of neurologic (brain and spinal cord) disability.

Predisposing Factors All the risk factors for ischemic heart disease resulting from atherosclerosis also apply to CVA; in addition, a history of transient ischemic attacks, gout, and postural hypotension (blood pressure below normal on standing) have been found to increase the risk.

Warning Signs of Stroke

Although many stroke victims have little advance warning of an impending crisis, there are some warning signals of stroke that should be recognized. The American Heart Association encourages everyone to be aware of the following signs:

- Sudden, temporary weakness or numbness of the face, arm, and leg on one side of the body
- Temporary loss of speech or trouble in speaking or understanding speech
- Temporary dimness or loss of vision, particularly in one eye
- Unexplained dizziness, unsteadiness, or sudden falls
- Many major strokes are preceded by "little strokes," warning signals like the above, experienced days, weeks, or months before the more severe event

Prompt medical or surgical attention to these symptoms may prevent a fatal or disabling stroke from occurring.

Symptoms

Strokes are classified according to their course of progression. A transient ischemic attack (TIA) lasts only a few seconds to hours and is referred to as a "little stroke." A progressive stroke or stroke in evolution, begins with slight neurologic impairment that gradually worsens within a day or two. In a completed stroke, the damage is maximal in the beginning. The symptoms for the completed stroke generally occur suddenly, with unconsciousness and heavy breathing caused by paralysis of a portion of the soft palate. The pupils are sometimes unequal, with the larger one being on the side of the hemorrhage or occlusion. Paralysis usually involves one side of body, skin is sweaty, and speech disturbances are present. If caused by a thrombosis, onset may be more gradual, with generalized symptoms such as headache, vomiting, mental impairment, convulsions, fever, and disorientation.

Prevention

Primary prevention involves elimination or reduction of any predisposing factors possible. For secondary prevention, the box above gives the warning signs for a stroke published by the American Heart Association. These should be learned, and if any signs are present in anyone, medical help should be sought immediately.

Treatment

Following the stroke, anticonvulsants may be used to prevent seizures; stool softeners to avoid straining, which increases intracranial pressure; corticosteroids to minimize swelling; and analgesics to relieve headache, but not aspirin if hemorrhagic CVA has occurred. Surgery may be performed to improve cerebral circulation for patients with thrombotic or embolic CVA.

SUMMARY

The table summarizes relevant data on cardiovascular and cerebrovascular diseases.

Disease	Special Characteristics	Predisposing Factors	Common Symptoms	Prevention/ Control
Atherosclerosis (AS), a form of arteriosclerosis	Atheromas form on lining of arteries. Most common in aortic, coronary, and cerebral arteries. Progressive narrowing of lumen causes decrease in blood flow to tissue in area. Clot may block vessel completely and result in MI, CVA, or other tissue damage, depending on location. One theory of cause is reaction to injury.	Age, sex, family predisposition, hyperlipidemia, hypertension, smoking, and diabetes mellitus definite. Stressful lifestyle, aggressive personality, obesity, lack of exercise, and use of oral contraceptives possible. Cholesterol a major component of atheromatic plaque. LDL strongly related to atherosclerosis. HDL disposes of cholesterol.	Angina pectoris (severe, constricting pain in chest, often radiating to left shoulder and down arm), TIAs, and other symptoms, depending on location of plaques.	Prevention depends upon controlling or eliminating risk factors as much as possible with medical care and a healthful lifestyle. Condition can be reversed with diet, exercise.
Treatment	HDL levels can be improved by right diet and regular exercise if AS is not too far advanced. For most cases, quitting smoking, healthful diet, weight control, and exercise can optimize lipid levels and reduce risk of AS. Nitroglycerine often prescribed for angina.			
Hypertension	Essential hypertension is most common, cause unknown. Secondary hypertension results from another identifiable cause. Malignant hypertension can occur in either form. Blood pressure rises quickly, causing damage to arteries; 140/90 or below generally considered normal.	Family history, race, stress, obesity, high-fat or high-sodium diet, tobacco use, oral contraceptive use, sedentary lifestyle, and aging.	No symptoms until another serious disease occurs as a result of high blood pressure, such as renal failure, MI, or stroke.	Controlling or eliminating risk factors; yearly blood pressure check.
Treatment	For essential hypertension, regular exercise and low-fat diet may be all that is needed. In some cases, salt restriction and weight reduction may be necessary also. Treatment for secondary hypertension depends on cause.			
Coronary artery disease (CAD)	Insufficient supply of blood to the heart usually caused by AS and/or clot in coronary arteries.	Same as for AS.	Angina is the classic symptom. Described as a squeezing or tightness in chest. May also have pain in left arm, neck, jaw, or shoulder blade; nausea, vomiting, fainting, sweating, cold hands or feet. Often after physical or emotional stress. May have only one symptom or many.	Same as for atherosclerosis.
Treatment	See atherosclerosis.			

Continued.

Disease	Special Characteristics	Predisposing Factors	Common Symptoms	Prevention/ Control
Myocardial infarct (MI)	Reduced blood flow to heart causing ischemia, necrosis. Death in 4 to 6 minutes if heart stops beating and CPR is not administered.	Same as for AS.	Indigestion may be only sign. More often, pain in center of chest under sternum described as heavy, crushing, or squeezing and may radiate to left arm, jaw, neck, or shoulder. May also be vomiting, sweating, difficulty in breathing. Also see symptoms for AS.	Same as for AS.
Treatment	CPR, drugs, cardioversion and pacemaker, depending on case.			
Rheumatic heart disease	Results from rheumatic fever that may follow streptococcal infection in childhood. Thought to be an allergic reaction of body to antibodies manufactured to fight streptococci. Months or years later, damage to the heart may become apparent.	Children who are undernourished and living in crowded conditions are more susceptible. Lowered resistance may be involved.	Rheumatic fever: joint pain and fever; transient chorea may occur. Rheumatic heart disease: inflammation of heart, congestive heart failure, and damage to one or more heart valves.	Early antibiotic treatment of any streptococcal infection can prevent rheumatic heart disease.
Treatment	Emphasis is on aggressive treatment of rheumatic fever. Treatment for rheumatic heart disease varies, depending on presenting heart problems.			
Congestive heart failure	Inability of heart to maintain circulation. Usually left, because of damaged left ventricle but may happen in right ventricle. Many causes.	MI, hypertension, mitral or aortic stenosis, and other conditions that weaken heart.	Fatigue, dyspnea, enlarged neck veins, enlarged liver, cold-like symptoms with dry cough; swelling of ankles.	Same as for AS.
Treatment	Bed rest, diuretics to reduce blood volume, digitalis to strengthen myocardial contractility, vasodilators to increase cardiac output—use depending on patient condition. Once heart failure is treated, underlying cause is sought, treated.			
Thrombophlebitis	Inflammation of a vein accompanied by formation of a thrombus. Most often occurs in a leg. Involvement of deeper veins more serious—may lead to embolism, which can travel to lungs and be fatal.	Many factors—anything causing a change in lining of vein. May result from surgery, childbirth, obesity, heredity, aging, excessive platelets, overproduction of fibrinogen, oral contraceptives, prolonged bed rest.	Heat, pain, swelling, redness, tenderness and hardness along length of vein. Possible pain, fever, chills, malaise, and cyanosis for deep vein.	Same as for AS.
Treatment	Bed rest with leg or arm elevated. Anticoagulants, antiinflammatory drugs, moist soaks, and antiembolism stockings may also be prescribed.			

SUMMARY TABLE Cardiovascular disease—cont'd

Disease	Special Characteristics	Predisposing Factors	Common Symptoms	Prevention/ Control
Varicose veins	Accumulation of blood in veins because of defective valves. Most often in legs but may be rectal (hemorrhoids).	Heredity, prolonged standing, varied amounts of pressure (hemorrhoids), pregnancy.	May be none; dull aching, fatigability, pain in feet and ankles, cramps at night.	Same as for AS.
Treatment	Antiembolism stockings, prescribed exercise, rest and elevation of affected leg. Surgery only in severe cases.			
Congenital heart defects	Any heart abnormality present from birth. Include ventricular septal defect, patent ductus arteriosum, atrial septal defect, pulmonary stenosis, coarctation of aorta, aortic stenosis, tetralogy of Fallot. Most occur during first trimester.	Cause unknown in over 90% of cases. Possible genetic and environmental. (Conditions affecting mother, e.g. rubella, drinking, age.)	Depend on type of defect—cyanosis, easy tiring. May be none until adult; may be found during surgery for other heart disease.	Keeping pregnant women as healthy as possible would help; until cause is identified, defects will continue to occur.
Treatment	Rest, oxygen, and various drugs may offer relief; if not, surgery may be considered as many effective techniques of correcting congenital heart defects have been developed.			
Cerebrovascular accident (stroke)	Caused by sudden impairment of circulation in one or more blood vessels supplying the brain; three types: TIA, progressive, and completed. Third most common cause of death in United States.	Same as for AS plus history of TIAs, gout, postural hypotension.	May be none. Generally sudden unconsciousness, heavy breathing, unequal pupil size, paralysis on one side, sweaty skin, speech disturbances. Can be more gradual with headache, vomiting, mental impairment, convulsions, fever, disorientation.	Same as for AS.
Treatment	Anticonvulsants, stool softeners, corticosteroids, and analgesics. Surgery if necessary to improve circulation.			

QUESTIONS FOR REVIEW

1. What caused the change in emphasis from infectious to noninfectious disease?
2. What route does the blood take in circulating through the heart?
3. What is the pathway for the electrical impulses that cause the heart to beat?
4. What are the possible causes of heart block?
5. What treatment is there for heart block?

6. What is AS?
7. Which arteries are most frequently affected by AS?
8. What is the reaction-to-injury theory of atherogenesis?
9. What are the end results of uncontrolled AS?
10. Which risk factors for AS can and cannot be changed?
11. What is the connection between AS and cholesterol?
12. What are the lipoproteins in the blood?
13. How are hypertension, smoking, and diabetes mellitus related to AS?
14. What symptoms may be present in AS?
15. What is the significance of the levels of HDL and LDL in a person's blood?
16. What factors are thought to have a relationship to AS, although more evidence needs to be gathered?
17. What is balloon angioplasty?
18. What is the difference between essential hypertension, secondary hypertension, and malignant hypertension?
19. What damage may occur in the body if a person has untreated hypertension?
20. What are considered safe limits for systolic and diastolic blood pressure readings?
21. What are the risk factors for hypertension?
22. Why do individuals with hypertension often neglect to take their medication?
23. How can blood pressure be lowered without drugs?
24. What is the usual cause of coronary artery disease?
25. What are the symptoms of coronary artery disease?
26. What is the difference between the symptoms of angina and those of a MI?
27. What risk factors are associated with congestive heart failure?
28. Why does rheumatic heart disease occur in some who have had rheumatic fever and not in others?
29. What is the progression from rheumatic fever to rheumatic heart disease?
30. What danger is present when thrombophlebitis occurs in a deep vein?
31. What factors may lead to thrombophlebitis?
32. What factors are associated with varicose veins?
33. What congenital heart defects are covered in this chapter?
34. What might be the cause of each of the heart defects named in response to question 33?
35. What treatments can be used for the heart defects named in response to question 33?
36. What is a CA?
37. What are the risk factors for CA?
38. Why is a transient ischemic attack a significant predisposing factor for a stroke?
39. What measures are used in treatment of stroke?

FURTHER READING

Alberta, Mark J., Christina Bertels and Deborah V. Dawson. "An Analysis of Time of Presentation after Stroke." *Journal of the American Medical Association,* Jan 5, '89, 263:65-68.

"Aspirin and Stroke." *Harvard Medical School Health Letter,* May '90, 15:1-2.

Ayanian, John Z. and Arnold M. Epstein. "Differences in the Use of Procedures between Women and Men Hospitalized for Coronary Heart Disease." *New England Journal of Medicine,* July 25, '91, 325:221-225.

Bailey, L. L. et al. "Bless the Babies: One Hundred Fifteen Late Survivors of Heart Transplantation During the First Year of Life." *Journal of Thoracic Cardiovascular Surgery,* May '93. 105 (5):805-814.

Bandimon, J. J. et al. "Coronary Atherosclerosis. A Multi-factorial Disease." *Circulation,* Mar. '93, 87 (3 Suppl) 113-116.

Barrett-Connor, Elizabeth. "Estrogen and Coronary Heart Disease in Women." *Journal of the American Medical Association,* Apr. 10, '91, 265:1861-1867.

Biller, J. and B. B. Love. "Diabetes and Stroke." *Medical Clinics of North America.* Jan., '93, 77 (1):95-110.

Burke, Laura J. "Bradycardia: When Is It Life Threatening?" *Nursing,* Sept. '88, 10:102-104.

Cohn, Jeffrey P. "Making a Stand against Leg Cramps." *FDA Consumer,* Mar. '88, 22: 12-15.

Colditz, G. A. et al. "Cigarette Smoking and Risk of Stroke in Middle-Aged Women." *New England Journal of Medicine,* Apr. 14, '88, 310:937-941.

Cooper, Gerald R. and Gary L. Mers. "Blood Lipid Measurements: Variations and Practical Utility." *Journal of the American Medical Association,* Mar. 25, '92, 267:1652-1660.

Crawford, Patricia. "The Nutrition Connection: Why Doesn't the Public Know?" *American Journal of Public Health,* Sept. '88, 78:1147-1148.

"Defining, Treating Borderline Hypertension Continues to Challenge Clinicians, Researchers." *Journal of the American Medical Association,* Aug. 14, '91, 266:767-768.

Downey, Anne M. et al. "Heart Smart—A Staff Development Model for a School-Based Cardiovascular Health Intervention." *Health Education,* Apr-May '88, 19:12-20.

Elnicki, M. and T. A. Kotchen. "Hypertension: Patient Evaluation, Indications for Treatment." *Geriatrics,* Apr. '93. 48 (4):47-50, 59-62.

Fackelmann, Kathy. "The African Gene?" *Science News,* Oct. 19, '91, 140:254-255.

Feinstein, A.R. et al. "Changes in Dyspnea-Fatigue Ratings as Indicators of Quality of Life in the Treatment of Congestive Heart Failure." *American Journal of Cardiology,* '89, 64:1, 50-55.

Fiebach, Nicholas H. et al. "Differences between Women and Men in Survival after Myocardial Infarction: Biology or Methodology? *Journal of the American Medical Association,* Feb. 23, '90, 263 (8):1092-1096.

"Final Report on the Aspirin Component of the Ongoing Physicians' Health Study." *New England Journal of Medicine,* Aug. '89, 321:129-135.

Fisher, Elliott S. et al. "Risk of Carotid Endarterectomy in the Elderly." *American Journal of Public Health,* Dec. '89, 79:1617-1620.

Fuster, Valentin et al. "The Pathogenesis of Coronary Artery Disease and the Acute Coronary Syndromes." (First of Two Parts). *New England Journal of Medicine,* Jan. 23, '92, 326:242-250.

Genest, J.J., Jr. et al. "Familial Lipoprotein Disorders in Patients with Premature Coronary Artery Disease." *Circulation,* June '92, 85(6):2025-2033.

Gillman, M.W. and R.C. Ellison. "Childhood Prevention of Essential Hypertension." *Pediatric Clinics of North America,* Feb. '93, 40 (1):179-194.

Goldberg, R.J. et al. "The Impact of Age on the Incidence and Prognosis of Initial Acute Myocardial Infarction: The Worcester Heart Attack Study." *American Heart Journal,* Mar. '89, 117:543-549.

Goldsmith, Marsha. "Lipid Particles May Help Solve Puzzle Regarding Genesis of Some Cardiovascular Diseases." Jan. 15, '92, 267:336-337.

Grundy, S.M. and A.G. Bearn (eds.). *The Role of Cholesterol in Atherosclerosis: New Therapeutic Opportunities,* Philadelphia: Hanley & Belfus, 1988.

Gunby, Phil. "Cardiovascular Diseases Remain Nation's Leading Cause of Death." *Journal of the American Medical Association,* Jan. 15, '92, 267:335-336.

Guthrie, James F. et al. "Tips on Managing Anorectal Disorders." *Patient Care,* Dec. 15, '88, 23:31-38.

Hobson, R.W. II. et al. "Efficacy of Carotid Endarterectomy for Asymptomatic Carotid Stenosis." *New England Journal of Medicine,* Jan. 28, '93, 328 (4):221-227.

Hosking, S.W. et al. "Anorectal Varices, Haemorrhoids, and Portal Hypertension." *Lancet,* Feb. 18, '89, 1:349-352.

Houston, M.C. "New Insights and New Approaches for the Treatment of Essential Hypertension: Selection of Therapy Based on Files, Quality of Life, and Subsets of Hypertension." *American Heart Journal,* Apr. '89, 117:911-951.

"How Can We Prevent Strokes?" *Harvard Medical School Health Letter,* Aug. '89, 14:1-4.

Iles, Christopher G. et al. "Relation between Coronary Risk and Coronary Mortality in Women of the Renfrew and Paisley Survey: Comparison with Men." *Lancet,* Mar. 21, '92, 39 (895):702-706.

Iso, Hiroyasu et al. "Serum Cholesterol Levels and Six-Year Mortality from Stroke in 350,977 Men Screened for the Multiple Risk Factor Intervention Trial." *New England Journal of Medicine,* Apr. 6, '89, 320:904-910.

Jessup, Mariell. "Managing Congestive Heart Failure." *Geriatrics,* 1988, 43:11, 35-42.

Kamberg, Mary Lane. "Stroke: The Brain Disrupted." *Current Health 2,* Feb. '89, 15:3-9.

Kannel, D. "Hypertension: Impact of Risk Factors." *Consultant,* 1988, 20:104.

Kereiakes, D.J. et al. "Favorable Early and Long-Term Prognosis following Coronary Bypass Surgery Therapy for Myocardial Infarction: Results of a Multicenter Trial." *American Heart Journal,* 1989,118:199.

Kritz-Silverstein, Donna, Deborah L. Wingard, and Elizabeth Barrett Connor. "Employment Status and Heart Disease Risk Factors in Middle-Aged Women: The Rancho Bernardo Study." *American Journal of Public Health,* Feb. '92, 82:215-219.

Kulbertus, H.E. "Treatment of Congestive Heart Failure: Pharmacological Principles." *Cardiology,* 1988, 75:Suppl. 1.

Lerman, Amir et al. "Circulating and Tissue Endothelin Immunoreactivity in Advanced Atherosclerosis." *New England Journal of Medicine,* Oct. 3, '91, 325:997-1001.

Lerner, D.J. and W.B. Kannel. "Patterns of Coronary Heart Disease, Morbidity, and Mortality in the Sexes: A 26-Year Follow-up of the Framingham Population." *American Heart Journal,* 1986, 111:383.

Mack, Wendy J. and David H. Blankenhorn. "Factors Influencing the Formation of New Human Coronary Lesions: Age, Blood Pressure, and Blood Cholesterol." *American Journal of Public Health,* Sept. '91, 81:1180-1184.

MacMahon, Stephen et al. "Blood Pressure, Stroke, and Coronary Heart Disease: Part 1, Prolonged Differences in Blood Pressure: Prospective Observational Studies Corrected for the Regression Dilution Bias." *Lancet,* Mar. 31, '90, 335:765-774.

McCallum, Jack. "The Cruelest Thing Ever." *Sports Illustrated,* June 30, '86, 64:20-24.

Oliver, Gregory C. "Colon and Rectal Surgery." *Journal of the American Medical Association,* May 19, '89, 261:2833-2834.

Orencia, A. et al. "Effect of Gender on Long-term Outcome of Angina Pectoris and Myocardial Infarction / Sudden Unexpected Death." *Journal of the American Medical Association,* May 12, '93, 269 (18):2392-2397.

Palca, Joseph. "Getting to the Heart of the Cholesterol Debate." *Science,* 1988, 247:1170.

Peele, S. "The Conflict between Public Health Goals and the Temperance Mentality." *American Journal of Public Health,* June '93, 83 (6):805-810.

Pfeffer, M.A., J.M. Pfeffer and G.A. Lamas. "Development and Prevention of Congestive Heart Failure Following Myocardial Infarction." *Circulation,* May '93, 87 (5 Suppl): IV120-125.

Pollner, Fran. "Rethinking Cholesterol." *Harvard Health Letter,* June '92, 17:6-9.

"Preliminary Report of the Stroke Prevention in Atrial Fibrillation Study." *New England Journal of Medicine,* Mar. 22, '90, 322:863-868.

"Progress against Mortality from Stroke." *Statistical Bulletin,* Apr.-June '89, 70:18-28.

"Psychosocial Influences on Mortality of Patients with Coronary Heart Disease." (Editorial) *Journal of the American Medical Association,* Jan. 22/29, '92, 267:559-560.

Rader, Daniel J. and H. Bryan Brewer, Jr. "Lipoprotein(a): Clinical Approach to a Unique Atherogenic Lipoprotein." *Journal of the American Medical Association,* Feb. 26, '92, 267:1109-1112.

Razay, G. et al. "Alcohol Consumption and Its Relation to Cardiovascular Risk Factors in British Women." *British Medical Journal,* Jan. 11, '92, 304 (6819):80-83.

Reed, D. "Which Risk Factors Are Associated with Atherosclerosis?" *Circulation,* Mar. '93, 87 (3 suppl):1154-1155.

Regnstrom, Jan and Jan Nilsson, et al. "Susceptibility to Low-Density Lipoprotein Oxidation and Coronary Atherosclerosis in Man." *Lancet,* May 16, '92, 339:1183-1186.

Robinson, K. et al. "When Does the Risk of Acute Coronary Heart Disease in Ex-Smokers Fall to That in Non-Smokers? A Retrospective Study of Patients Admitted to Hospital with a First Episode of Myocardial Infarction or Unstable Angina." *British Heart Journal,* July 16, '89, 62:1.

Rocchini, A.P. "Adolescent Obesity and Hypertension." *Pediatric Clinics of North America,* Feb. '93, 40 (1):81-92.

Rocella, Edward J. "The Good News about Hypertension." *Statistical Bulletin,* 1988, 70:20.

Scanu, A.M. "Lipoprotein (a)—A potential Bridge between the Fields of Atherosclerosis and Thrombosis." *Archives of Pathology and Laboratory Medicine,* 1988, 112:1045.

Sempos, Christopher et al. "Divergence of the Recent Trends in Coronary Mortality for the Four Major Race Sex Groups in the United States." *American Journal of Public Health,* 1988, 70:1422.

"Sounding Out Clots." *Harvard Medical School Health Letter,* Jan. '90, 15:2-3.

Stamler, Rose et al. "Primary Prevention of Hypertension by Nutritional Hygienic Means." *Journal of the American Medical Association,* Oct. 6, '89, 262:1801-1807.

Stampfer, Meir J. et al. "A Prospective Study of Moderate Alcohol Consumption and the Risk of Coronary Disease and Stroke in Women." *New England Journal of Medicine,* Aug. 4, '88, 319:267-273.

Stampfer, Meir J. et al. "Postmenopausal Estrogen Therapy and Cardiovascular Disease." *New England Journal of Medicine,* Sept. 12, '91, 325:756-762.

Steinberg, Daniel and Joseph L. Witztum. "Lipoproteins and Atherogenesis." *Journal of the American Medical Association,* Dec. 19, '90, 264:3047-3052.

Steinberg, Daniel et al. "Beyond Cholesterol." *New England Journal of Medicine,* Apr. 6, '89, 320:915-924.

Tolman, Jayne. "Dietary Control of Hypertension: What Should We Be Teaching?" *Health Education,* Oct./Nov. '88, 19:61-63.

Weber, M.A. "Hypertension as a Risk Factor Syndrome: Therapeutic Implications." *American Journal of Medicine,* Apr. 23, '93. 94 (4A):24S-31S.

Williams, Daniel P. "Body Fatness and Risk for Elevated Blood Pressure, Total Cholesterol, and Serum Lipoprotein Ratios in Children and Adolescents." *American Journal of Public Health,* Mar. '92, 82:358-363.

Williams, Redford B. et al. "Prognostic Importance of Social and Economic Resources among Medically Treated Patients with Angiographically Documented Coronary Artery Disease." *Journal of the American Medical Association,* Jan. 22/29, '92, 267:520-524.

Wing, Steve et al. "Geographic and Socioeconomic Variation in the Onset of Decline of Coronary Heart Disease Mortality in White Women." *American Journal of Public Health,* Feb. '92, 82:204-209.

Wong, N.D. et al. "Risk Factors for Long-Term Coronary Prognosis after Initial Myocardial Infarction: The Framingham Study." *American Journal of Epidemiology,* Sept. '89, 130(3):469-480.

Yeater, R.A. "Hypertension and Exercise: Where Do We Stand?" *Post Graduate Medicine,* Apr. '92. 91 (5):429-436.

Chapter *13*

Cancers with the Highest Fatality Rates

O B J E C T I V E S

1 Define the term *cancer*.

2 State the difference between a benign tumor or neoplasm and a malignant tumor or neoplasm.

3 Define common terminology used to describe cancer.

4 Explain the theory of oncogenesis.

5 Identify five ways in which cancer cells differ from normal cells.

6 Identify five risk factors for cancer.

7 Explain the role of pain in cancer.

8 Identify means of primary and secondary prevention for cancer.

9 State the traditional methods for treating cancer.

10 Describe three newer methods of treating cancer.

11 Explain why lung cancer is increasing although smoking rates have dropped.

12 State possible reasons for the high rate of colorectal cancer in the United States.

13 Distinguish among the four types of mastectomy.

14 State the factors that have been found to be linked to breast cancer in women.

15 Distinguish between Hodgkin's disease and non-Hodgkin's lymphoma.

16 Explain the difference in rate of stomach cancer between Japanese and Americans.

17 Describe and identify predisposing factors, symptoms, prevention, and treatment for the cancers in this chapter.

INTRODUCTION

Cancer is the second leading cause of death in the United States. It is estimated that one out of three Americans alive today will develop cancer, and over half a million are expected to die in 1993 of cancer* (Table 13-1). Our increased longevity has led to an increased incidence of cancer and other disorders that are more common among older adults. But cancer is also a leading cause of death in children, second only to accidental death. Table 13-2 lists various cancer sites and their relationship to age.

Cancer is not one but many different diseases characterized by an uncontrolled growth and spread of cells. Although it may seem at times that no progress has been made against this dreaded disease, there has been a gain in the survival rate when all cancers are considered together. In the early 1900s, a diagnosis of cancer was believed to be a death sentence, and in those days it usually was, since many cancer patients had little hope of survival. During the years since the beginning of the century, advances have been made slowly but surely, and today, the overall survival rate for cancer is 50%. Cancer statistics are generally based on information that is at least 5 years old and for this reason do not reflect the recent advances in treatment and lifestyle changes. Even though the number of deaths from lung cancer is still increasing, it should start to decrease as more and more people stop smoking and as other carcinogens are identified and removed from the environment.

CANCER TERMINOLOGY

People often believe that the words *neoplasm* and *tumor* are synonymous with cancer, but that is not the case. *Neoplasm* literally means a "new thing formed," and the

---

*Statistics are from the American Cancer Society's *Cancer Facts and Figures—1993,* unless otherwise indicated.

TABLE 13-1 Estimated new cancer cases and deaths for 1993 (according to fatality rate)

Site	Cases	Rank	Deaths	Rank	Survival Rate (%) Local	Distant
Lung	170,000	2	149,000	1	46	01
Colorectal	152,000	3	57,000	2	89	06
Breast	183,000	4	46,300	3	93	18
Prostate	165,000	5	35,000	4	91	28
Pancreas	27,700	10	25,000	5	08	01
Lymph tissues		7		6		
Hodgkin's,	7,900		1,500		—	—
non-Hodgkin's lymphoma	43,000		20,500		—	—
Stomach	24,000	12	13,600	7	—	—
Leukemia		13		8		
Lymphocytic	12,600		5,400		—	—
and granulocytic	11,700		7,300		—	—
Ovary	22,000	14	13,300	9	89	18
Liver and biliary ducts	15,800	16	12,600	10	—	—
Brain and CNS	17,500	15	12,100	11	—	—
Kidney and other urinary	27,200	11	10,900	12	85	09
Esophagus	11,300	20	10,200	13	—	—
Uterus and unspecified	31,000	8	5,700	14	94	26
Cervix	13,500		4,400		89	14
Bladder	52,300	6	9,900	15	90	09
Multiple myeloma	12,800	17	9,400	16	—	—
Skin		1		17		
Melanoma	32,000		6,800		90	14
Basal and squamous cell	700,000		2,300		—	—
Oral (lip, tongue, mouth,	20,600	9	3,900	18		
pharynx)	9,200		3,800		76	19
Larynx	12,600	19	3,800	19	—	—
Bone	2,000	21	1,050	20	—	—
Thyroid	12,700	18	1,050	21	—	—
Testis	6,600	22	350	22	—	—

Adapted from figures in the American Cancer Society: *Cancer Facts and Figures—1993.*

word *tumor* means "a swelling." Both words are used when referring to cancer, but unless the word *malignant* ("a bad kind") is used with them, it is not cancer. The term *benign* ("a good kind") is used to indicate a noncancerous growth. Figure 13-1 shows *A,* benign, and *B,* malignant growths.

In one sense, benign neoplasms or tumors may not be good at all. They are only good because they are not malignant. However, benign tumors do continue to grow and, depending upon their location, can cause pain and damage. Like malignant tumors, benign tumors can also cause death if they are in an inoperable location. A malignant neoplasm or tumor does mean cancer, but it does not mean certain death.

One main difference between benign tumors and malignant tumors is that malignant tumors metastasize (spread) through the circulatory and lymphatic systems and invade surrounding tissue (Figure 13-2). Benign tumors are generally encapsulated and do not spread to other parts of the body, although a benign tumor occasionally may turn into a malignant tumor.

TABLE 13-2 Cancer sites and relationships to age

Cancer Site	Relationship to Age
Respiratory system	Among men, rates exceptionally high at ages 45-64 years compared with other cancers; in both sexes rates increase with age through 65-74 years
Digestive system	Low rates under 45 years; large increases extend through very advanced ages
Breast (female)	Rates highest of all cancers among women at ages 25-54 years
Male genital organs	High rates at ages 64 and over; large increases with age among older men
Female genital organs	Rates are significant at ages 35-54, but rate increases into older ages
Urinary organs	Very low rates under age 55 years; large increases through advanced ages
Leukemia	Compared with other cancers in children, a significant rate, but still a low rate; marked increases in rate starting at 35-44 years
Other lymph and blood tissues	Rare among children and young adults; age gradient starts in middle adult years

From Shapiro, 1983.

FIGURE 13-1 Diagram of benign versus malignant growth. **A,** A "typical" benign neoplasm is cohesive, expands from the center, has a smooth border, and is often encapsulated. **B,** A malignant neoplasm is less cohesive, has an irregular border, and invades adjacent tissue. Malignant cells are also capable of metastasis *(dotted arrow).*

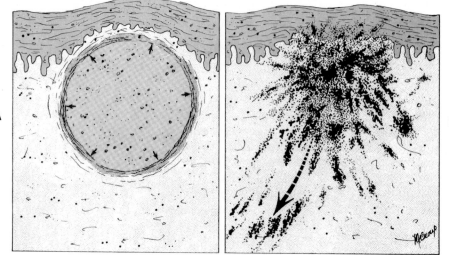

FIGURE 13-2   A, How cancer spreads. Movement of cells is integral to the entire process of metastasis. **B,** Scientists have identified a protein that causes cancer cells to grow arms, or pseudopodia, enabling them to begin to move to other parts of the body.

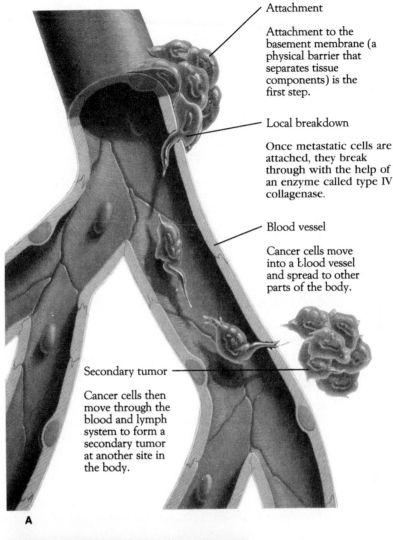

Attachment

Attachment to the basement membrane (a physical barrier that separates tissue components) is the first step.

Local breakdown

Once metastatic cells are attached, they break through with the help of an enzyme called type IV collagenase.

Blood vessel

Cancer cells move into a blood vessel and spread to other parts of the body.

Secondary tumor

Cancer cells then move through the blood and lymph system to form a secondary tumor at another site in the body.

A

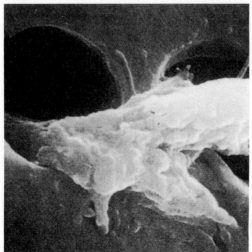

B

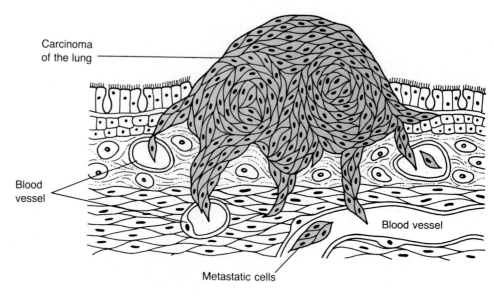

Carcinoma of the lung

Blood vessel

Blood vessel

Metastatic cells

FIGURE 13-3 Portrait of a cancer. The ball of cells is a carcinoma, developing from epithelial cells lining the interior surface of a human lung. Unless destroyed by the immune system, the mass of cells grows, invading surrounding tissues, eventually penetrating into lymphatic vessels and blood vessels, both of which are plentiful within the lung. These vessels carry metastatic cancer cells.

IDENTIFICATION OF CANCER BY TISSUE

Malignancies may be classified by the tissue in which they occur or by location and sometimes both, as in osteosarcoma (occurring in the bone). The following terms are used to identify cancers according to the tissue in which they occur.

CARCINOMA—EPITHELIUM

Carcinoma arises from the epithelial tissue that forms the outer surface of the body and lines the body cavities and principal tubes and passageways leading to the exterior. About 85% of all tumors occur in epithelial tissue. A drawing of a cancer is shown in Figure 13-3.

SARCOMA—CONNECTIVE TISSUE

Sarcoma arises from connective tissue cells such as those found in bone, cartilage, and tendons. Only 2% of malignant tumors are of this type.

MELANOMA—SKIN CELLS WITH MELANIN

Melanoma arises from the melanin-containing cells of the skin. This type of cancer has been rare, but it is becoming more common.

NEUROBLASTOMA—CNS

Neuroblastoma originates in immature cells of the central nervous system (CNS). A rare form of cancer, it is found mostly in children.

ADENOCARCINOMA—DUAL CONNECTION

Adenocarcinoma derives from cells from both the epithelium and endocrine glands.

HEPATOMA—LIVER

Hepatoma originates in cells of the liver; mortality is high.

LEUKEMIA—BLOOD CELLS

Leukemia is malignant growth of white blood cells and blood-forming tissue cells.

TABLE 13-3 Cancer staging—the TNM system*

T = Primary Tumor

T0	No evidence of a primary tumor
Tx	Evidence of tumor in some tests but unable to assess because of location, type, etc.
TIS	Tumor in situ (localized)
T1–T4	Increasing degrees of size and involvement

N = Nodal Involvement

N0	No lymph node involvement
N1–N3	Increasing number and range of lymph nodes
Nx	Unable to assess lymph node involvement

M = Metastases

M0	No evidence of metastases to distant points
M1–M3	Increasing degrees of metastases, including some to distant nodes

*Staging varies for each specific form of cancer, but these are general principles.

There are many forms of leukemia, and they are classified by the dominant cell type. Leukemia occurs in both children and adults.

LYMPHOMA—LYMPHATIC, OTHER IMMUNE SYSTEM TISSUES

Lymphoma is malignant growth of cells in the lymphatic tissues or other immune system tissues.

GRADING AND STAGING

The terms used in classifying tumors are grading and staging. In grading, the tumor cells are classified by grades I to IV, depending on their degree of difference from normal cells and growth rate. Because cancer cells tend to differ in different cancers and even in the same cancer, this system has not been as useful as staging.

Staging is often done by the TNM system (Table 13-3) and is used to quantify the extent of the cancer. The staging system allows oncologists (physicians who specialize in treating cancer) to discuss patient needs for various types of therapy according to the characteristics of the specific case.

CANCER CELLS

New cells are being produced constantly in each of us. Each cell has a prescribed function, but in the case of cancer, something happens and the cell does not develop in the expected manner. Cancer research today is zeroing in on these "lawless" cells and the genes that may cause their development. A current theory is that within each cell there are a number of protooncogenes, which, if altered, could cause the development of oncogenes, which in turn activate the development of cancer cells. It is thought that carcinogenic (cancer-causing) substances may convert the protooncogenes into oncogenes. There will have to be a more thorough understanding of cell development and regulation before we determine whether or not this theory is true.

Cancer cells differ from normal cells in a number of ways. Some of those ways are:

They are less likely to survive than normal cells because they lack the machinery necessary to sustain life.

They have higher nutrient demands since they are unable to make their own food.

They lack cellular cohesiveness. They do adhere to each other to some extent, but it is easier for them to break off and travel.

They grow and reproduce at an abnormal rate. Normal cells multiply by dividing into two cells, which are each capable of reproducing themselves; cancer cells may divide into three, four, or five different cells in a haphazard way.

They lack contact inhibition. They do not know when to stop growing as normal cells do.

PREDISPOSING FACTORS

Even though the search for the cause and a cure for malignant growths has produced no final answers, we do know many predisposing factors related to cancer, and many carcinogenic substances have been identified in the environment. The best prevention at present lies in avoidance or elimination of these factors and carcinogens in our lives whenever possible. Some genetic factors may increase susceptibility to

---

CONTEMPORARY CONCERNS

Heredity and Cancer

A few cancers tend to run in families. Although no gene has been identified that passes on cancer, it is believed that something inherited makes persons more susceptible to certain cancers when they are subjected to the right environmental stimuli.

If close relatives had breast cancer, a woman's risk is greater, but women need to remember that 75% of those who get breast cancer have no family history of the disease. It is therefore important for women to perform self-exams at least once a month and have mammograms.

Researchers now recognize a genetic factor in prostate cancer. A man's chances increase with the closeness and number of relatives who have had it. Men who know of relatives who have had or have prostatic cancer need to learn what screening tests are available and at what ages to have them.

Only 5% of ovarian cancers are thought to have a genetic relationship. However, the cancer is so deadly that physicians pay close attention to any woman with a family history of the disease.

People with one or two first-degree relatives who have or have had cancer of the colon have a risk that is two to four times higher than those who don't. Physicians should be informed, and strict adherence to screening procedures should be adopted.

Factors That May Increase Susceptibility to Cancer

Heredity. If cancer is prevalent in the family history, tests for early detection should be performed at recommended ages and intervals.

Occupation. Certain occupations bring employees into contact with carcinogenic agents and should be avoided. Possible occupational exposures to cancer are shown in Table 13-4.

Tobacco Use. Tobacco use can lead to cancer of the mouth and lungs. It is believed that the carcinogens in tobacco tar may be responsible for other forms of cancer.

Diet. The American Cancer Society makes the following recommendations on diet:
- Avoid obesity.
- Reduce total fat intake.
- Eat more high-fiber foods.
- Include foods rich in vitamins A and C in your daily diet.
- Include cruciferous vegetables (broccoli, cabbage, kale, etc.) in your diet.
- Avoid smoked, salt-cured, and nitrate-cured foods.
- Limit alcohol to moderate consumption.

Sun exposure. Ultraviolet (UV) radiation from the sun or tanning beds can trigger cancer, particularly for people with light complexions. Using a sunscreen may help, but it does not always prevent cancer.

cancer. Although these cannot be changed, being aware of them can lead to earlier detection and thus increase the chances of surviving cancer. (See box above.) Scientists believe that most, if not all, cancer can be cured if caught in the early stages.

Symptoms Many associate cancer with pain, but in cancer, pain does not usually occur until the later stages. Approximately 20% to 40% of cancer patients have no pain at all. The amount of pain, the time of onset, and the severity all differ, depending upon the location and size of the cancer and its pattern of growth. For example, a tumor located in the brain has very little space to grow before it compresses nerves and blood vessels. Individuals with cancer become more susceptible to infections, which can also cause pain. Cancer patients also tend to lose interest in eating and may be nauseous because of chemotherapy. For this reason, they become malnourished and lose weight. Most patients also have a mild anemia.

Primary Prevention The best prevention is a healthy lifestyle and avoidance of environmental carcinogens and the other risk factors associated with cancer (Table 13-4). No smoking, a varied diet, moderation in alcohol (if at all) and staying out of the sun or using a sunscreen are all preventive measures.

Secondary Prevention For the most part, secondary prevention measures will be dealt with as each type of cancer is discussed. In general, it is important that everyone know cancer's seven warning signals, developed by the American Cancer Society (ACS). They are

TABLE 13-4 Occupational exposures and cancer

Cancer Sites (Causal Agent)	Work or Exposure
Lung	
Bischloro-methylether	Ion exchange resins producers
Chromium	Ore and pigment manufacturers
Mustard gas	Poison gas producers
Lung, pleura (asbestos)	Asbestos, insulation; miners, shipyard workers
Lung and skin (arsenic)	Smelter and pesticide workers
Lung and nasal (nickel)	Nickel refiners
Lung and skin (polycyclic hydrocarbons)	Mineral oil and tar workers
Skin (ultraviolet [UV] light)	Outdoor workers; fishing
Liver	
Vinyl chloride	Vinyl chloride workers
Alcohol	Brewery workers
Bladder	
Aromatic amines	Dye and rubber workers
Leukemia	
Benzene	Glue and varnish workers
Nasal	
Isopropyl alcohol	Isopropyl alcohol manufacturers
Wood dust	Furniture workers
Multiple sites	
Ionizing radiation	Radium dial painters, uranium miners

Adapted from American Cancer Society, 1986.

1. **C** hange in bowel or bladder habits
2. **A** sore that does not heal
3. **U** nusual bleeding or discharge
4. **T** hickening or lump in breast or elsewhere
5. **I** ndigestion or difficulty in swallowing
6. **O** bvious change in a wart or mole
7. **N** agging cough or hoarseness

If any of these lasts more than 5 days, a doctor should be consulted immediately.

Treatment Traditional treatments for cancer include surgery, chemotherapy, radiation, hormones, or a combination of these. Table 13-5 gives some examples of treatment for selected sites.

Researchers are working all the time to find better methods of treating cancer. One area of study is based on the belief that cancer cells have the ability to inactivate the immune system. The drug interleukin-2 is one that has been used to boost the immune system and produce more "killer" cells. It has been effective against some forms of cancer when the usual therapy has not been effective. However, there have been severe side effects associated with this drug.

Researchers are also working with monoclonal antibodies to strengthen the

TABLE 13-5 Examples of treatment of site-specific cancers

Usual Treatment	Site
Surgery	Colon Breast Ovary Lung Thyroid Skin Uterus
Chemotherapy	Lymphoma Leukemia Choriocarcinoma Ovary Breast
Radiation	Breast (all have been combined with surgery) Uterus or cervix Lymphomas Lung Combined with surgery in many sites.
Hormones	Breast Prostate Endometrium

Adapted from King, Fenoglio, & Lefkowitch, 1983.

immune response. The idea is for these "clones" of antibodies to carry toxic substances to cancer cells and destroy them much as the antibodies that our bodies produce destroy pathogenic organisms. The problem comes in producing monoclonal antibodies that will be attracted only to cancer cells and attaching a chemical to them that will destroy cancer cells while leaving normal cells unharmed. Monoclonal antibody treatment for cancer has recently been approved for human trials.

Among the less "scientifically" oriented forms of therapy is the emphasis on the mind-body connection. Most doctors now agree that patients' attitude can make a significant difference in their recovery. One physician who has investigated this area is Dr. Bernie Siegel, a surgeon in the eastern United States who has operated on thousands of cancer patients. He began to wonder not about cancer causation but about why some people considered to be terminally ill somehow survived. Dr. Siegel founded a group called E-Cap (an acronym for exceptional cancer patients).

The group soon branched into many groups in many parts of the country. In these groups, newly diagnosed cancer patients are joined by "survivors" who talk about their experiences and encourage the others to express their feelings. Dr. Siegel found that those who survived took their diagnosis as a challenge and had the attitude "I can beat this" rather than accepting it as a death sentence. He believes that patients should use traditional cancer treatments but also attend these groups. Although group leaders think that the groups are beneficial, it would be difficult to prove the benefits of group therapy for cancer because having a control group is not feasible (who could withhold beneficial treatment from a cancer patient?).

SUMMARY OF BASIC INFORMATION ON CANCER

Cancer is the second leading cause of death in the United States. However, cancer is many diseases, not just one. Overall survival rates have increased, and by 1993 one half of those diagnosed with cancer were cured. A number of different words and terms are used to describe cancer, its location, and its severity or spread. These developed so that physicians specializing in cancer (oncologists) could discuss patient needs for treatment.

Cancer cells differ from other cells: they (1) are less likely to survive, (2) have a higher nutrient demand, (3) lack cellular cohesiveness, (4) grow and reproduce at a different rate, and (5) lack contact inhibition.

Heredity, occupation, tobacco use, diet, and sun exposure are some factors that have been linked to cancer. For many people with cancer, there is no pain, and if pain does occur, the cancer is generally in a late stage.

Primary prevention of cancer is based on reducing or eliminating risk factors. Secondary prevention involves identifying high-risk groups, screening, visiting a

FIGURE 13-4 Nine deadliest cancers.

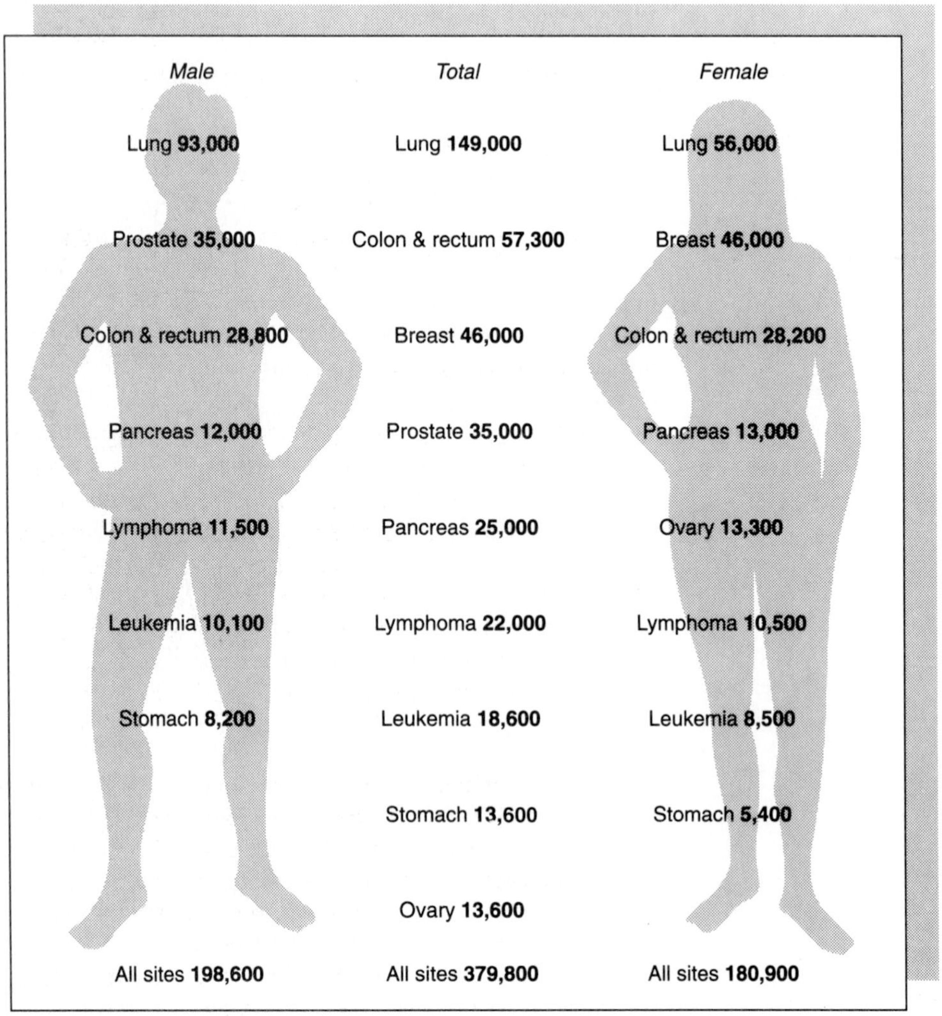

Male	Total	Female
Lung **93,000**	Lung **149,000**	Lung **56,000**
Prostate **35,000**	Colon & rectum **57,300**	Breast **46,000**
Colon & rectum **28,800**	Breast **46,000**	Colon & rectum **28,200**
Pancreas **12,000**	Prostate **35,000**	Pancreas **13,000**
Lymphoma **11,500**	Pancreas **25,000**	Ovary **13,300**
Leukemia **10,100**	Lymphoma **22,000**	Lymphoma **10,500**
Stomach **8,200**	Leukemia **18,600**	Leukemia **8,500**
	Stomach **13,600**	Stomach **5,400**
	Ovary **13,600**	
All sites **198,600**	All sites **379,800**	All sites **180,900**

doctor if an individual has any of the seven warning signs of cancer, and following guidelines for diagnostic tests for detecting various types of cancer.

The traditional treatments for cancer are surgery, radiation, and chemotherapy, used singly or in combination. New drugs and other methods for treating cancer are being developed. They include boosting the immune system, monoclonal antibodies, emphasis on the mind–body connection, and group therapy.

THE DEADLIEST CANCERS

Of all the diseases labeled with the dreaded name of cancer, nine have earned the epithet deadliest (Figure 13-4). The reasons range from difficulty of detection, as with ovarian cancer, to resistance to treatment, as with pancreatic cancer. A clinical description and prognosis for each cancer, the predisposing factors, symptoms, prevention measures, and treatment are discussed.

LUNG CANCER

Cancer of the lungs has become the most common killing cancer for both sexes, with 170,000 new cases and 149,000 deaths estimated for 1993. In the past, there were more cases in men than women, who are catching up quickly; lung cancer now exceeds breast cancer in deaths among women. Figure 13-5 shows a steady increase in deaths for both sexes over a 30-year period. The cancer usually develops in the walls of the bronchial tubes and may appear as an ulcer, nodule, or small flattened lump, or on the surface, blocking air tubes. It may also invade the surface of the tubes and extend to lymphatics and blood vessels (Figure 13-6). The prognosis is poor, with a 5-year survival rate of 46% when the cancer is still localized but less than 1% if the cancer has spread to distant sites. Unfortunately, only 16% of lung cancers are discovered in the early stage.

Predisposing Factors   Of those who develop lung cancer, 83% are smokers, and the chances for persons who smoke to get lung cancer increase with the number of years they have been smoking and the number of cigarettes they smoke per day. There are also carcinogenic agents that many of us are exposed to, such as automobile exhaust gases,

FIGURE 13-5 Thirty-year trends in age-adjusted death rates from lung cancer per 100,000 population— 1957-59 to 1987-89.

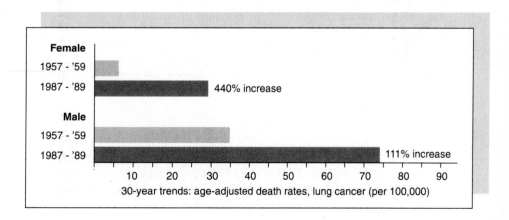

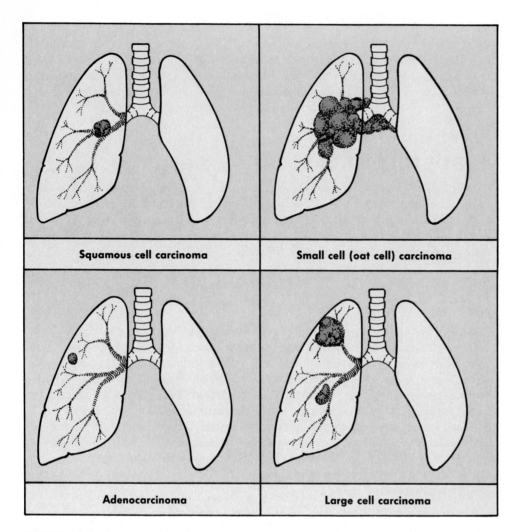

Squamous cell carcinoma

Small cell (oat cell) carcinoma

Adenocarcinoma

Large cell carcinoma

FIGURE 13-6   Common sites of lung cancer.

residential radon gas and radioactive dust, asbestos, sidestream smoke, and other pollutants in the air (Figure 13-7). Persons who are not or who have never been smokers may develop lung cancer if they have a history of long-time exposure to passive and / or sidestream smoke or environmental / occupational hazards other than tobacco smoke. Moreover, smokers exposed to one or more of these other carcinogens are even more likely to develop lung cancer.

Symptoms   In the early stages there are generally no symptoms. Late-stage symptoms include smoker's cough, wheezing, labored or difficult breathing, coughing up of blood, chest pain, fever, weakness, weight loss, and anorexia. Because lung tumors may alter the production of hormones that regulate body function, there may also be gynecomastia and bone and joint pain. Once the cancer has metastasized, there may be other symptoms, depending upon the structures involved.

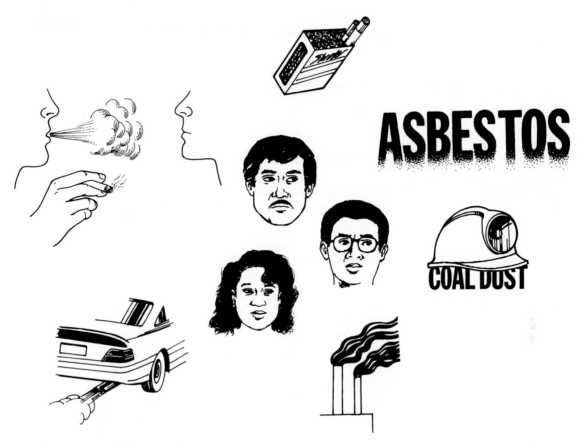

FIGURE 13-7   Risk factors for lung cancer.

Primary Prevention   Cigarette smokers have up to twenty times or even greater risk than nonsmokers of developing lung cancer. If smoking is discontinued, the chances for exsmokers to develop lung cancer quickly approach those of nonsmokers, providing that the cancer process has not already begun before they stop. Persons working in an industrial situation where they are exposed to particulates in the air should be sure proper measures are taken to prevent inhaling them constantly. A relationship between asbestosis and lung cancer has been proved, and it is suspected that exposure to materials in other industries might also increase the risk of lung cancer.

Secondary Prevention   Individuals at high risk for lung cancer should consult their doctors about having a lung X-ray exam during routine physicals. Cancer that shows up in an X-ray film is usually far advanced, but a lesion can still be detected by X ray up to 2 years before symptoms appear. Analysis of the types of cells in the sputum and fiberoptic examination of the bronchial tubes can also aid in detecting lung cancer.

Treatment   Depending upon the stage of the cancer, treatment could be surgery, radiation, chemotherapy, or a combination of these. Several drugs in combination have been

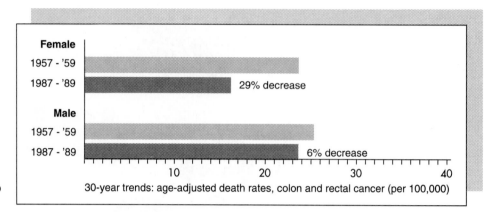

FIGURE 13-8 Thirty-year trends in age-adjusted death rates from colon and rectum cancer per 100,000 population—1957-59 to 1987-89.

found to induce remission in some kinds of lung cancer. Immunotherapy and laser therapy are both being used experimentally.

COLORECTAL CANCER

For the second most common cancer in the United States, colorectal cancer, 152,000 new cases are predicted for 1993, with an estimated 57,000 deaths for the same year. There has been a decrease in colorectal cancer death rates for men and women over a 30-year period (Figure 13-8). Colorectal cancer develops slowly and remains localized for a long time. With improved diagnostic techniques, the 5-year survival rate is now over 91% for colon cancer and 85% for rectal cancer when detected in the localized state. However, there is only 7% survival if distant metastasis is present.

Predisposing Factors   Colorectal cancer is more likely in those with a history of this kind of cancer in the family, polyps in the rectum, and/or ulcerative colitis. The role of diet in the development of colorectal cancer has not been scientifically proved, but there is enough evidence of a relationship between soft diet and cancer of the colon and/or rectum for doctors to advise including as many fresh fruits, vegetables, and whole grains in the diet as possible.

Symptoms   Symptoms of colorectal cancer depend on the location of the tumor, as shown in Figure 13-9.

Primary Prevention   Studies have shown that individuals who are 40% or more overweight run a substantially higher risk of developing colorectal cancer. Maintaining an ideal weight can reduce the risk of cancer as well as other chronic diseases. Although the evidence at this time is not consistent, a number of studies have shown a relationship between high-fat, low-fiber diets and colorectal cancer. Since low-fat, high-fiber diets are recommended by most doctors and prominent groups such as the ACS, it would

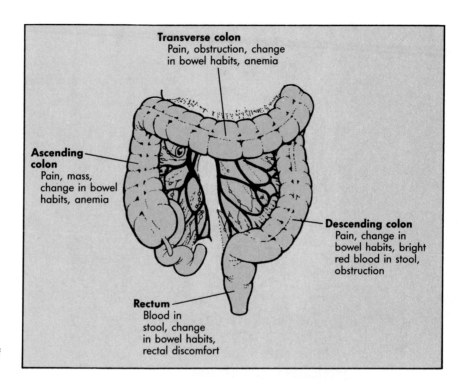

Transverse colon
Pain, obstruction, change
in bowel habits, anemia

Ascending colon
Pain, mass,
change in bowel
habits, anemia

Descending colon
Pain, change in
bowel habits, bright
red blood in stool,
obstruction

Rectum
Blood in
stool, change
in bowel habits,
rectal discomfort

FIGURE 13-9 Sites of colorectal cancers.

be wise to adopt the eating habits that offer the best chance of reducing the risk for colorectal cancer.

Secondary Prevention

Digital examination can detect almost 50% of the tumors in the anus, rectum or lower sigmoid, where over 50% of the tumors occur. The ACS recommends that everyone over 40 should have this exam once a year.

A hemoccult or "hidden blood" test can detect blood in the stools. This test can be performed at home and sent to a lab for diagnosis. The ACS recommends this test be performed annually after age 50.

Proctosigmoidoscopy involves the use of an instrument that can be inserted into the anus, allowing the physician to examine the areas of concern. This examination can detect 50% of all colorectal cancers. The ACS recommends undergoing this examination every 3 to 5 years after the age of 50. Other procedures may be used to confirm the diagnosis or whether there are indications that a problem exists that has not been identified by the above tests. Only a tumor biopsy can verify colorectal cancer.

Treatment

Surgery, sometimes combined with radiation, is the most effective treatment for colorectal cancer, and different procedures are used depending on the location of the tumor. If the surgery requires removal of a part of the colon so that feces cannot travel through the rectum, a **colostomy** may be performed, which involves making an opening in the abdominal wall and attaching a pouch to collect the feces (Figure 13-10).

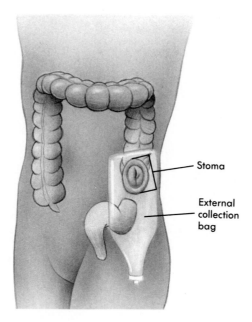

FIGURE 13-10 Colostomy site and pouch.

BREAST CANCER

One in nine women presently living will be diagnosed as having breast cancer. For 1993, 183,000 new cases and 46,300 deaths are estimated, although death rates for men and women increased in the 30-year period shown in Figure 13-11.

Historically, more women have developed breast cancer than any other kind of cancer, and more women have died from breast cancer than any other disease. However, lung cancer has now become the number one killer from cancer for both men and women. Although breast cancer may occur in men, it does so rarely. The distribution of sites for breast cancer is shown in Figure 13-12.

The 5-year survival rate for localized breast cancer has improved from 78% in the 1940s to 93% today because of earlier diagnosis and new treatment methods. If the cancer has spread regionally, the survival rate is 71%. If metastasis has occurred in distant parts of the body, the survival rate is 18%. The disease may develop at

FIGURE 13-11 Thirty-year trends in age-adjusted death rates from breast cancer per 100,000 population— 1957-59 to 1987-89.

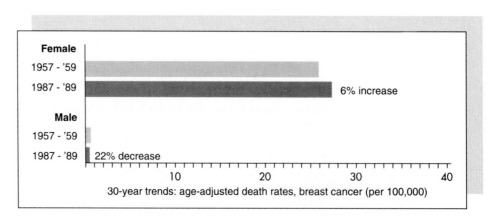

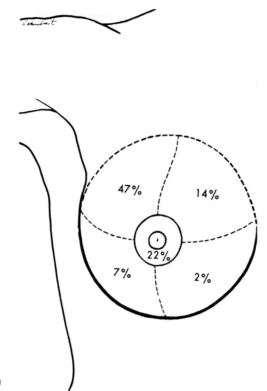

FIGURE 13-12 Distribution of carcinomas in the breast.

any time of life, but it is uncommon before age 35. Breast cancer occurs more often in the left breast than in the right, and 50% occur in the upper outer quadrant. Growth rates can vary. Slow-growing breast cancer can take up to 8 years before it can be detected by self-examination.

Predisposing Factors

There are a number of factors that place a woman at *high risk.* These include:
- A family history of breast cancer
- Long menstrual cycles or early menses
- Late menopause (after age 50)
- First pregnancy after age 30
- History of endometrial, ovarian, or colon cancer
- Higher education and socioeconomic class
- Constant stress or unusual disturbances in home or work life
- Never giving birth, or late age at first live birth
- Obesity (40% above normal)

If a woman has been pregnant before the age of 20, has had multiple pregnancies, is Indian or Asian, and/or is of lower socioeconomic class, she is at a *reduced risk* for developing breast cancer.

Symptoms

A woman is far more likely to discover a sign of breast cancer than her doctor, since she knows her own body better, and by self-examination at least once a month, she can detect changes. A lump or mass in the breast that has not been there before is one sign. Noncancerous cysts often form in women's breasts, but the only way to be certain is to seek a medical diagnosis. A change in breast symmetry or size is suspect, as is a change in skin temperature or color, such as a small warm, hot, or pink spot. Dimpling or sores on the skin need to be investigated, as does any unusual drainage or bloody discharge from the nipple. Scaliness, pain, or tenderness of the nipple may also indicate cancer. Pain should always be reported to the doctor, but it is generally not a sign of breast cancer unless the tumor is advanced.

Primary Prevention

At present it is thought that a high-fat diet may be a factor in the development of breast cancer. Obesity should be avoided. The planning of pregnancies should take the risk factors into consideration. The rest of the risk factors cannot be controlled now, although any woman who is susceptible because of them needs to take all steps possible to prevent cancer.

Secondary Prevention

The ACS recommends the monthly practice of breast self-examination (BSE) by women 20 years and older (Figure 13-13). From ages 20 to 40, a physical examination should be done by a doctor at least every 3 years. A baseline mammogram is recommended for women ages 35 to 39, a mammogram every 1 to 2 years between 40 and 49, and every year after age 50. A mammogram is shown in Figure 13-14.

Treatment

Breast cancer may be treated in a number of ways, depending upon the extent of the cancer. Radiation therapy, chemotherapy, hormone manipulation, or surgery may be used singly or in combination. However, for most breast tumors, surgery would generally be selected, particularly if the tumor has not metastasized to distant locations. Breast reconstruction after surgery for removal of a breast has had good results. There are basically four types of breast surgery or mastectomy. They are:

FIGURE 13-13 Breast self-examination. Breasts can be examined, **1,** in a shower, **2,** in front of a mirror, or **3,** lying down.

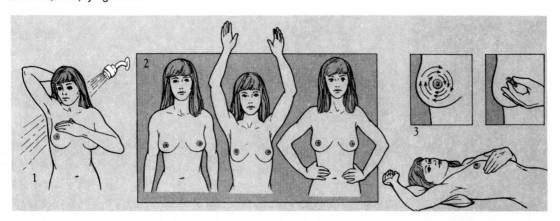

Symptoms

Primary Prevention

Secondary Prevention

Treatment

F

Predisposing Factors

FIGURE 13-17 Thirty-year trends in age-adjusted death rates from pancreatic cancer per 100,000 population—1957-59 to 1987-89.

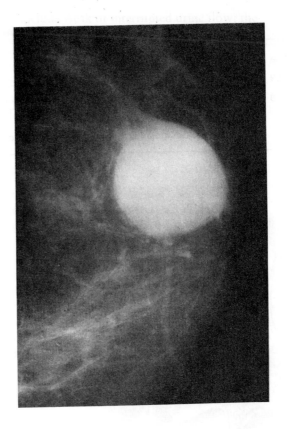

FIGURE 13-14 Mammogram.

1. *Radical mastectomy,* in which the entire affected breast, the chest muscles underneath, and the lymph nodes in the armpit are removed. If there is any chance that the cancer has spread or metastasized, then this procedure is preferred.

2. *Modified radical mastectomy,* in which the entire affected breast and the lymph nodes in the armpit are removed. However, the chest muscles are left intact.

3. *Total or simple mastectomy,* which involves complete removal of the breast but not the lymph nodes or chest muscles.

4. *Partial or segmental mastectomy* (also called lumpectomy or local excision), in which only a portion of the breast is removed, including the cancer and a surrounding portion of breast tissue.

Chemotherapy may be used after surgery to eliminate any remaining cancer cells. Treatment by radiation is sometimes used before or after surgery for additional therapy. Other forms of treatment are used, depending upon the individual case and the woman's response to traditional therapies.

PROSTATE CANCER

Cancer of the prostate is among the top three killers of men, with 165,000 new cases and 35,000 deaths estimated for 1993. About one man in 10 will develop prostate cancer at some time during his life. Better methods of screening and diagnosis have been a factor in the increased incidence. There has been a 17% increase

FIGURE 13-15 Thirty-year trend in age-adjusted death rates for cancer of the prostate—1957-59 to 1987-89.

1!

1!

FIGURE 13-16 Cancer of the prostate.

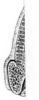

in th
the 5
it is
occu
over

Predisposing Factors

No p
of th
whic
rate
some
influ
facto
wher
since
high-
cance
relati

exposure to certain industrial chemicals, and chronic alcohol abuse have all been implicated by various studies. A recent study at Harvard suggested that drinking two or more cups of coffee a day may also be a cause. Cancer of the pancreas also appears frequently in diabetics.

Symptoms

Early signs are vague and nonspecific. In the later stages jaundice, weight loss, and abdominal or low back pain are the most common symptoms. Fever, skin lesions (usually on the legs), and emotional disturbances may also be present.

Primary Prevention

Eliminating as many of the risk factors as possible is the best course to follow to minimize the chances of pancreatic cancer. The relationship to smoking has become clear-cut. Smokers who develop the disease do so 15 years earlier than those who are nonsmokers. Avoiding the carcinogenic substances that have been linked to pancreatic cancer may provide protection against other cancers also.

Secondary Prevention

There is as yet no method to detect pancreatic cancer before symptoms occur.

Treatment

Surgery, radiation, and chemotherapy may be used but are rarely effective. Different surgical techniques have been tried with little success.

LYMPHATIC CANCER
HODGKIN'S DISEASE

This rare form of cancer involves the tissues of the lymphatic system, mainly in the lymph nodes and spleen. There are 7900 new cases estimated for 1993 and 1500 deaths. The disease occurs more often in people 20 to 40 (average age of 32) and in people between the ages of 55 and 70. It follows a variable but relentlessly progressive course and is ultimately fatal if untreated, but recent advances in treatment make Hodgkin's disease potentially curable even in advanced cases. The overall 5-year survival rate is 77% when diagnosed in the early stages. Figure 13-18 shows the

FIGURE 13-18 Thirty-year trend in Hodgkin's disease—1957-59 to 1987-89.

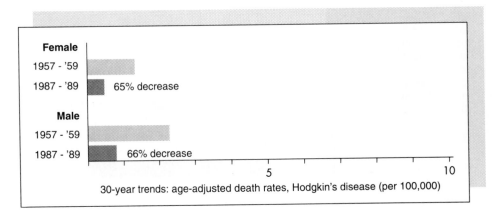

Female

1957 - '59

1987 - '89   65% decrease

Male

1957 - '59

1987 - '89   66% decrease

5   10

30-year trends: age-adjusted death rates, Hodgkin's disease (per 100,000)

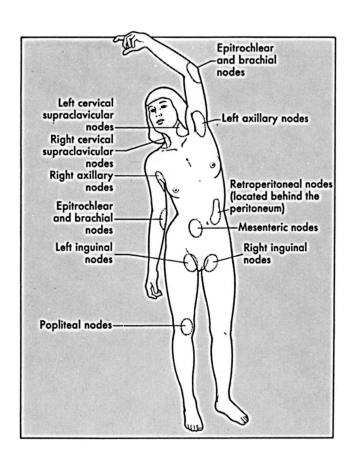

FIGURE 13-19 Sites for Hodgkin's disease.

decrease in death rates that occurred over a 30-year period from 1957-59 to 1987-89. The sites which are involved in Hodgkin's disease are shown in Figure 13-19.

Predisposing Factors   The cause of Hodgkin's disease is unknown.

Symptoms   The first sign is usually a painless enlargement of lymph nodes in the neck or armpits. Most of the other symptoms are due to this enlargement and the invasion of other body organs by the proliferating lymphoid tissue or impairment of the effectiveness of the immune system. These symptoms include a feeling of malaise, fever, loss of appetite, weight loss, night sweats, and itching. Other symptoms may occur, depending on which lymph nodes or organs become involved.

Prevention   Unknown.

Treatment   If the disease is diagnosed in an early stage, radiation may cure it. If it is more advanced and involves many organs, then chemotherapy is usually recommended. Bone marrow transplants and monoclonal antibody treatment are being tested.

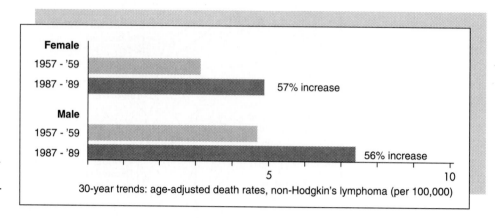

FIGURE 13-20 Thirty-year trend for non-Hodgkin's lymphoma—1957-59 to 1987-89.

NON-HODGKIN'S LYMPHOMA

Any cancer of the lymphoid tissue that is not diagnosed as Hodgkin's disease is referred to as non-Hodgkin's lymphoma. These cancers vary in degree, with some being more dangerous than others, depending on their nature. Figure 13-20 shows a steady increase in death rates from non-Hodgkin's lymphoma from 1957-59 to 1987-89. Forty-three thousand new cases are estimated for 1993, and 20,500 deaths. The peak incidence is higher than that of Hodgkin's disease, with about 25% occurring between the ages of 50 to 59 and the greatest incidence between 60 to 69. The overall 5-year survival rate is 51%.

Predisposing Factors

In most cases, the cause is unknown. Suppression of the immune system, viruses, and chromosomal abnormalities have been suspected. One kind, Burkitt's lymphoma (Figure 13-21), found only in Africa, is thought to be caused by the Epstein-Barr virus, and it is suspected that infection with human immunodeficiency virus (HIV) increases the risk for developing non-Hodgkin's lymphoma. It is also more common in organ transplant patients and other patients with autoimmune diseases such as rheumatoid arthritis and systemic lupus erythematosus.

Symptoms

There is usually a painless swelling of one or more lymph nodes in the groin or neck areas. There may also be enlargement of the liver and spleen. Other symptoms are abdominal pain, intestinal bleeding, and vomiting of blood. When different organs become involved, the symptoms vary. Spread of the disease impairs the immune system, so the patient may die from infections or an uncontrolled spread of other cancers.

Prevention

Unknown.

Treatment

Radiation, chemotherapy, and bone marrow transplants may be used alone or together, depending upon the stage and location of the cancer.

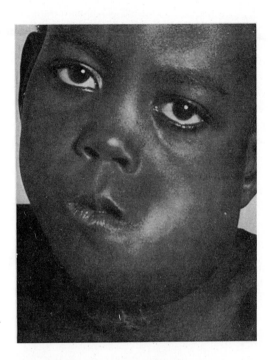

FIGURE 13-21   Burkitt's lymphoma.

STOMACH CANCER

Stomach cancer develops in the lining of the stomach. It is estimated that there will be 24,800 new cases and 13,600 deaths from stomach cancer in 1993. Stomach cancer usually develops after the age of 40 and is twice as common in men as in women. There are geographical variations in incidence, with a very high rate in Japan of 80 to 90 cases per 100,000, compared to less than 10 per 100,000 in the United States. In the last 50 years, the incidence of stomach cancer has shown a dramatic decrease worldwide, but the reason for this is unknown. Figure 13-22 shows the decrease in death rates over a 30-year period in the United States.

Predisposing Factors   The cause of stomach cancer is unknown, but it is thought that diet plays a part, and recent research indicates that *Helicobacter* (formerly *Campylobacter*) bacteria may

FIGURE 13-22   Thirty-year trends in age-adjusted death rates from stomach cancer per 100,000 population—1957-59 to 1987-89.

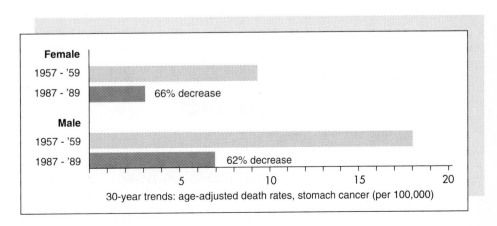

Female
1957 - '59
1987 - '89   66% decrease
Male
1957 - '59
1987 - '89   62% decrease

5   10   15   20

30-year trends: age-adjusted death rates, stomach cancer (per 100,000)

also be involved. Having gastritis, anemia, and belonging to blood group A seem to increase the risk. Eating a great deal of smoked, pickled, or salted food may also be a factor in the development of stomach cancer.

Symptoms Generally there are no symptoms until the cancer is in an advanced state. When they do appear, they are similar to those for peptic ulcer, and people tend to treat themselves with antacids for the fullness feeling, nausea, and eventual vomiting.

Prevention Unknown.

Treatment Gastrectomy, or removing all or part of the stomach, is the only effective treatment. If the condition is inoperable, then radiation therapy and anticancer drugs can help relieve symptoms and prolong survival.

LEUKEMIA

Leukemia is a chronic or acute disease characterized by unrestrained growth of white blood cells (leukocytes). There are many different types of leukemia, which are classified according to the dominant cell type and severity of the disease. Although leukemia is often thought of as primarily a childhood disease, leukemia strikes many more adults (26,700 cases per year, compared with 2600 in children). For 1993 it is estimated that there will be 29,300 new cases and 18,600 deaths. Efforts to treat leukemia have been more successful than for most other cancers. Although the 5-year survival rate for all types is only 37%, this is due to very poor survival for some types while the rates have improved significantly for others. For acute lymphocytic leukemia, the 5-year survival rate has improved from 4% in the 1960s to 51% in the mid-1980s. For children, the 5-year survival rate for acute lymphocytic leukemia has improved from 4% to 73% for the same period. Cancer death rates for males and females for leukemia have remained almost the same over the 30-year period (Figure 13-23).

FIGURE 13-23 Thirty-year trends in age-adjusted death rates from leukemia—1957-59 to 1987-89.

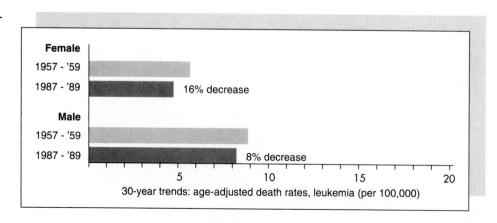

Predisposing Factors The causes of leukemia are unknown. Among the possible factors are viruses, radiation, and certain chemicals.

Symptoms Cold symptoms that do not clear up within two weeks, fatigue, weight loss, repeated infections, and easy bruising are the warning signs for leukemia.

Prevention Unknown.

Treatment The traditional treatments for leukemia are chemotherapy and bone marrow transplant.

OVARIAN CANCER

Twenty-two thousand new cases of ovarian cancer were estimated in the United States for 1993 and 13,300 deaths. Because ovarian cancer is often asymptomatic, it may be far advanced before detection. The 5-year survival rate for localized ovarian cancer is 89%, but that drops to 18% when it has spread to distant sites. Over a 30-year period, death rates for ovarian cancer have decreased (Figure 13-24).

Predisposing Factors Ovarian cancer is rare in women under 40 and occurs more in women of higher socioeconomic status and in single women. Women who have never had children are twice as likely to develop ovarian cancer. If a woman has had breast cancer, her chances of developing ovarian cancer double. Risk increases with age, with the highest rates for women over 60. The highest incidence rates for ovarian cancer come from the industrialized nations, except for Japan.

Symptoms As was indicated earlier, ovarian cancer is often symptomless until it is advanced. If symptoms do occur, there may be abdominal swelling and discomfort, vague pain, bloating, nausea, anorexia, or heartburn. These symptoms are related to the location of the cancer in the ovaries. There may also be frequent urination, constipation, pelvic discomfort, distention, and weight loss.

Primary Prevention Unknown.

FIGURE 13-24 Thirty-year trends in age-adjusted death rates from ovarian cancer—1957-59 to 1987-89.

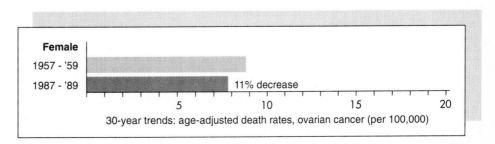

Female

1957 - '59

1987 - '89   11% decrease

5   10   15   20

30-year trends: age-adjusted death rates, ovarian cancer (per 100,000)

Secondary Prevention   Yearly pelvic examinations after the age of 40 may lead to early detection. With early detection, 90% live 5 years or longer.

Treatment   Treatment for ovarian cancer varies a great deal, with different combinations of surgery, chemotherapy, and radiation. If the cancer is only on one side in adolescents or young women, a more conservative approach may be used. In other cases, more aggressive therapy may be used, including hysterectomy and removal of the fallopian tubes and ovaries on both sides, along with multiple biopsies of other organs and lymph nodes. In some cases, remissions have been achieved with drug combinations.

SUMMARY

The table provides a summary of relevant data concerning the nine major cancers just discussed.

SUMMARY TABLE	The nine deadliest cancers			
Disease	**Special Characteristics**	**Predisposing Factors**	**Common Symptoms**	**Prevention**
Lung cancer	Most common cancer in the United States, 170,000 new cases, and most deaths, 149,000, estimated for 1993; 5-year survival 46%;* more in men, but women catching up; in 1987, for first time, caused more deaths than breast cancer in women.	Cigarette smoking; history of smoking 20 or more years; exposure to certain industrial substances; residential radon exposure; exposure to sidestream smoke.	Persistent cough, sputum streaked with blood, chest pain, recurring pneumonia or bronchitis, fever, weakness, weight loss, anorexia, bone and joint pain, gynecomastia (all late stage symptoms).	No smoking; chest x-ray exam; sputum analysis; fiberoptic exam of bronchi.
Treatment	Traditional treatment; immunotherapy and laser therapy are being used experimentally.			
Colorectal cancer	Second most common cancer, 152,000 new cases, second highest number of deaths, 57,000 estimated for 1993; 5-year survival 89%; develops slowly, remains localized for long time; equal number of deaths among men, women.	Personal or family history of cancer; polyps of colon or rectum; inflammatory bowel disease, high-fat and/or low-fiber diet; 40% or more over ideal weight.	Pallor, malnutrition, fluid in abdomen, enlarged liver, swollen lymph glands, black, tarry stools, cramping, rectal bleeding, and feeling of pressure in abdomen (colon); in rectum, change in bowel habits, with diarrhea or alternating periods of diarrhea, constipation; blood or mucus in stools;	Maintain ideal weight; low-fat, high-fiber diet; digital exam, hemoccult test and proctoscopy as recommended by doctor.

*5-yr survival rates are for early diagnosis (cancer localized).

SUMMARY TABLE   The nine deadliest cancers—cont'd

Disease	Special Characteristics	Predisposing Factors	Common Symptoms	Prevention
Colorectal cancer—cont'd			sense of incomplete evacuation. In late stages, pain, feeling of fullness, constant ache in rectal or sacral area.	
Treatment	Surgery the most effective; colostomy may be necessary.			
Breast cancer	1 in 9 women will develop breast cancer; 183,000 new cases, 46,300 deaths estimated for 1993; 5-year survival, 93%; incidence rate has steadily increased, but death rate stable with improved treatment methods.	Family history of breast cancer; long menstrual cycles; early menses or late menopause; first pregnancy after age 35; white race, middle or upper socioeconomic level; constant stress in home or work life.	A lump, thickening, swelling, dimpling, skin irritation, distortion of the breast; retraction, scaliness, pain, or tenderness of nipple.	Stress management, self-examination, mammograms.
Treatment	Radiation therapy, chemotherapy, hormone manipulation, or surgery; 4 types of mastectomy: radical, modified radical, total or simple, and partial or segmental (lumpectomy).			
Prostatic cancer	Among top three killers of men; 165,000 new cases, 35,000 deaths for 1993; 91% survival rate.	Highest in African-American males; cause unknown, many possibilities being investigated.	Weak or interrupted urine flow, need to urinate frequently, especially at night; blood in urine; pain or burning on urination; continuing pain in lower back, pelvis, or upper thighs; symptoms in advanced stages only.	Rectal exam yearly for men over 40; ultrasound for men at high risk.
Treatment	Surgery to remove male hormone of testicle, 72% retain potency; administration of female hormone, chemotherapy, radiation.			
Pancreatic cancer	Incidence increasing steadily over past 20 years; over 27,700 new cases, 25,000 deaths estimated for 1993; 5-year survival rate 8%.	Smoking, sex (30% more in men) and race (65% more in African-Americans); chronic drinking, coffee, diets high in fat and protein, food additives, certain industrial chemicals.	No symptoms until advanced stages, then jaundice, weight loss, abdominal or low back pain.	No smoking; avoid suspected carcinogens such as coffee, food additives, alcohol, high-fat, high-protein foods.
Treatment	Traditional treatments rarely successful.			
Hodgkin's disease	Involves lymphatic tissue mainly in lymph nodes, spleen; fatal if untreated; recent advances leading to	Unknown.	Enlargement of lymph nodes in neck or armpits; malaise; fever; loss of appetite, weight; night sweats.	Unknown.

Continued.

SUMMARY TABLE The nine deadliest cancers—cont'd

Disease	Special Characteristics	Predisposing Factors	Common Symptoms	Prevention
Hodgkin's disease—cont'd	a cure; 7,900 new cases, 1,500 deaths estimated for 1993.			
Treatment	Radiation or chemotherapy; bone marrow transplant, monoclonal antibodies being tested.			
Non-Hodgkin's lymphoma	Any cancer of lymphoid tissue other than Hodgkin's disease; 43,000 new cases, 20,500 deaths estimated for 1993.	Unknown.	Swelling of lymph nodes in groin or neck; enlarged liver and spleen; abdominal pain, intestinal bleeding, vomiting of blood.	Unknown.
Treatment	Traditional treatment.			
Stomach cancer	Develops in stomach lining; 24,000 new cases, 13,600 deaths estimated for 1993; incidence increased dramatically in last 50 years.	Cause unknown; diet, bacteria may be factors; gastritis, anemia and belonging to blood group A may also be factors.	Feeling of fullness, nausea and vomiting in last stages.	Unknown.
Treatment	Gastrectomy only effective treatment; if inoperable, chemotherapy and radiation therapy to relieve symptoms, prolong survival.			
Leukemia	Unrestrained growth of white blood cells; many different types; survival dramatically improved for some types; estimate for 1993: 24,300 new cases, 9700 deaths.	Unknown, possibly a virus, radiation, or heredity.	Cold symptoms lasting beyond 2 weeks; fatigue, weight loss, repeated infections, easy bruising.	Unknown.
Treatment	Chemotherapy, bone marrow transplant.			
Ovarian cancer	22,000 new cases, 13,300 deaths estimated for 1993; detection usually in advanced stages.	Rare in women under 40; more in higher socioeconomic status and single women; twice as likely in women who have never had children and in those who have had endometrial cancer; risk increases with age, highest in women 65-84.	Often none until advanced; if symptoms, abdominal swelling and discomfort, vague pain, bloating, nausea, anorexia, or heartburn.	Yearly pelvic exams after age 40.
Treatment	Different combinations of surgery, chemotherapy, radiation. May include hysterectomy, removal of the fallopian tubes, ovaries on both sides; remissions have occurred with combinations of drugs.			

5-year survival rates given are for cancer that is localized, unless otherwise stated.

QUESTIONS FOR REVIEW

1. How does cancer compare with heart disease in number of deaths?
2. What is the survival rate for cancer today?
3. Why is the number of deaths from lung cancer increasing when there are fewer people smoking today?
4. Define the following: neoplasm, tumor, benign neoplasm, malignant tumor.
5. Identify each step in the current theory of cancer development stated in the text.
6. Define the following: carcinoma, sarcoma, melanoma, neuroblastoma, adenocarcinoma, hepatoma, leukemia, lymphoma.
7. What is meant by staging a cancer, and why is it done?
8. In what five ways do cancer cells differ from regular cells?
9. What factors can increase the susceptibility to cancer, and how can they be changed?
10. What is the significance of pain as a symptom of cancer?
11. What are the best means of primary prevention for cancer?
12. What are the seven warning signals for cancer developed by the ACS?
13. What traditional methods are used to treat cancer?
14. What other methods of treating cancer are being studied scientifically?
15. What is meant by the mind-body connection in reference to curing cancer (or any other disease)?
16. What does E-Cap stand for, and how did the group get started?
17. Why is it difficult to research some alternative cancer treatments scientifically?
18. What are the common symptoms of lung cancer in the early stages and in the later stages?
19. What steps can be taken to reduce the risk of lung cancer?
20. Why is the prognosis for lung cancer so poor?
21. What two factors have helped to improve the 5-year survival rate for colorectal cancer?
22. What are the predisposing factors for colorectal cancer?
23. What are the symptoms for colorectal cancer?
24. How can the risk of colorectal cancer be reduced?
25. What means are available for diagnosing colorectal cancer?
26. What surgery may be performed for advanced stages of colorectal cancer?
27. What percentage of women who are alive today will develop breast cancer if the present rates continue?
28. What factors may put a woman at high risk for breast cancer?
29. What factors cause a woman to be at lower risk for breast cancer?
30. Why is a woman more likely to discover a sign of breast cancer than a doctor or nurse?
31. What are the signs for breast cancer?
32. What steps can be taken to lower the risk of breast cancer?
33. What secondary prevention methods for breast cancer are recommended by the ACS?
34. Describe the four types of breast surgery used for cancer.
35. What two factors could you indicate as playing a part in the rise of cancer of the prostate?
36. What races have the highest and lowest incidence of prostatic cancer? What theories can be given for the cause of this?

37. What symptoms are associated with cancer of the prostate?
38. Which men should have a digital rectal exam and which should have ultrasound screening for prostatic cancer?
39. What kind of treatment may be used for prostatic cancer?
40. Why is the 5-year survival rate for pancreatic cancer so low?
41. What risk factors are associated with pancreatic cancer?
42. What are the symptoms of pancreatic cancer?
43. What is Hodgkin's disease?
44. What are the symptoms of Hodgkin's disease?
45. What is non–Hodgkin's lymphoma?
46. What factors have been linked with non–Hodgkin's lymphoma?
47. What are some of the unique characteristics of stomach cancer?
48. What can be done to reduce the risk of stomach cancer?
49. Why is stomach cancer generally not diagnosed until an advanced stage?
50. What is leukemia?
51. When efforts to treat leukemia are considered so successful, why is the 5-year survival rate still so low?
52. What are the symptoms of leukemia?
53. What is the treatment for leukemia?
54. Why is the death rate high for ovarian cancer?
55. Which women are most at risk for ovarian cancer?

FURTHER READING

American Cancer Society. *Cancer Facts and Figures—1993*. Atlanta: American Cancer Society, 1993.

"An International Association between Helicobacter Pylori Infection and Gastric Cancer." *Lancet,* May 29, '93, 341(8857):1359-1362.

Blot, William J., Susan S. Devesa et al. "Rising Incidence of Adenocarcinoma of the Esophagus and Gastric Cardia." *Journal of the American Medical Association,* Mar. 13, '91, 265:1287-1289.

Burnstein, M. J. "Dietary Factors Related to Colorectal Neoplasms." *Surgical Clinics of North America.* Feb. '93. 73(1):13-29.

Butturini, Anna and Robert P. Gale. "Age of Onset and Type of Leukemia." *Lancet,* '89, 2:789-791.

Cabanes, P.A., R.J. Salmon et al. "Value of Axillary Dissection in Addition to Lumpectomy and Radiotherapy in Early Breast Cancer." *Lancet,* May 23, '92, 339:1245-1248.

Cassileth, Barrie. "Survival and Quality of Life among Patients Receiving Unproven as Compared with Conventional Cancer Treatment." *New England Journal of Medicine,* Apr. 25, '91, 324(17):1180-1185.

Congressional Office of Technology Assessment. *Unconventional Cancer Treatments*. Washington, D.C.: Government Printing Office, 1991.

Cramer, Daniel W. et al. "Galactose Consumption and Metabolism in Relation to the Risk of Ovarian Cancer." *Lancet,* July 8, '89, 2:66-71.

Ezzell, Carol. "Cancer Gene May Be Relatively Common." *Science News,* May 16, '92, 141:324.

Fackelmann, Kathy A. "Hints of a Chlorine-Cancer Connection." *Science News,* July 11, '92, 142:23.

Farrow, Diana C., William C. Hunt and Jonathan M. Samet. "Geographic Variation in the

Treatment of Localized Breast Cancer." *New England Journal of Medicine,* Apr. 23, '92, 326:1097-1101.

Fisher, Bernard et al. "Eight-Year Results of a Randomized Clinical Trial Comparing Total Mastectomy and Lumpectomy with or without Irradiation in the Treatment of Breast Cancer." *New England Journal of Medicine,* Mar. 30, '89, 320:822-888.

Gunby, Phil. "Battles against Many Malignancies Lie Ahead as Federal 'War on Cancer' Enters Third Decade." *Journal of the American Medical Association,* Apr. 8, '92, 267(14):1891.

Hamann, Philip. "Monoclonal Antibodies in Cancer Treatment" (Personal Interview), Sept. '92.

Hand, R. et al. "Staging Procedures, Clinical Management, and Survival Outcome for Ovarian Carcinoma." *Journal of the American Medical Association,* Mar. 3, '93, 269(9):1119-1122.

Harris, Jules E. "The Treatment of Cancer in an Aging Population." *Journal of the American Medical Association,* July 1, '92, 268:96-97.

Higginson, J. "Changing Concept in Cancer Prevention: Limitation and Implications for Future Research in Environmental Carcinogenesis." *Cancer Research,* Mar. 15, '88, 48:1381-1389.

Ingle, James N. "Assessing the Risk of Recurrence in Breast Cancer." *New England Journal of Medicine,* Feb. 1, '90, 322:329-331.

King, M. C., S. Rowell and S. M. Love. "Inherited Breast and Ovarian Cancer. What Are the Risks? What Are the Choices." *Journal of the American Medical Association,* Apr. 21, '93, 269(15):1975-1980.

Kinlen, L. J. et al. "Rural Population Mixing and Childhood Leukemia: Effects of the North Sea Oil Industry in Scotland, Including the Area near Dounreay Nuclear Site." *British Medical Journal,* Mar. 20, '93, 306(6880):743-748.

Lacey, Loretta Pratt et al. "An Urban Community-Based Cancer Prevention, Screening and Health Education Intervention in Chicago." *Public Health Reports,* Nov.-Dec. '89, 104:536-541.

Link, Mitchell G. "Living with Leukemia." *Current Health 2,* Apr. '93, 19:13-15.

Lippert, Joan. "Why Doctors Miss Breast Cancer." *New Woman,* May '92, 5:122-127.

London, Stephanie J. "Prospective Study of Relative Weight, Height, and Risk of Breast Cancer." *Journal of the American Medical Association,* Nov. 24, '89, 262:2853-2858.

Marwick, Charles. "First Infection-Fighting Monoclonal Antibodies Scrutinized by FDA Advisory Committee Members." *Journal of the American Medical Association,* Oct. 16, '91, 266:2052.

Marwick, Charles. "*Helicobacter:* New Name, New Hypothesis Involving Type of Gastric Cancer." *Journal of the American Medical Association,* Dec. 5, '90, 264:2724-2725.

Marx, Jean. "New Genes May Shed Light on Cell Growth Control." *Science,* July 24, '92, 257:484-485.

Michielutte, Robert et al. "Development of a Community Cancer Education Program: The Forsyth County, NC, Cervical Cancer Prevention Project." *Public Health Reports,* Nov.-Dec. '89, 104:542-551.

Modan, Baruch. "Diet and Cancer: Causal Relation or Just Wishful Thinking?" *Lancet,* July, 18, '92, 340:162-164.

Morris, Robert D, Anne-Marie Audet et al. "Chlorination, Chlorination By-Products, and Cancer: A Meta analysis." *American Journal of Public Health,* July '92, 82:955-963.

Olsen, Geary W. et al. "A Case-Control Study of Pancreatic Cancer and Cigarettes, Alcohol, Coffee, and Diet." *American Journal of Public Health,* Aug. '89, 79:1016-1019.

Pienta, K. J. and P. S. Esper. "Risk Factors for Prostate Cancer." *Annals of Internal Medicine,* May 15, '93, 118(10):793-803.

Pollak, Richard D. "The Science of Cancer." *Public Interest,* Winter '92, 106:122-134.

Raloff, Janet. "Ovarian Cancer: Homing in on the True Risks." *Science News,* Jan. 23, '93, 143:54.

Riela, A. et al. "Increasing Incidence of Pancreatic Cancer among Women in Olmsted County, Minnesota, 1940 through 1988." *Mayo Clinic Proceedings,* Sept. '92, 67(9):839-845.

Samet, J. M. "The Epidemiology of Lung Cancer." *Chest,* Jan. '93, 103(1 Suppl.):20S-29S.

Schapira, D. V. "Variation in Body Fat Distribution and Breast Cancer Risk in the Families of Patients with Breast Cancer and Control Families." *Cancer,* May 1, '93, 71(9):2764-2768.

Sellers, Thomas A., Lawrence H. Kushi et al. "Effect of Family History, Body-Fat Distribution, and Reproductive Factors on the Risk of Postmenopausal Breast Cancer." *New England Journal of Medicine,* May 14, '92, 326:1323-1329.

Siegel, Bernie S. *Love, Medicine and Miracles.* New York, 1986: Harper and Row.

Sigurdsson, Helgi et al. "Indicators of Prognosis in Node-Negative Breast Cancer. *New England Journal of Medicine,* Apr. 12, '90, 1045-1053.

Waldmann, Thomas A. "Monoclonal Antibodies in Diagnosis and Therapy." *Science,* June 21, '91, 252:1657-1662.

Zahm, S. H. et al. "Use of Hair-Coloring Products and the Risk of Lymphoma, Multiple Myeloma, and Chronic Lymphocytic Leukemia." *American Journal of Public Health,* July '92, 82(7):990-997.

Zapka, Jane G. et al. "Breast Cancer Screening by Mammography: Utilization and Association Factors." *American Journal of Public Health,* Nov. '89, 79:1499-1502.

Zheng, T. et al. "Epidemiology of non-Hodgkin's Lymphoma in Connecticut, 1935-1988." *Cancer,* Aug. 15, '92, 70(4):840-849.

Other Cancers

1 Explain the association between hepatitis B, cirrhosis, and liver cancer.

2 State the connection between multiple myeloma and the immune system.

3 Identify measures that can be used in secondary prevention of uterine, cervical, and testicular cancer.

4 Compare squamous cell and basal cell cancer with malignant melanoma.

5 Explain the ABCD method for identifying malignant melanoma.

6 State the way in which tobacco may lead to oral cancer.

7 Describe and give symptoms, predisposing factors, prevention, and treatment for the types of cancer in this chapter.

Death rates for other cancers

Male	Total	Female
Liver **6,800**	Liver **12,600**	Liver **5,800**
Oral **4,975**	Oral **7,700**	Uterus **10,100**
CNS **6,600**	CNS **12,100**	Oral **2,725**
Esophageal **7,600**	Kidney **10,900**	CNS **5,500**
Kidney **6,500**	Esophageal **10,200**	Multiple myeloma **4,600**
Bladder **6,500**	Bladder **9,900**	Kidney **4,400**
Multiple myeloma **4,800**	Multiple myeloma **9,400**	Bladder **3,400**
Melanoma **4,200**	*Melanoma **6,800**	Esophageal **2,600**
Laryngeal **3,000**	Uterus **10,100**	Melanoma **2,600**
Bone **600**	Laryngeal **3,800**	Laryngeal **800**
Thyroid **450**	Bone **1,050**	Thyroid **600**
Testicular **350**	Thyroid **1,050**	Bone **450**
	Testicular **350**	
All sites **52,375**	All sites **95,950**	All sites **43,575**

*About 2,300 non melanoma skin cancer deaths will occur in 1993.

LIVER CANCER

Liver cancer may arise in liver cells or, frequently, be the result of metastasis from other parts of the body. There were 15,800 new cases and 12,600 deaths estimated for cancer of the liver and biliary (bile) system for 1993. For the 30-year period shown in Figure 14-1 there has been a slow, steady decrease in death rates for both men and women from primary and unspecified cancer of the liver. Cancer of the liver is more prevalent in men, and, as with many cancers, it becomes more common as people get older. The disease is usually fatal within a year.

Predisposing Factors

Exposure to hepatitis B seems to be closely linked to primary liver cancer. This cancer may also be associated with cirrhosis of the liver. Whether cirrhosis leads to cancer or whether alcoholism and the subsequent malnutrition predispose the liver to develop cancer is unclear. Either way, alcoholism is a high-risk factor. There have been some indications that exposure to certain environmental carcinogens may result in liver cancer. These substances include the chemical compound aflatoxin (a mold that grows on rice and peanuts), androgens, and oral estrogens.

Symptoms

The most common signs of liver cancer are weight loss, loss of appetite, and lethargy. There may also be pain in the upper abdomen. In the later stages of disease there is jaundice and ascites (fluid in the abdomen).

Primary Prevention

Avoidance of hepatitis B, not sharing needles used for injections, and use of alcohol in moderation (if at all) reduce the risk of developing cancer of the liver.

Secondary Prevention

A physical exam can detect an enlarged liver, and ultrasound scanning can detect abnormal areas in the liver, but a liver biopsy is the only way to confirm the diagnosis. These tests are not performed routinely.

Treatment

In primary liver cancer, if cirrhosis is not also present and the cancer is in only one lobe of the liver, the tumor can be removed surgically, possibly leading to a cure.

FIGURE 14-1 Thirty-year trend in age-adjusted death rates from liver cancer per 100,000 population—1957-59 to 1987-89.

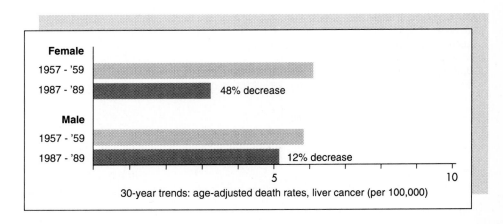

Female
1957 - '59
1987 - '89   48% decrease

Male
1957 - '59
1987 - '89   12% decrease

5   10

30-year trends: age-adjusted death rates, liver cancer (per 100,000)

A liver transplant may be considered if the disease has not spread, and there is chemotherapy that can help the patient survive longer. There is no cure for secondary liver cancer, but survival can still be prolonged with chemotherapy.

CANCER OF THE CENTRAL NERVOUS SYSTEM

About 17,500 new cases and 12,100 deaths for cancers of the central nervous system (brain and spinal cord) were estimated in 1993. Because tumors of the spinal cord are rare, they will not be discussed, and the following material deals with brain cancer, unless stated otherwise. Cancer in the brain may be a primary growth arising from tissues within the brain or a secondary growth (metastasis) spread by the bloodstream from cancer elsewhere in the body, most often the lungs or breasts. People around the age of 50 and children are the most common victims. Figure 14-2 shows an increase in deaths from brain cancer over a 30-year period, but the rates have leveled off.

Predisposing Factors   Unknown.

Symptoms   Depending upon the location of the tumor, there may be muscle weakness, loss of vision, speech difficulties, epileptic seizures, headache, vomiting, visual disturbances, impaired mental functioning, personality changes, loss of coordination, and hydrocephalus. These symptoms are insidious and vary depending on site, size, and method of expansion.

Prevention   Unknown.

Treatment   When possible, removal of the tumor through surgery is the best treatment, but many malignant tumors in the brain are inaccessible, or surgery may be too invasive to allow removal. Chemotherapy and radiation may be used, and corticosteroids may be prescribed to reduce swelling and relieve symptoms. Treatment is mostly

FIGURE 14-2 Thirty-year trend in age-adjusted death rates from brain cancer per 100,000 population— 1957-59 to 1987-89.

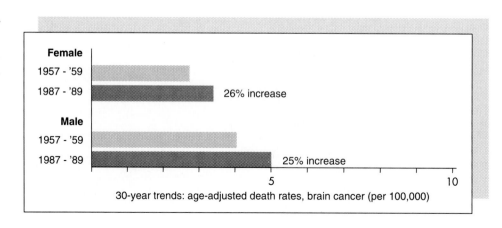

Female
1957 - '59
1987 - '89   26% increase

Male
1957 - '59
1987 - '89   25% increase

5   10
30-year trends: age-adjusted death rates, brain cancer (per 100,000)

symptomatic, and if the growth cannot be removed completely, 1-year survival is less than 20%.

KIDNEY CANCER

Tumors of the kidney usually occur in older adults and may affect either one or both kidneys. With early detection, 5-year survival rates are 85%. However, about 30% are not diagnosed until the cancer has metastasized. Kidney cancer death rates have been increasing in males faster than in females. (Figure 14-3). For 1993, 27,200 new cases and 10,900 deaths are expected.

Predisposing Factors

The cause of kidney cancer is unknown, but exposure to environmental pollutants may be a factor. It is twice as common in men as in women and usually strikes after age 40, with most of the cases being detected between ages 50 and 60.

Symptoms

Hematuria (blood in the urine) is the most common early sign of kidney cancer. In some individuals, pain or a palpable mass may be the first symptom. Most patients do not have all three. Other symptoms include fever, hypertension, hypercalcemia, and urinary retention. When the disease is more advanced, weight loss, edema in the legs due to the enlargement of lymph nodes, nausea, and vomiting occur.

Primary Prevention

Unknown.

Secondary Prevention

The best prevention is a yearly cancer check after age 40. A doctor should be consulted at the first sign of hematuria, unusual pain, or a lump.

Treatment

Surgery to remove the affected parts is the only chance of relieving symptoms or being cured. Anticancer drugs and radiation have had little effect on this cancer. The individual can survive with one kidney, providing the noncancerous one is healthy, and there is the possibility of a transplant if both kidneys are diseased.

FIGURE 14-3 Thirty-year trend in age-adjusted death rates from kidney cancer per 100,000 population— 1957-59 to 1987-89.

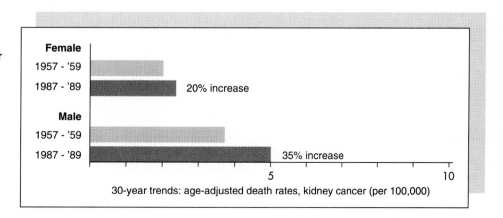

Female
1957 - '59
1987 - '89   20% increase
Male
1957 - '59
1987 - '89   35% increase

5   10

30-year trends: age-adjusted death rates, kidney cancer (per 100,000)

UTERINE CANCER (Corpus or body of uterus)

Uterine cancer is primarily a postmenopausal disease with a median age at diagnosis of 61 years. It is the most common invasive cancer of the female genital tract. The cancer begins in the lining of the uterus (endometrium) and generally spreads to the cervix and vagina as well as other parts of the body through the lymphatic system. Thirty-one thousand new cases and 5700 deaths were estimated for 1993. The death rates for uterine cancer decreased steadily between the years 1957 to 1959 and 1987 to 1989 (Figure 14-4). The 5-year survival rate is 94% if discovered in an early stage (Table 13-1).

Predisposing Factors

Uterine cancer seems linked to a number of predisposing factors. These include:

Multiple sex partners

Never had children

History of infertility

Early menarche

Late menopause

Obesity

Family history of endometrial cancer

Failure to ovulate

History of uterine polyps

Tamoxifen or unopposed estrogen therapy

Women with one or more of these factors have an increased chance of developing uterine cancer, but none has been identified as the underlying cause of the disease.

Symptoms

A bloody discharge at any time other than the menstrual period may be a sign of uterine cancer. The discharge could be watery and blood streaked at first but gradually becomes more bloody. Other symptoms such as weight loss and pain do not occur until the cancer is in an advanced stage.

Primary Prevention

There is a greater risk of developing cancer of the endometrium if unopposed estrogen therapy is used to allay the symptoms of menopause. Women should maintain their ideal weight, which reduces the risk not only for cancer of the uterus but also for diabetes and many other disorders.

FIGURE 14-4 Thirty-year trend in age-adjusted death rates from uterine cancer (cervix not included) per 100,000 population—1957-59 to 1987-89.

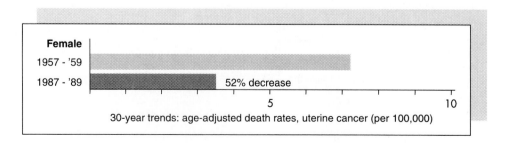

Female

1957 - '59

1987 - '89   52% decrease

5   10

30-year trends: age-adjusted death rates, uterine cancer (per 100,000)

Secondary Prevention

The Pap smear is highly effective for diagnosing cancer of the uterine cervix but only partially effective in detecting cancer of the body of the uterus. The American Cancer Society (ACS) advises an annual test for women who have reached the age of 18 and over. Women 40 and over should have an annual pelvic exam, and if they are at high risk for endometrial cancer, an endometrial tissue sample should be evaluated.

Treatment

Depending on the extent of the disease when diagnosed, treatment generally involves surgery or radiation or both. Hormonal therapy may be used if there are precancerous endometrial changes.

CERVICAL CANCER (Neck of uterus)

Cervical cancer usually occurs between ages 30 and 50. Until the advent of the Pap test, it was most common cancer of the female genitalia. For 1993, 13,500 new cases and 4400 deaths are expected. Deaths from cervical cancer decreased steadily from 1957 to 1959 to 1987 to 1989 (Figure 14-5). The 5-year survival rate is 89% for localized cancer.

Predisposing Factors

Multiple sex partners, multiple pregnancies, intercourse at a young age, smoking, herpes simplex virus 2, human papillomavirus, and other bacterial or viral infections have been related to the development of cervical cancer.

Symptoms

Depending on the type of cancer, there may be no symptoms, or there may be vaginal bleeding, vaginal discharge, and pain and bleeding after intercourse. Symptoms for advanced stages include pelvic pain, anorexia, weight loss, painful urination, lower extremity edema, and anemia.

Primary Prevention

Long-lasting monogamous sexual relationships, planned family size, deferral of intercourse until young adulthood, and avoidance of genital herpes and other viral or bacterial infections that affect the reproductive system are the best measures for prevention.

Secondary Prevention

The American Cancer Society recommends a Pap test every year for females who have been or are sexually active or over the age of 18. If the test is negative for 3

FIGURE 14-5 Thirty-year trend in age-adjusted death rates from cervical cancer per 100,000 population—1957-59 to 1987-89.

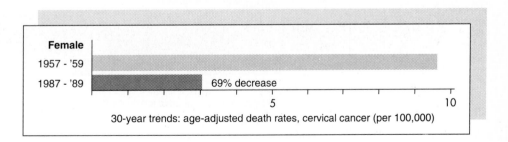

Female

1957 - '59

1987 - '89   69% decrease

5   10

30-year trends: age-adjusted death rates, cervical cancer (per 100,000)

consecutive years, the frequency of the exam should be left to the discretion of the physician.

Treatment

The treatment for cervical cancer depends upon the stage of the cancer. If there is no indication of spread, the treatment may include removing the cancerous part by surgery, using a laser to destroy it or performing cryosurgery (subjecting tissues to extreme cold). Hysterectomy is performed only if the cancer has metastasized. If the cancer has metastasized, chemotherapy may be added to the treatment regimen.

ESOPHAGEAL CANCER

About 11,300 new cases and 10,200 deaths for esophageal cancer are estimated for 1993. There was a small increase in death rates (Figure 14-6) for the period 1957 to 1959 through 1987 to 1989. The disease occurs mostly in people over 50 and is more common in men than in women, in blacks than in whites.

Predisposing Factors

The cause of cancer of the esophagus is unknown, but a high alcohol consumption and smoking are thought to be factors.

Symptoms

Initially the symptoms are nonspecific—a vague sense of pressure and fullness, and indigestion. Difficulty in swallowing, first with solids and later with fluids, occurs and becomes progressively worse until it is even difficult to swallow saliva. When the food cannot pass, vomiting and weight loss occur (40 to 50 pounds in 2 to 3 months), but, as with most cancers, there is no pain until the disease is far advanced. The spilling over of vomited food into the trachea leads to frequent respiratory infections and some hoarseness.

Primary Prevention

Moderation in drinking and no smoking may reduce the risk of esophageal cancer.

FIGURE 14-6 Thirty-year trend in age-adjusted death rates from esophageal cancer per 100,000 population—1957-59 to 1987-89.

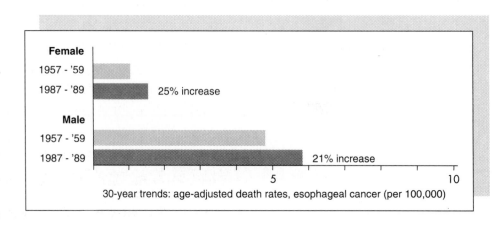

Female
1957 - '59
1987 - '89   25% increase
Male
1957 - '59
1987 - '89   21% increase
5   10
30-year trends: age-adjusted death rates, esophageal cancer (per 100,000)

Secondary Prevention   Tests to determine cancer of the esophagus would be performed only if a problem is suspected. They include a barium swallow and X-ray examinations, endoscopy, and biopsy.

Treatment   Removal of the esophagus provides the best hope of cure, but it involves radical surgery. Most of the esophagus is removed, and the stomach, or sometimes part of the colon, is pulled up into the chest to connect to the remaining upper portion of the esophagus. When the patient is too old or debilitated to survive this surgery, or the disease has spread, radiation and chemotherapy can cause regression of the cancer, relief of some of the symptoms, and occasionally a cure. Sometimes a tube is inserted into the stomach through the abdomen to allow the person to take in liquid or semisolid food.

BLADDER CANCER

The American Cancer Society estimated 52,300 new cases of bladder cancer and 9900 deaths for 1993. Over a 30-year period (Figure 14-7) there was a decrease in death rates. Bladder cancer occurs more often in people over age 50 and at an increasing rate as people get older. It has been more common in men than in women but this is changing.

Predisposing Factors   Smoking is considered to be the greatest risk factor, with smokers experiencing twice the risk of nonsmokers. Other environmental carcinogens may be risk factors for bladder cancer. Among these are 2-naphthylamine, benzidine, tobacco, nitrates, saccharin, alcohol, and coffee. Rubber workers, cable workers, weavers, aniline dye workers, hairdressers, petroleum workers, spray painters, and leather finishers are all at risk.

Symptoms   Generally the first symptom is blood in the urine, usually unaccompanied by pain. There may also be bladder irritability, urinary frequency, nocturia (increased urination at night), and dribbling.

FIGURE 14-7 Thirty-year trend in age-adjusted death rates from bladder cancer per 100,000 population—1957-59 to 1987-89.

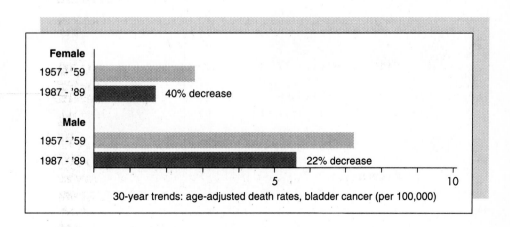

30-year trends: age-adjusted death rates, bladder cancer (per 100,000)

Primary Prevention   Selecting a job that does not entail exposure to known carcinogens and avoidance of other carcinogenic agents greatly reduce the risk of bladder cancer.

Secondary Prevention   Bladder cancer can be diagnosed by the use of a cystoscope. This is a slender tube that has a lens and light, and it can be inserted through the urethra, and into the bladder to enable the physician to examine the bladder wall.

Treatment   Traditional cancer treatments are used. For a more advanced case, a cystectomy (bladder removal) may be performed, and urine collected through a stoma (mouth-like opening) in the abdomen.

MULTIPLE MYELOMA

Multiple myeloma is a malignancy of plasma cells in the bone marrow. These cells are a type of B lymphocyte that function in making antibodies. When the cancerous cells begin to proliferate, they produce excessive amounts of one kind of antibody while production of the other antibodies is impaired (Figure 14-8). Thus the individual becomes particularly susceptible to infection. There has been a steady increase in multiple myeloma as shown in Figure 14-9. For 1993 the estimates were 12,800 new cases and 9400 deaths. Only about 20% of patients survive for 4 years or longer from the time of diagnosis.

FIGURE 14-8   Multiple myeloma.

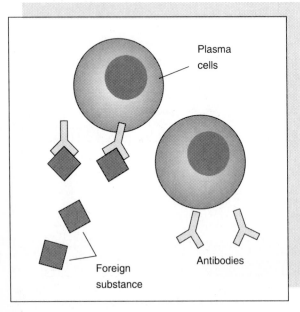

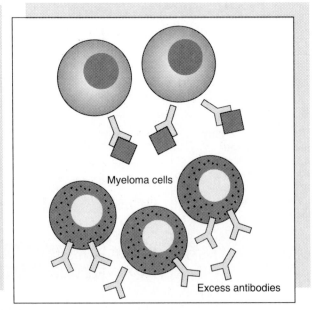

(a)   (b)

FIGURE 14-9 Thirty-year trend for multiple myeloma—1955-57 to 1987-89.

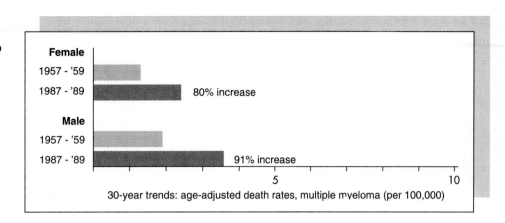

Predisposing Factors Unknown.

Symptoms Severe, constant back pain is the earliest symptom of multiple myeloma. Exercise causes an increase in the pain. There may also be arthritic symptoms, fever, malaise, anemia, and pathologic fractures. As the disease worsens, the patient is particularly susceptible to infection; there may also be a decrease in renal function or renal failure along with other symptoms of vertebral compression.

Prevention Unknown.

Treatment Chemotherapy and radiation are the treatments used for this cancer. Bone marrow transplant has been effective in some cases.

SKIN CANCER

Most skin cancers are either basal cell carcinoma or squamous cell carcinoma, which are highly curable. Skin cancer is the most common of all cancers. Over 732,000 new cases of skin cancer will be diagnosed in the United States in 1993. One in every seven Americans is affected. Malignant melanoma is the most dangerous form of skin cancer and can spread swiftly throughout the body if untreated, resulting in death. About 32,000 Americans develop malignant melanoma each year with about 6500 deaths annually (Figure 14-10). The 5-year survival rate is 91% for melanoma that is discovered early. If it has metastasized regionally, 5-year survival drops to 54%, and distant metastasis results in only a 13% survival rate. There has been a steady increase in melanoma since 1957 (Figure 14–10). There are more than 700,000 new cases of basal cell and squamous cell cancer each year and 2000 deaths. There has been a steady decrease in death rates from skin cancers other than melanoma for the 30-year period from 1957 to 1959 through 1987 to 1989 (Figure 14-11).

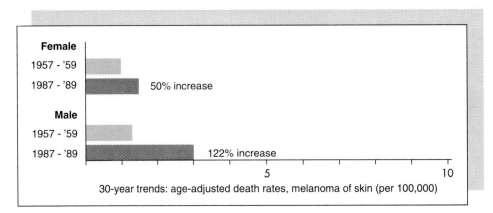

FIGURE 14-10 Thirty-year trend in age-adjusted death rates from melanoma of the skin per 100,000 population—1955-57 to 1987-89.

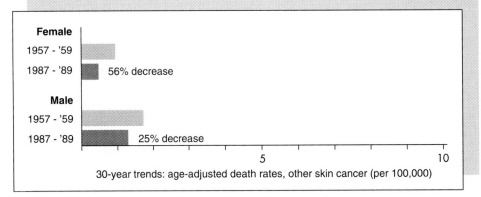

FIGURE 14-11 Thirty-year trend in age-adjusted death rates from basal cell and squamous cell skin cancer per 100,000 population—1955-57 to 1987-89.

Predisposing Factors

Risk factors for skin cancer include excessive exposure to ultraviolet radiation, fair skin, and occupational exposure to coal, tar, pitch, and creosote. Most of the 732,000+ new cases diagnosed each year are due to sun exposure.

Symptoms

The ACS has developed an ABCD method for identifying malignant melanoma:

*A*symmetry, or one half does not match the size or color of the other half.

*B*order irregularity (edges of the mole are irregular, notched, blurred, or ragged).

*C*olor changes or variation (melanomas are often mottled with various shades of brown, black, tan, red, blue, and white occurring on a single mole).

*D*iameter greater than 6 mm (larger than the size of a common pencil eraser).

These various characteristics of melanoma are illustrated in Figure 14-12.

Any unusual lesions on the hands, face, or other exposed parts of the body that do not heal should be checked by a doctor.

Primary Prevention

The risk of skin cancer can be reduced with less exposure to the sun and by using sun screens, umbrellas, and hats with wide brims or visors. Exposure to the sun between 10 A.M. and 3 P.M., when the sun's rays are strongest, should be avoided.

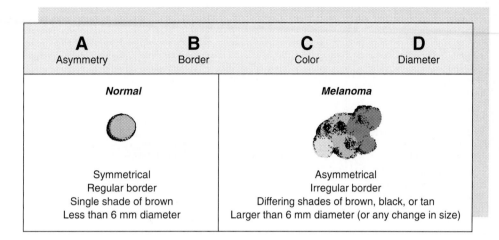

| **A** | **B** | **C** | **D** |
| Asymmetry | Border | Color | Diameter |

Normal	*Melanoma*
Symmetrical	Asymmetrical
Regular border	Irregular border
Single shade of brown	Differing shades of brown, black, or tan
Less than 6 mm diameter	Larger than 6 mm diameter (or any change in size)

FIGURE 14-12 Melanoma characteristics.

Tanning beds should not be used because the same kind of ultraviolet rays are used. The damage is not immediately apparent, so overexposure occurs more easily. Check for moles regularly and note original size and color of any moles.

Secondary Prevention

Skin cancer is completely curable when treated in its earliest stages. A doctor should examine any mole that changes in size, shape, or color, or becomes ulcerated and does not heal. A dry scaly patch or pimple that persists, an inflamed area with a crusting center, or a waxy, pearly nodule are all considered to be warning signs.

Treatment

There are four methods of treatment for skin cancer: surgery, radiation therapy, electrodesiccation (tissue destruction by heat), or cryosurgery (tissue destruction by freezing). Melanoma generally occurs in places where it is visible and easily removed. In some cases, it may occur between the toes, on the scalp or in other areas of the body where it is not easily seen. Surgery is the basic treatment since the lesions are easy to excise when discovered early. However, the chance of metastasis is greater as the depth of the lesion increases. Removal of nearby lymph nodes is sometimes necessary. Plastic surgery may be needed for large areas.

ORAL CANCER

Cancerous growths may appear on the lips, tongue, or anywhere else in the mouth. They may appear benign in early stages as just a small lump, but they develop into sores that do not heal and if not removed will metastasize. For 1993 it is estimated that there will be 29,800 new cases of oral cancer and 7700 deaths. The 30-year trend shown in Figure 14-13 shows a decrease in cases of oral cancer for men but no change for women.

Predisposing Factors

Smoking is considered a major factor, especially in combination with alcohol. Loose dentures are also associated with oral cancer, but a great threat today is the increased use of smokeless tobacco, particularly by those under 21. There are three forms of

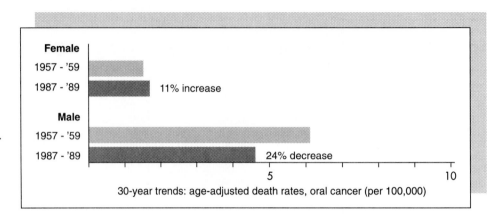

FIGURE 14-13 Thirty-year trend in age-adjusted death rates from oral cancer per 100,000 population—1955-57 to 1987-89.

smokeless tobacco, plug, leaf, and snuff. It is the "dipping snuff" that is now causing the greatest concern. This product is made by processing tobacco into a coarse, moist powder that is placed between the cheek and gum. The nicotine and other carcinogenic substances are absorbed through the oral tissue. According to the ACS, oral cancer occurs several times more frequently among those using smokeless tobacco, and the risk may increase 50 times for those who are long-time users.

Symptoms   A sore on the lip, tongue, or any other part of the mouth that does not heal within 2 weeks, painful whitish plaques, or velvety red lumps all could indicate a potential cancerous growth.

Primary Prevention   No one should use tobacco, and there should be only moderate use of alcohol, if any. Loose-fitting dentures need to be corrected immediately.

Secondary Prevention   Dentists should check for any warning signs during annual checkups. Physicians should check the oral cavity during visits.

Treatment   Cancerous lesions in the oral cavity take a long time to develop and should be recognized before metastasizing. If diagnosed early, most can be removed by surgery, never to occur again. Unfortunately, because the public does not receive adequate health education or because doctors fail to examine patients thoroughly, the cancer has sometimes infiltrated nearby tissue or spread to other parts of the body before it is diagnosed.

LARYNGEAL CANCER

Cancer of the larynx is approximately five times more common in males than in females. Malignant tumors of the larynx are classified as intrinsic (within the larynx) and extrinsic (outside the larynx). Ninety-five percent of the latter are squamous cell carcinomas, although any kind of carcinoma or sarcoma may occur in or on

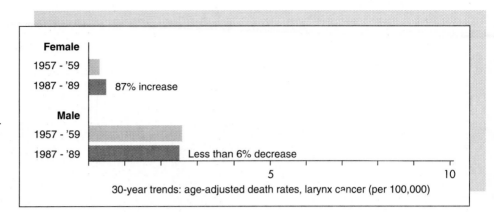

FIGURE 14-14 Thirty-year trends in age-adjusted death rates from laryngeal cancer per 100,000 population—1955-57 to 1987-89.

the larynx. For 1993, 12,600 new cases and 3800 deaths were expected. The 30-year trend shows no change in death rates for men, but a steady increase for women (Figure 14-14). In the United States laryngeal cancer does not generally occur until the fourth decade and occurs most often in individuals over the age of 60.

Predisposing Factors

The exact cause of laryngeal cancer is unknown but more occurs in those who smoke and are heavy drinkers. An increased incidence of exposure to asbestos has also been discovered in those with cancer of the larynx. Other environmental factors may also play a part in its development.

Symptoms

Persistent hoarseness is often the first symptom and may be followed by pain, difficulty in swallowing, and coughing up blood. The symptoms are dependent upon the location of the cancer on or in the larynx. If it is on the vocal cords, there may be symptoms before it has had a chance to spread. However, if the cancer occurs in another location, symptoms may not appear until it has grown large enough to cause symptoms.

Primary Prevention

To prevent this disease, people should not use tobacco in any form and drink moderately, if at all. Older buildings need to be checked for asbestos and, if found, this should be removed immediately (this is occurring in most states). Any environmental substances known to be carcinogenic should be avoided.

Secondary Prevention

If hoarseness continues for more than a week with no known cause, a doctor should be consulted. A laryngoscopy can be performed to check the vocal cords.

Treatment

If the lesion is identified early, there is an 85% to 90% chance of cure by radiation alone. If it is found during the later stages, partial or total removal of the larynx may be necessary. Radiation and surgery together have increased the 5-year survival rate by 50%. Chemotherapy may also be used in combination with the other two therapies. Treatment is aimed at eliminating the cancer and preserving speech.

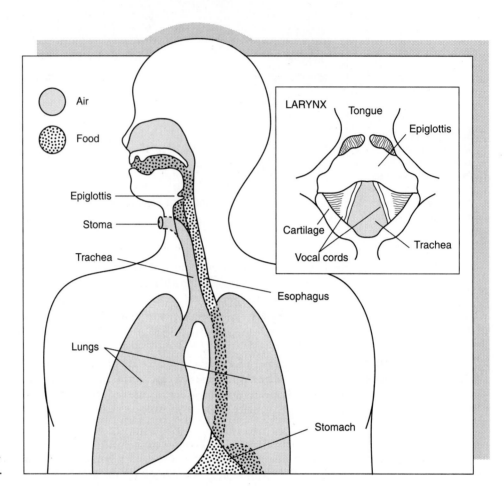

FIGURE 14-15 Location of stoma in larynx.

If speech is lost, the patient is taught how to speak by use of a stoma, or hole, in the neck. Figure 14-15 shows the relationship of such a stoma to the normal structures.

BONE CANCER

Bone cancer is rare. Less than 1% of all cancers are found in the bone, and most of these are metastases from other sites. The most common form, osteosarcoma, is found most often in the leg bones of children and young adults. Two thousand new cases and 1050 deaths from bone cancer were estimated for 1993.

Predisposing Factors

The cause of primary bone cancer is unknown.

Symptoms

Symptoms are dependent on the location of the affected bones. One of the most common signs is pain that may not be disabling but becomes worse at night.

Prevention   Unknown.

Treatment   Includes radiation, chemotherapy, and surgery (amputation may be necessary).

THYROID CANCER

This cancer is also rare, accounting for just over 1% of all cancers. The cause is generally unknown, although this kind of cancer has been associated with high doses of radiation. The estimate for 1993 is 12,700 new cases and 1050 deaths. Cancer of the thyroid gland occurs more than twice as often in women.

Predisposing Factors   Unknown except for radiation exposure.

Symptoms   A nodule on the neck is generally the first sign. Routine examination cannot distinguish a benign from a malignant growth, and other techniques such as imaging, biopsy, or actual removal of the nodule for microscopic examination are necessary for diagnosis.

Prevention   Avoiding exposure to radiation.

Treatment   Cancer of the thyroid has one of the highest cure rates of all cancers. Physicians differ on the best treatment to use, but traditional forms of therapy (radiation, chemotherapy, and surgery) are used alone or in combination.

TESTICULAR CANCER

About 6600 males, generally between ages 15 and 40, are afflicted with testicular cancer annually, and there are approximately 350 deaths. The 5-year survival rate is 96% if the cancer is localized. If it has metastasized, the 5-year survival rate is only 54%. Although the number of new cases per year and the death rate are among the lowest now, the incidence of this kind of cancer has been increasing in recent years. It is the leading cancer killer for boys and men in the 15- to 40-year age group.

Predisposing Factors   The cause of testicular cancer is unknown except that the incidence is higher in men with undescended testicles and in male children of women exposed to exogenous estrogen (diethylstilbestrol) during pregnancy. The relationship remains even if there has been surgery to correct the condition.

Symptoms   Self-examination or examination by a physician can lead to the detection of a lump that may range in size from a pea to a grapefruit. As with many cancers, there is

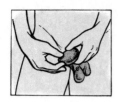

FIGURE 14-16 Testicular self-examination.

no pain, although there may be a feeling of heaviness. If the tumor produces hormones, there may be gynecomastia and nipple tenderness. In the later stages, there may be urethral obstruction, shortness of breath, weight loss, and fatigue.

Primary Prevention   Unknown.

Secondary Prevention   The most common and effective means of early detection is self-examination. Young men should be educated on how to detect a tumorous growth in the testicles (Figure 14-16).

Treatment   Traditional cancer treatment is used. The intensity of the treatment depends upon the stage and type of the tumor. Most surgeons remove just the testis(es) involved and leave the scrotum to be used for a prosthetic testicular implant at a later date, if desired.

SUMMARY

The table summarizes relevant data concerning the forms of cancer discussed in this chapter.

SUMMARY TABLE Other cancers					
Site	**Special Characteristics**	**Predisposing Factors**	**Common Symptoms**	**Prevention**	**Treatment**
Liver	15,800 new cases, 12,600 deaths estimated for 1993; more prevalent in men; incidence increases with age; usually fatal within a year.	Exposure to hepatitis B; alcoholism; exposure to certain environmental carcinogens.	Weight loss, loss of appetite, lethargy, pain in upper abdomen, jaundice, ascites.	Avoidance of hepatitis B, moderation in use of alcohol.	Surgical removal of involved tissue, chemotherapy; liver transplant possible.
Brain and CNS	17,500 new cases, 12,100 deaths estimated	Unknown for primary brain cancer.	Depend upon location; may be muscle	Unknown for primary brain cancer.	Surgical removal of the tumor if possible, chemo-

SUMMARY TABLE Other cancers—cont'd					
Site	**Special Characteristics**	**Predisposing Factors**	**Common Symptoms**	**Prevention**	**Treatment**
	for 1993; often a metastasis; people around age 50 and children most common victims.		weakness, loss of vision, speech problems, epilepsy, headache, vomiting, visual disturbances, impaired mental function, hydrocephalus.		therapy, radiation, and possibly corticosteroids to reduce swelling and relieve symptoms. Many brain tumors when diagnosed are inaccessible or too far advanced to be curable.
Kidney	Usually occurs in older adults; 5-year survival over 50%; twice as common in men; usually strikes between ages 50, and 60; 27,200 new cases and 10,900 deaths for 1993.	Cause unknown; exposure to environmental pollutants may be factor.	Blood in urine, pain or palpable mass, fever, hypertension, hypercalcemia, urinary retention; more advanced symptoms: weight loss, edema in legs, nausea, vomiting.	Avoidance of environmental pollution.	Surgery to remove tissue involved or whole kidney; chemotherapy not effective; patient can survive on one kidney; possibility of kidney transplant if both affected.
Uterus	Usually affects postmenopausal women ages 50 to 60; 31,000 new cases, 5700 deaths for 1993.	Early age at first intercourse; multiple sex partners; never had children; abnormal uterine bleeding; obesity; hypertension; diabetes; family history of endometrial cancer; history of uterine polyps; estrogen therapy.	Bloody discharge between periods.	No estrogen therapy if possible; maintain ideal weight; avoid diabetes; Pap smear if over 20; regular pelvic exams; biopsy at menopause if at risk.	Removal of uterus (hysterectomy) and other involved structures; radiation, hormonal therapy to inhibit recurrence, lengthen survival.
Cervix	Steady decrease; 13,500 new cases, 4400 deaths estimated for 1993.	Multiple sex partners; multiple pregnancies; intercourse at young age; herpes simplex virus 2, other genital infections.	None or vaginal bleeding; vaginal discharge; pain, bleeding after intercourse.	Long-lasting monogamous sexual relations, planned family size, deferral of intercourse until young adulthood, avoidance of genital herpes and other genital infections.	Removal of involved tissue or hysterectomy if metastasized; cryosurgery, laser destruction of tissue.

Continued.

SUMMARY TABLE Other cancers—cont'd

Site	Special Characteristics	Predisposing Factors	Common Symptoms	Prevention	Treatment
Esophagus	11,300 new cases, 10,200 deaths estimated for 1993; more common in men than in women, in blacks than in whites.	Cause unknown; high alcohol consumption, smoking may be factors.	Difficulty in swallowing; vomiting, weight loss; pain during later stages.	No smoking, moderation in drinking.	Surgery, radiation, chemotherapy depending upon the stage of cancer, condition of patient.
Bladder	Occurs more in people over 50; 52,300 new cases, 9900 estimated for 1993.	Tobacco, coffee, nitrates, other environmental chemicals; many occupations cause exposure to risk factors.	Blood in urine, pain, urinary frequency, nocturia, dribbling.	Job selection, no tobacco, moderation in coffee drinking.	Surgery; may involve bladder removal and replacement by abdominal opening for external urine collection; radiation, chemotherapy may also be used.
Bone marrow (multiple myeloma)	Cancer of plasma cells in bone marrow; 12,800 new cases, 9400 deaths for 1993.	Unknown.	Severe, constant back pain; arthritic symptoms; fever, malaise; pathologic fractures.	Unknown.	Chemotherapy, radiation.
Skin	Basal cell, squamous cell most common; malignant melanoma most deadly; most new cases due to sun exposure; 732,000 new cases estimated skin cancer for 1993: 32,000 melanoma; 8500 melanoma deaths each year—increasing.	Excessive sun exposure, fair skin, exposure to coal, tar, pitch, creosote.	Asymmetry; border irregularity; color changes or variation; diameter greater than 6 mm; lesion that does not heal.	Less sun exposure; sun screens, hats with wide brims, umbrellas; no tanning beds; check moles; check with doctor if A, B, C, or D occurs.	Surgery generally successful; radiation and/or chemotherapy may be used in case of metastasis.
Oral cavity	Cancers on lips, tongue, mouth, or pharynx; 29,800 new cases 7700 deaths estimated for 1993.	Smoking; use of smokeless tobacco; excess use of alcohol; loose dentures.	Sore that bleeds easily, does not heal; red or white patch; lump or thickening; difficulty in chewing, swallowing, moving tongue or jaw (late changes).	No tobacco use; moderation in alcohol use; regular dental checkups for early detection.	Surgery successful if identified early; radiation, chemotherapy if metastasized.

	SUMMARY TABLE Other cancers—cont'd				
Site	Special Characteristics	Predisposing Factors	Common Symptoms	Prevention	Treatment
Larynx	Nine times more common in males; intrinsic or extrinsic; mainly squamous cell; 12,600 new cases, 3800 deaths expected for 1993; most often in individuals over 60.	Unknown; more in smokers, heavy drinkers.	Persistant hoarseness, followed by pain, difficulty swallowing, and coughing up blood.	No tobacco use, moderation in drinking if at all, environmental carcinogens removed, avoided.	Radiation if discovered early; surgery, chemotherapy for metastasized lesions.
Bone	Rare, most metastases from other sites; 2000 new cases, 1050 deaths estimated for 1993.	Unknown.	Dependent on location; may have pain that worsens at night.	Unknown.	Radiation, chemotherapy, surgery.
Thyroid	Rare, associated with high doses of radiation; 12,700 new cases estimated for 1993; 1050 deaths.	Unknown except for radiation connection.	Nodule on neck.	Avoid exposure to radiation.	Radiation, chemotherapy, and surgery.
Testis	About 6600 men aged 15–40 diagnosed annually, 350 deaths; incidence increasing; 96% survival when found early.	Unknown.	Heaviness or a lump.	Self-examination.	Surgery, radiation, chemotherapy.

QUESTIONS FOR REVIEW

1. Why is the survival rate for cancer of the liver usually so short?
2. What factors are linked to the development of liver cancer?
3. What behavioral changes could reduce the risk of liver cancer?
4. What symptoms may occur in brain cancer?
5. What treatments may be used for brain cancer?
6. What are the common symptoms for kidney cancer?
7. Why was the development of the Pap test so important?
8. What recommendation does the ACS make for taking the Pap test?
9. What group of women are most likely to have cancer of the uterus?
10. What are the symptoms of uterine cancer?
11. What three factors play an important role in the primary prevention of uterine cancer?

12. What methods may be used to detect early uterine cancer?
13. What is a hysterectomy?
14. What are the predisposing factors for cervical cancer?
15. What are the symptoms for esophageal cancer?
16. What measures can be taken to reduce the risk of esophageal cancer?
17. Describe the treatment for esophageal cancer.
18. At what age is bladder cancer more likely to occur?
19. What is likely to be the first symptom of bladder cancer?
20. What environmental carcinogens are known to be factors in the development of bladder cancer?
21. What surgical technique may be performed for advanced cases of bladder cancer?
22. What is multiple myeloma?
23. What are the symptoms for multiple myeloma?
24. What are the two most common types of skin cancer?
25. Why is malignant melanoma the most dangerous type of skin cancer?
26. What is thought to be the major cause of skin cancer?
27. What is the ABCD method for identifying malignant melanoma?
28. What are the warning signs for basal cell and squamous cell skin cancer?
29. Why does oral cancer have a high number of new cases each year but a comparatively low death rate?
30. For what kind of lesions on the lips, tongue, or in the mouth should a doctor or dentist be consulted?
31. What are the risk factors for oral cancer?
32. Why is laryngeal cancer more common in males?
33. What is meant by intrinsic or extrinsic in reference to cancer of the larynx?
34. What factors may play a part in the development of laryngeal cancer?
35. What are the symptoms of cancer of the larynx?
36. What process may be used to detect laryngeal cancer?
37. What surgery may be performed if laryngeal cancer is not diagnosed in an early stage?
38. What treatment may be used for bone cancer?
39. What is often the first sign of cancer of the thyroid?
40. At what age does testicular cancer most often occur?
41. What condition is related to the development of testicular cancer?
42. What are the signs of testicular cancer?
43. What is the procedure for secondary prevention of testicular cancer, and how is it performed?
44. What procedure may be used if surgery is performed for testicular cancer?

FURTHER READING

Baron, John A. and E. Robert Greenberg. "Could Aspirin Really Prevent Colon Cancer?" *New England Journal of Medicine*, Dec. 7, '91, 325:1644-1646.

Bayer, S.R. and A.H. DeCherney. "Clinical Manifestations and Treatment of Dysfunctional Uterine Bleeding." *Journal of the American Medical Association*, Apr. 14, '93, 269(14):1823-1828.

Black, Peter McL. "Brain Tumors." *New England Journal of Medicine*, May 23, '91, 324:1471-1476.

Brooks, Anne Marie. "Smokeless Tobacco: Who Wants a Spitting Image?" *Current Health 2,* Oct. '91, 18:11-13.

Brownson, Ross C., John S. Reif et al. "An Analysis of Occupational Risks for Brain Cancer. *American Journal of Public Health,* Feb. '90, 80:169.

Chen, Z. et al. "Prolonged Infection with Hepatitis B Virus and Association between Low Blood Cholesterol Concentration and Liver Cancer." *British Medical Journal,* Apr. 3, '93, 306(6882):890-894.

Choi, S.Y. and H. Kahyo. "Effect of Cigarette Smoking and Alcohol Consumption in the Aetiology of Cancer of the Oral Cavity, Pharynx, and Larynx." *International Journal of Epidemiology,* Dec. '91, 20:878-885.

De-Stefani, E.F. Oreggia, S. Rivero, and L. Fierro. "Hand-Rolled Cigarette Smoking and Risk of Cancer of the Mouth, Pharynx, and Larynx." *Cancer,* Aug. 1, '91, 70:679-682.

Dunbar, C.E. and A.W. Nienhuis. "Multiple Myeloma. New Approaches to Therapy." *Journal of the American Medical Association,* May 12, '93, 269(19):2412-2416.

Elliott, Paul, Michael Hills et al. "Incidence of Cancers of the Larynx and Lung Near Incinerators of Waste Solvents and Oils in Great Britain." *Lancet,* Apr. 4, '92, 339:854-858.

Fackelmann, Kathy A. "Pregnancy Protection for Brain Cancer?" *Science News,* Oct. 31, '92, 142:299.

Fackelmann, Kathy A. "Vitamin A–Like Drug May Ward Off Cancers." *Science News,* May 30, '92, 141:358.

Glass, Andrew G. "The Emerging Epidemic of Melanoma and Squamous Cell Skin Cancer." *Journal of the American Medical Association,* Oct. 20, '89, 262:2097-2100.

Green, D.M. "Effects of Treatment for Childhood Cancer on Vital Organ Systems." *Cancer,* May 15, '93, 71(10):3299-3305.

Ikeda, K. et al. "Risk Factors for Tumor Recurrence and Prognosis after Curative Resection of Hepatocellular Carcinoma." *Cancer,* Jan. 1, '93, 71(1):19-25.

"Induction Chemotherapy plus Radiation Compared with Surgery plus Radiation in Patients with Advanced Laryngeal Cancer." *New England Journal of Medicine,* June 13, '91, 324:1685-1690.

Jankowski, J. et al. "Oncogenes and Onco-suppressor Gene in Adenocarcinoma of the Oesophagus. *Gut,* Aug. '92, 33(8):1033-1038.

Karagas, M.R. et al. "Risk of Subsequent Basal Cell Carcinoma and Squamous Cell Carcinoma of the Skin among Patients with Prior Skin Cancer." *Journal of the American Medical Association,* June 24, '92, 267(24):3305-3310.

Kato, I., A.M. Nomura, G.N. Stemmermann, and P.H. Chyou. "Prospective Study of the Association of Alcohol with Cancer of the Upper Aerodigestive Tract and Other Sites." *Cancer Causes and Control,* Mar. '92, 3:145-151.

Lane, Joseph M. and Andrew E. Rosenberg. "Case Records of the Massachusetts General Hospital: Case 4-1991." *New England Journal of Medicine,* Jan. 24, '91, 324:251-259.

La Vecchia, C., E. Negri and S. Franceschi. "Education and Cancer Risk." *Cancer,* Dec. 15, '92, 70(12):2935-2941.

Layde, Peter M. "Smoking and Cervical Cancer: Cause or Coincidence?" *Journal of the American Medical Association,* Mar. 17, '89, 261:1631-1633.

Lord, Mary. "Underground Medicine." *U.S. News and World Report,* May 11, '92, 112:62-71.

MacKie, Rona M., T. Freudenberger and T.C. Aitchison. "Personal Risk-Factor Chart for Cutaneous Melanoma." *Lancet,* Aug. 26, '89, 2:487-490.

McKenna, James P., Lisa M. Fornataro-Clerici et al. "Laryngeal Cancer: Diagnosis, Treatment and Speech Rehabilitation." *American Family Physician,* July '91, 44:123-129.

Moore, S. et al. "Treating Bladder Cancer: New Methods, New Management." *American Journal of Nursing,* May '93, 93(5):32-39.

Muscat, J.E. and E.L. Wynder. "Tobacco, Alcohol, Asbestos, and Occupational Risk Factors for Laryngeal Cancer." *Cancer,* May 1, '92, 69:2244-2251.

Patchell, Roy A., Phillip A. Tibbs et al. "A Randomized Trial of Surgery in the Treatment of Single Metastasis to the Brain." *New England Journal of Medicine,* Feb. 22, '90, 322:494-500.

Ritchie, J.P. "Detection and Treatment of Testicular Cancer." *CA Cancer Journal (Clinical),* May '93, May-June, 43(3):151-175.

Sessions, R.B. and B.J. Davidson. "Thyroid Cancer." *Medical Clinics of North America.*

Slattery, Martha L. et al. "Cigarette Smoking and Exposure to Passive Smoke Are Risk Factors for Cervical Cancer." *Journal of the American Medical Association,* Mar. 17, '89, 261:1593-1598.

Slingluff, C.L. Jr., R.T. Vollmer and H.F. Seigler. "Multiple Primary Melanoma: Incidence and Risk Factors in 283 Patients." *Surgery,* Mar. '93, 113(3):330-339.

Tebbi, C.K. "Treatment Compliance in Childhood and Adolescence." *Cancer,* May 15, '93, 71(10):3441-3449.

Thompson, Larry. "Healy Approves an Unproven Treatment (Gene Therapy for Brain Cancer)." *Science,* Jan. 8, '93, 259:172.

Tiollais, Pierre and Marie-Annick Buendia. "Hepatitis B Virus." *Scientific American,* Apr. '91, 264:116-122.

Van Wijngaarden, W.J. and I.D. Duncan. "Rationale for Stopping Cervical Screening in Women over 50." *British Medical Journal,* Apr. 10, '93, 306(6883):967-971.

Weinstock, Martin A. "The Epidemic of Squamous Cell Carcinoma." *Journal of the American Medical Association,* Oct. 20, '89, 262:2138-2139.

Ziegler, Jan. "The Dilemma of Estrogen Replacement Therapy." *American Health,* Apr. '92, 11:68-71.

Chapter 15

Chronic Respiratory, Digestive, and Excretory Diseases

RESPIRATORY DISEASES

There is nothing so terrifying as the inability to fill the lungs with air. The lodged object in the windpipe, the smothering effect of thick smoke, and the inability of the drowning victim to gain air are all experiences that cause terror because of insufficient oxygen. Thousands of people are stricken every year with chronic lung diseases that can produce the terror of suffocation. As with many chronic diseases, most common disorders of the respiratory system could be prevented with changes in lifestyle and the environment. Figure 15-1 shows the structures of the respiratory system.

Chronic bronchitis and emphysema cause years of suffering for their victims that may lead to constant discomfort, overwhelming disability, and, eventually, death. Asthma, which was discussed in Chapter 3, results in much of the same kind of suffering because of the inability of the victim to get enough air. However, asthma differs from chronic bronchitis and emphysema since there is no strong relationship between asthma and smoking as there is for chronic bronchitis and emphysema. These three disorders are often grouped under the acronym COPD, for chronic obstructive pulmonary disease, or COLD, for chronic obstructive lung disease, and two or more may be present in the same person at the same time. Each disorder interferes with the functioning of the respiratory system, making it increasingly difficult for the individual to breathe.

Normal respiration requires efficient action of the diaphragm, a clear route to the lungs, healthy bronchial tubes, and effective diffusion of gases. Oxygen that is inhaled must be diffused across the alveolar-capillary membrane into the blood, and at the same time, carbon dioxide is being diffused from the blood across the same membranes, into the lungs for exhalation.

Air usually enters the body through the nose. During periods of exertion, it may enter through the mouth, but the nose is a preferable point of entry for several reasons. First, the cilia (fine hairs in the nasal passages) protect against dust and other particles from the air. Next, particles that may slip through the cilia are caught in the thick, sticky, mucous lining of the nasal passages, allowing only clean air to pass to the lungs. Third, air is warmed in the nasal cavity, and, finally, moisture is added.

Air passes from the nose backward and downward through the pharynx to the larynx. The larynx contains the vocal cords, which the air passes through on its way to the trachea. The trachea branches into the right and left bronchial tubes, which in turn branch into bronchioles, which ultimately end in alveolar sacs.

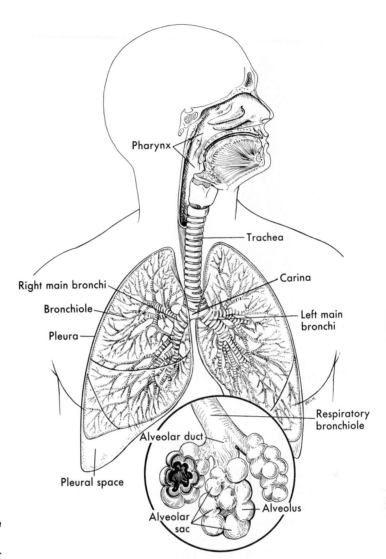

FIGURE 15-1 Structures of the respiratory system. The circle denotes the alveoli where oxygen and carbon dioxide are exchanged.

The two chronic diseases discussed in this section of the chapter involve processes that cannot or fail to function efficiently because of a respiratory disorder.

CHRONIC BRONCHITIS

When a productive cough is present for at least 3 months of 2 successive years with no other cause, the diagnosis is chronic bronchitis. The cough is the result of irritation and inflammation of the bronchial tubes, leading to excess production of mucus and the inability of the cilia, paralyzed by pollutants, to remove the irritants. Figure 15-2 shows the damage that can occur in chronic bronchitis.

Predisposing Factors   Chronic bronchitis is caused by, and progresses because of, environmental pollutants (waste of factories, carbon and tar of smoke—household or tobacco), infections,

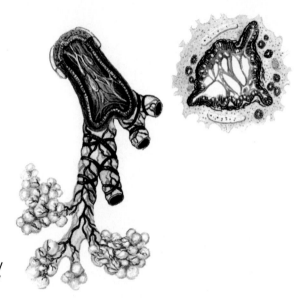

FIGURE 15-2 Airway obstruction caused by chronic bronchitis.

and allergies. Smoking is by far the most important factor. In a smoker, the cilia become paralyzed and are unable to sweep the impurities and foreign particles from the bronchi. Smoking also causes increased mucus production, destruction of alveolar walls, and an abnormal formation of fibrous tissue around the bronchioles.

Symptoms   A productive cough and shortness of breath on exertion are the first signs of chronic bronchitis. Most individuals have no symptoms until middle age. The coughing gradually gets worse and the amount of mucus secretion increases. Environmental pollutants lead to hyperplasia of the mucous glands, hypertrophy of smooth muscle, and increased thickening of the bronchial wall. The excess secretion of mucus leads to plugging of the small airways. Residual lung volume increases, vital capacity decreases, and there is wheezing and shortness of breath. As the symptoms worsen, the increased demands on the heart from lack of sufficient oxygen lead to death from *cor pulmonale* (failure of right ventricle caused by disorders of the lungs, pulmonary vessels, or chest wall).

Prevention   The best means of prevention are nonuse of tobacco products, living and working where there is low exposure to environmental pollutants, and treatment of allergies.

Treatment   A person with chronic bronchitis should not smoke, and if living or working in an area of high environmental pollution, relocation is advisable. Bronchodilators may be used to relieve bronchospasm and help to remove excess mucus. Ultrasonic and mechanical nebulizers may be used to loosen secretions, diuretics for edema, and oxygen for difficulty in breathing.

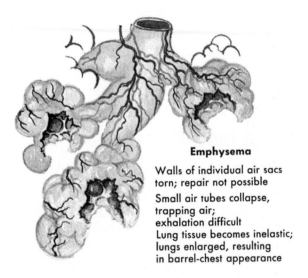

Emphysema

Walls of individual air sacs torn; repair not possible

Small air tubes collapse, trapping air; exhalation difficult

Lung tissue becomes inelastic; lungs enlarged, resulting in barrel-chest appearance

FIGURE 15-3 Airway obstruction caused by emphysema.

EMPHYSEMA

Emphysema is sometimes divided into four different types according to its anatomic location in one or both lungs. The term will be used loosely in this discussion to apply to all types. In emphysema, the walls of the alveoli are destroyed, causing an enlargement of total air space as alveoli coalesce to form one saccule. The alveoli also lose their elasticity, and the process of breathing becomes exceedingly difficult as air exchange becomes more and more difficult. The destruction of alveoli that occurs in emphysema is pictured in Figure 15-3. Because of the struggle to breathe, the chest becomes barrel shaped, respiratory movements are diminished, and expiration is difficult and prolonged. It is a dreaded disease because those with emphysema do not die quickly but live for years, fighting for every breath.

Predisposing Factors

Smoking and a deficiency of alpha-antitrypsin (hereditary) are the major predisposing factors for emphysema. The hereditary factor is rare, but if present, the trypsin may digest lung tissue, or so it is believed.

Symptoms

The disease has an insidious onset. Labored breathing and gasping for breath are the most common symptoms. Long-term signs include a chronic cough, anorexia, weight loss, "barrel chest," hypoxemia (too little oxygen in the blood), and heart failure *(cor pulmonale)*.

Prevention

No smoking and avoidance of other environmental pollutants as much as possible reduce the risk of getting emphysema. Once a person is diagnosed with emphysema, recommended are (1) eliminating as many respiratory irritants in their environment as possible by changing occupation (if there is exposure to these substances), and (2) moving to a part of the country that has less air pollution.

Treatment   Bronchodilators, *mucolytic* agents, weight reduction if obesity is present, oxygen for easier breathing, *no smoking,* and avoidance of air pollutants are included in the treatment. In some cases a process of massaging and pressure applied to the chest (chest physiotherapy) is used to help mobilize the mucus. Vaccination for influenza and pneumonia is advisable.

DIGESTIVE DISORDERS

From one meal to the next, our digestive systems function without ceasing and without our awareness until something goes wrong. As long as we ingest a well-balanced, nutritious diet, the process of digestion, which begins in the mouth, generally takes place efficiently and quietly. (For a theory about indigestion, see Did You Know? in this chapter.) But when a disease or disorder occurs in some part of the digestive tract (the mouth, esophagus, stomach, and intestines) or the organs that secrete digestive juices, the pleasure that most find in eating can change to discomfort, pain, and suffering. Figure 15-4 shows the structure of the gastrointestinal tract.

The teeth and tongue start the process of digestion by cutting, tearing, and kneading the food, while saliva adds lubrication and enzymes begin to break down starches. By the time the food is swallowed, it is a soft ball called a bolus. The bolus passes down the pharynx to the esophagus, where peristalsis moves it downward to the stomach.

The upper part of the stomach, or fundus, holds the food as it is delivered gradually to the lower part, or antrum. There the food is churned and mixed with enzymes and acids that continue the digestive process until the contents are reduced to a sticky liquid called chyme.

DID YOU KNOW?

Nonimaginary Digestive Discomfort

Many individuals with ulcer symptoms may be victims of nonulcer dyspepsia, or in simpler terms, indigestion. This does not explain why, for some people, the symptoms are there after every meal. One theory has been that some people may be more sensitive to internal events, picking up messages that most people don't get.

The first evidence of this theory was published in 1991 by researchers at the Autonomous University of Barcelona. A device was used that has an inflatable bag that can be passed into the stomach; also present were electronic sensors that can detect how much pressure a given volume of inflation creates and how tense the stomach wall becomes. The researchers discovered that patients with nonulcer dyspepsia were far more sensitive than others to what was taking place in their stomachs. Those with nonulcer dyspepsia reported feeling pain when at a level of inflation that produced no symptoms at all in the control group.

This discovery did not produce a cure for nonulcer dyspepsia, but at least those suffering with it now know that there is a reason for their discomfort, and they are not imagining it.

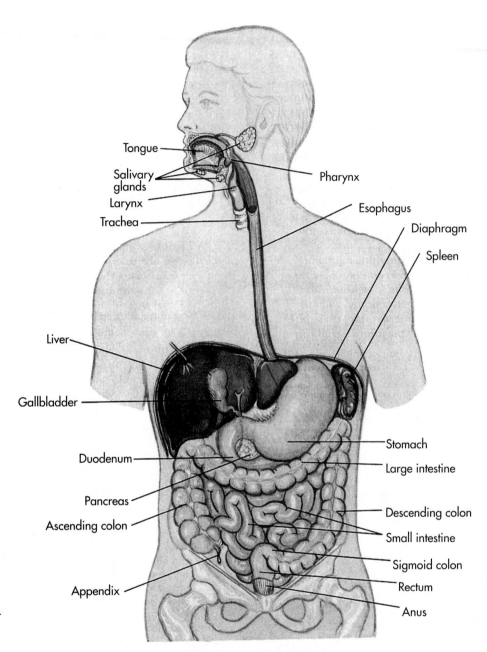

Tongue

Salivary glands

Larynx

Trachea

Pharynx

Esophagus

Diaphragm

Spleen

Liver

Gallbladder

Duodenum

Pancreas

Ascending colon

Appendix

Stomach

Large intestine

Descending colon

Small intestine

Sigmoid colon

Rectum

Anus

FIGURE 15-4 Location of the organs of the digestive system.

The chyme is released gradually into the first section of the small intestine, the duodenum, through the pyloric sphincter. The entry of the acid chyme into the duodenum brings about the discharge of bile from the gallbladder and the secretion of pancreatic juice by the pancreas.

The nutrients are absorbed into the blood from the small intestine, and the indigestible part of the chyme passes through the large intestine. Liquid is extracted along the way, and the remaining feces pass on out of the body. The disorders of the digestive system that will be discussed in this chapter occur in the stomach, intestines, liver, gallbladder, and pancreas.

PEPTIC ULCER

A peptic ulcer is a break or ulceration (sore) in the mucosal membrane (lining) of the lower esophagus, stomach, or upper part of the small intestine. About 80% of peptic ulcers are in the duodenum (duodenal ulcers), and most of the rest are in the stomach (gastric ulcers). Although several theories have been advanced over the years, a precise cause for the initial "break" or lesion has not been determined. Males are more likely to have an ulcer than females (ratio of 3.5:1). Figure 15-5 shows a deep ulcer in the wall of the duodenum.

Predisposing Factors

Duodenal Ulcers. Heredity is important in susceptibility to duodenal ulcers but does not seem to be a factor in gastric ulcers. Studies of identical twins have shown that 50% of the time, if one twin has a duodenal ulcer, the other has one too. In fraternal twins, the percentage drops to 14%. In general, people with duodenal ulcers tend to secrete excess acid and pepsin, respond more to stimuli of acid secretion, and have more rapid gastric emptying. The rapid emptying of the stomach's contents into the duodenum may result in exposing the duodenal mucosa to greater acidity.

The relationship between certain personality types and ulcers has not been confirmed. However, in many cases, stress, anxiety, and fatigue have been known to reactivate or aggravate an ulcer. Smoking, aspirin, and other NSAIDS have been implicated in ulcer formation, but there is not enough evidence to confirm this, although they are known irritants and, as with stress, may aggravate or reactivate an ulcer that is or has been present.

A bacterium recognized over 50 years ago and named *Campylobacter pylori* is now thought to be a major factor in the pathogenesis (beginning of disease) of ulcers. The organism, renamed *Helicobacter pylori,* has been found to be more prevalent in patients with duodenal or gastric ulcer than in matched controls. It was also found that people with *H. pylori* secreted more acid and gastrin (a hormone that stimulates the production of acid in the stomach) in response to a meal than did those who were not infected with *H. pylori* (Levi, S., I. Beardshall, I. Swift et al. "Antral *Helicobacter pylori,* Hypergastrinaemia, and Duodenal Ulcers: Effect of Eradicating the Organism." *British Medical Journal,* '89, 299:1504-1505).

Gastric Ulcers. People with gastric ulcers tend to have lower levels of gastric acid than normal. It is thought that these individuals may have a primary defect in their gastric mucosa, making it more susceptible to lesions. In 60% to 80% of the cases, gastritis is present along with an ulcer. Interestingly enough, when the ulcer heals, the gastritis persists, suggesting that the gastritis is primary and the ulcer secondary. Another theory is that the pyloric sphincter (lower valve of the stomach) may be weakened, allowing bile to reflux into the stomach. Cigarette smoking also decreases the effectiveness of the resting sphincter, increasing bile reflux. It is possible that bile acids seeping back into the stomach could damage the mucosal barrier, lead to chronic gastritis, cause increased acid penetration and eventually ulcers. Exogenous agents, in addition to smoking, that have been implicated in the for-

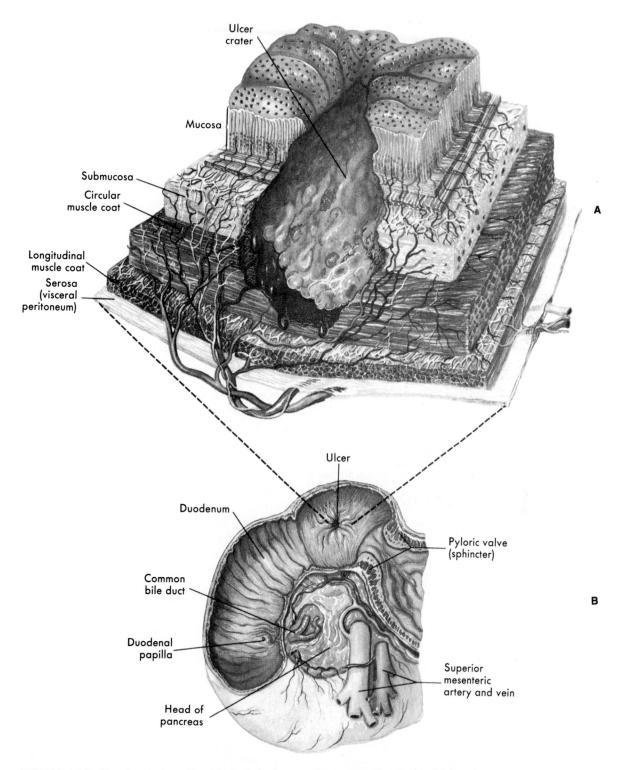

FIGURE 15-5 Duodenal ulcer. The illustration shows a deep ulceration in the duodenal wall, extending as a crater through the entire mucosa and into the muscle layers. **A,** A cut-away segment of the duodenal wall showing an ulcer crater. **B,** The position of the ulcer in the duodenum.

mation of gastric ulcers are aspirin and other NSAIDS, chronic alcohol consumption, caffeine, corticosteroids, and other drugs.

Symptoms   Heartburn, indigestion, and pain are the typical symptoms of peptic ulcers. For a gastric ulcer, the pain is in the left epigastrium and accompanied by a feeling of fullness immediately after eating. A duodenal ulcer causes discomfort in the midepigastrium 2 to 4 hours after eating; this is relieved by eating. Individuals with gastric ulcers tend to lose weight, since eating a large meal stretches the gastric wall, causing discomfort and pain. On the other hand, eating relieves the discomfort and pain from duodenal ulcers, and sufferers eat more in an effort to feel better. In both kinds of peptic ulcer, the symptoms range from none to severe back pain. An untreated ulcer may suddenly rupture and hemorrhage.

Prevention   Avoiding the use of nicotine, caffeine, alcohol, and aspirin-containing compounds and learning to manage stress are the best means of prevention. Medical advice should be sought for any persistent pain, heartburn, or indigestion.

Treatment   The treatment for peptic ulcer depends upon the severity of the symptoms. Antacids are sometimes sufficient to clear up the condition. Newer drugs are now available to help reduce the secretion of acid. If complications occur, surgery may be performed. Even after the ulcer is healed, renewed stress or alcohol use may lead to recurrence.

HIATAL HERNIA

When an organ protrudes or projects through the tissues that usually contain it, this protrusion is called a hernia. A hiatal hernia occurs when a defect in the diaphragmatic hiatus allows part of the stomach to protrude into the chest cavity at the gastroesophageal junction. The hernia may be direct, or "sliding," paraesophageal, or "rolling," or mixed. Figure 15-6 shows two types of hiatal hernia.

FIGURE 15-6 Two types of hiatal hernia shown with a normal stomach. **A,** Direct or sliding. **B,** paraesophageal or rolling.

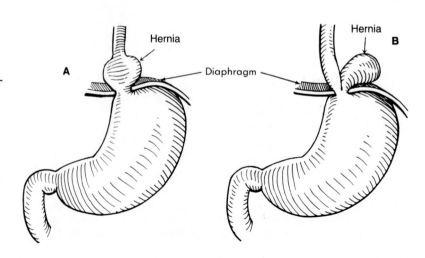

Predisposing Factors

Hiatal hernias increase in incidence with age and are more prevalent in women than in men. They usually result from muscle weakness that is common with aging or other factors, including esophageal cancer, trauma, surgical procedures, or congenital weakness of the diaphragmatic hiatus. Intraabdominal pressure, which may be from pregnancy, obesity, coughing, bending, straining, or extreme physical exertion, creates the conditions that allow the stomach to rise into the chest. This may be accompanied by reflux of stomach acids, which leads to the familiar condition of heartburn.

Symptoms

Many individuals with hiatal hernia never have symptoms. If there are symptoms they could include heartburn from 1 to 4 hours after eating and chest pain (retro- or substernal). Complications such as difficulty in swallowing, bleeding, severe pain, and shock may also occur.

Prevention

Since a number of different factors may lead to hiatal hernia, there is no single means of prevention. Avoidance of excessive weight gain during pregnancy and maintaining an ideal weight throughout life may reduce the risk, as would avoidance of other factors that cause intraabdominal pressure.

Treatment

Treatment is aimed at minimizing symptoms and avoiding complications. Surgery is not recommended initially since the hernia often recurs after surgery. The individual is given antiemetics and cough suppressants and told to avoid constrictive clothing, adjust the diet to ensure easy bowel movements, stop smoking if a smoker, use antacids, lose weight if overweight, and elevate the head of the bed. Drug therapy is also used to strengthen the cardiac sphincter tone. If these measures do not control the symptoms or if complications occur, surgical repair may be necessary.

CIRRHOSIS OF THE LIVER

The liver has an amazing capacity to repair itself after all kinds of damage. A healthy liver is shown in Figure 15-7 and cirrhosis of the liver in a 65-year-old man in Figure 15-8. The widespread destruction of cells and fibrotic regeneration that occur in cirrhosis lead to permanent loss of function. There are also many complications that can occur. Resistance to blood flow in the portal vein leads to portal hypertension. In order to reach the heart without going through the liver, the body opens up other pathways called collateral circulation. These new veins are often in the lower part of the esophagus, and as the pressure builds up, tend to hemorrhage, resulting in a life-threatening situation.

Predisposing Factors

The causes of cirrhosis of the liver can be identified as follows:

Alcoholism—30% to 50%

Bile duct disease—15% to 20%

Various types of hepatitis—10% to 30%

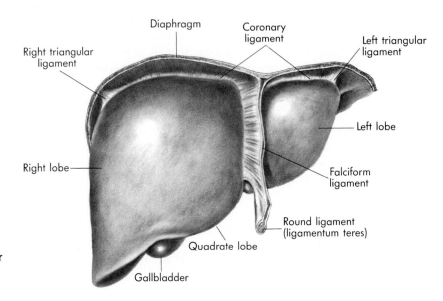

Diaphragm

Coronary ligament

Left triangular ligament

Right triangular ligament

Left lobe

Right lobe

Falciform ligament

Round ligament (ligamentum teres)

Quadrate lobe

Gallbladder

FIGURE 15-7 Anterior view of the liver structure.

FIGURE 15-8 Cirrhosis of the liver. **A,** Liver showing alcoholic cirrhosis in a 65-year-old man. **B,** Cut surface of liver showing damage caused by cirrhosis.

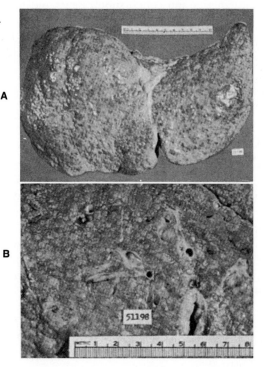

A

B

Miscellaneous disorders—5% to 10%

Unknown cause—10%

Symptoms

The early symptoms include anorexia, indigestion, nausea, vomiting, and hepatomegaly. There may be no symptoms, but a doctor can detect an enlarged liver. There may also be vascular hemangiomas, gynecomastia, and testicular atrophy. Later symptoms include edema, splenomegaly, hemorrhoids, esophageal varices, collateral veins about the umbilicus, and jaundice. As the disease continues, widespread damage to the body occurs, and death most frequently comes as a result of hepatic coma.

Prevention

Eating regular nutritious meals and using alcohol in moderation, if at all, greatly reduce the risk for developing cirrhosis of the liver. In addition, if there are any symptoms of disease such as nausea, indigestion, anorexia, and/or vomiting that are persistent, the individual should see a physician. (Contemporary Concerns in this chapter discusses liver damage from excess ingestion of vitamin A.)

Treatment

Therapy depends upon the cause and severity of the disease. The goal is to remove or alleviate the underlying cause and prevent further liver damage or treat complications.

GALLBLADDER DISEASE

Gallbladder disease is one of the most common causes of hospitalization among adults. It is usually caused by calculi or gallstones, which may irritate the gallbladder and/or clog the bile duct, causing pain and discomfort on the right side. Figure 15-9 shows the location of the gallbladder, liver, and pancreas.

CONTEMPORARY CONCERNS

When Too Much of a Good Thing Is Bad

Excess amounts of vitamin A can be deadly, and individuals taking it to improve their health wind up damaging it instead. In one study, 41 patients who had no other evident reason for liver disease were found to have abnormalities known to result from too much vitamin A. Seventeen had cirrhosis, 18 showed milder damage, and 6 died of liver failure.

Too much vitamin A can also cause itching, hair loss, dry skin and mouth, irritability, nausea or vomiting, bone and joint pains, fatigue, and chronic headache. Children are more sensitive to excess amounts than adults, and no one should take more than the recommended daily amount unless prescribed by a doctor.

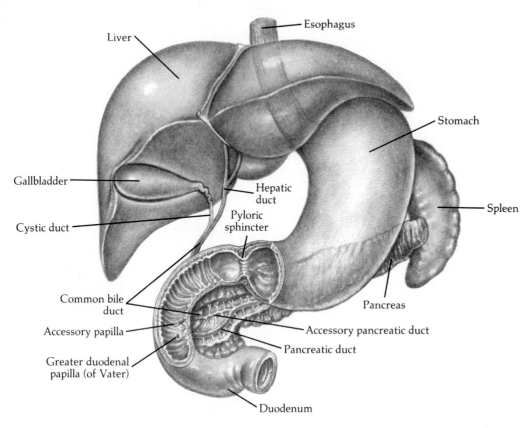

Liver

Esophagus

Stomach

Gallbladder

Hepatic duct

Pyloric sphincter

Cystic duct

Spleen

Common bile duct

Accessory papilla

Accessory pancreatic duct

Pancreatic duct

Pancreas

Greater duodenal papilla (of Vater)

Duodenum

FIGURE 15-9 Location of the liver, gallbladder, and pancreas, which are necessary organs of digestion.

Predisposing Factors Gallstones are formed from cholesterol, bilirubin, and calcium. They appear to arise because of a sluggish gallbladder, which may be caused by pregnancy, oral contraceptives, diabetes mellitus, celiac disease, cirrhosis of the liver, and pancreatitis. Or they may be the result of too much cholesterol in the bile (synthesized by the liver). Fasting for long periods may lead to the development of gallstones by causing bile to stagnate in the liver. Gallstones generally occur during middle age and are more common in women. Recent evidence indicates that heredity affects the formation of gallstones, and there is a strong correlation between gallstones and obesity. High levels of estrogens, use of oral contraceptives, and having many children also increase the risk.

Symptoms Gallbladder disease may be asymptomatic. However, symptoms may occur, particularly after eating a fatty meal. These may range from acute, sharp pain on the right side radiating to the back with nausea and vomiting, to mild discomfort in the abdominal area. The pain may be so severe that emergency room treatment is sought.

Prevention None known.

Treatment   Because it is believed that the gallbladder is not necessary to health, elective surgery is generally the treatment. Most doctors have felt that when there are gallstones present, then the gallbladder should be removed. In a few short years, removal of the gallbladder by laparoscopy has largely taken the place of major surgery. Although some physicians were afraid that complications might occur in a procedure that was so new, a study of 1518 laparoscopic cholecystectomies found that fewer complications were present using the new method than had been reported in previous studies of conventional gallbladder removal. Laparoscopic gallbladder surgery is referred to as "bandaid" surgery, since only a few "keyhole" incisions are necessary for the procedure.

EXCRETORY DISORDERS
KIDNEY DISEASE

The kidneys are part of the urinary tract, which contains the two kidneys, a ureter connected to each one, the bladder, and the urethra, which leads to the outside of the body (Figure 15-10). An individual can survive with only one kidney, but if both kidneys fail, the waste products of metabolism will build up in the blood, leading to discomfort, suffering, and, ultimately, death. The kidneys perform the life-sustaining functions of removing fluid and waste products from the blood and regulating internal body chemistry by selectively excreting or retaining various compounds.

FIGURE 15-10 Organs of the urinary system.

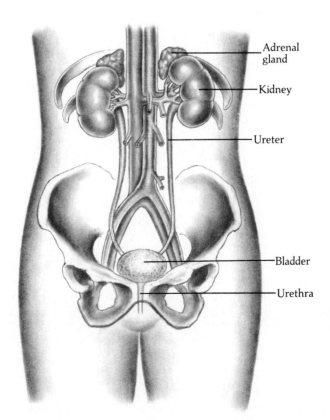

Adrenal gland

Kidney

Ureter

Bladder

Urethra

Within each kidney is an intricate mechanism to provide the filtering, reabsorption, and excretion functions. Over a million nephrons perform the operation; the actual filtering of the blood takes place in a glomerulus within each nephron. Blood flows from the aorta into the nephrons through the renal arteries and, after passing through the maze of tubules and other structures, returns to the lower vena cava through the renal veins. The liquid wastes extracted from the blood are carried by the ureter to the bladder for excretion through the urethra. When the glomeruli or other parts of the kidney do not function as they should, then kidney disease is the result.

CHRONIC RENAL FAILURE

Chronic renal failure is usually the end result of a gradually progressive loss of renal function that can be due to one or more different diseases. Occasionally, it is the result of a rapidly progressive disease of sudden onset. Few symptoms develop until after more than 75% of glomerular filtration is lost. Then the remaining normal tissue deteriorates progressively, and symptoms worsen as renal function decreases. If the condition continues unchecked, uremic toxins accumulate and produce potentially fatal physiologic changes in all major organ systems.

Predisposing Factors   Chronic glomerular disease (glomerulonephritis), chronic infections, congenital defects, vascular diseases, kidney stones, systemic diseases such as lupus erythematosus, drug overdose, and endocrine diseases.

Symptoms   Symptoms arise from the major changes that occur in all body systems. These include:

Cardiovascular—hypertension, arrhythmias, and congestive heart failure

Respiratory—increased susceptibility to infection, pulmonary edema, and pleurisy

Gastrointestinal—ulcers, colitis, and pancreatitis

Skin—yellow-bronze color, dry, scaly, itchy; thin, brittle fingernails

Neurologic—restless legs syndrome, pain, burning, and itching in legs and feet, muscle cramping, shortened memory span, and drowsiness

Blood—anemia and easy bruising

Skeletal—calcium-phosphorus imbalance, demineralization, and fractures

Prevention   Although some of the predisposing factors cannot be changed, attending to any infectious conditions when they occur and controlling hypertension could help avoid kidney problems in later years. Proper nutrition, avoiding the use of drugs, and a healthy lifestyle in general could also reduce the chances of chronic renal failure.

Treatment   Dialysis can eliminate or markedly decrease most symptoms. However, some may remain. A low-protein diet may be prescribed, fluid balance must be maintained, and a regular stool analysis may be required. Drug therapy often relieves some of the symptoms, and careful monitoring of serum potassium levels is necessary. Kidney transplant is also an option.

KIDNEY STONES

A stone or calculus that forms in the kidney usually consists of two or more of the following: uric acid, oxalates, and calcium phosphate. In the United States, kidney stones are more common in men and are rare in blacks and children.

Predisposing Factors Infections, as well as irritation and disease of the parathyroid glands, may cause the formation of stones. Other risk factors are a family history of kidney stones, dehydration, certain medications, and metabolic factors such as too much uric acid in the blood and diet.

Symptoms The usual symptom is pain, which can be excruciating. Depending on the location of the stone, the pain may be in the back, legs, or abdomen, and it may be dull or severe. Nausea and vomiting often accompany severe pain. There may also be chills and fever.

Prevention Particular attention to diet and medications is important if there is a family history of kidney stones. A physician should be consulted if a stone occurs to determine any underlying cause that can be eliminated to prevent recurrence.

Treatment If the stone is not too large to pass through the urinary tract, then measures are taken to promote natural passage. If the stone is not in the lower pelvic area, it can be crushed with a laser. If it is in the urethra, a cystoscope (tube with a light and crushing device attached) can be inserted to destroy the stone. Ultrasonic lithotripsy has been used in recent years. In this process, an ultrasonic probe is used through a telescopic tube to help break up the stones. And, as has been discussed with gallstones, a shockwave can be focused on the stones from outside the body, causing their disintegration. If these methods cannot be used because of placement or size of the stone, analgesics are administered to relieve pain, and surgery may be necessary.

IRRITABLE BOWEL SYNDROME

Irritable bowel syndrome is the most common disorder of the intestines, accounting for more than half of the patients seen by gastroenterologists. The condition is associated with psychological stress, but it may also result from physical factors. It is twice as common in women as in men.

Predisposing Factors Although irritable bowel syndrome is associated with psychological stress, it may also be due to physical factors such as diverticular disease (to be discussed next), lactose intolerance, abuse of laxatives, food poisoning, or colon cancer.

Symptoms In addition to the abdominal pain, diarrhea, and constipation, there may be mucus in the feces, a sense of incomplete evacuation of the bowels, excessive gas, and symptoms aggravated by certain foods.

Predisposing Factors The sacs may be formed when there is excess pressure on weak areas in the walls of the intestine; lack of fiber in the diet is thought to be a factor.

Symptoms If symptoms are present in diverticulosis, they tend to be the same as for irritable bowel syndrome. In diverticulitis, there may be fever, pain, tenderness, and rigidity of the abdomen over the intestine area that is involved.

Prevention Eating a diet high in fiber is thought to lower the risk of diverticular disease.

Treatment For cramps, a high-fiber diet, fiber supplements, and antispasmodic drugs may relieve the symptoms. Bed rest and antibiotics will usually take care of diverticulitis. If the symptoms are severe, treatment may include a liquid diet, intravenous feeding, or surgery to remove the diseased section of the intestine.

SUMMARY

The table summarizes relevant data on the chronic respiratory, digestive, and excretory diseases discussed in this chapter.

SUMMARY TABLE	Chronic respiratory, digestive, and excretory diseases			
Disease	**Special Characteristics**	**Predisposing Factors**	**Common Symptoms**	**Prevention**
Respiratory Disorders				
Chronic bronchitis	Presence of a productive cough for at least 3 mos. of 2 successive years; middle-age, older people, smokers, and those exposed to excess industrial and environmental pollutants; part of COPD, with emphysema, asthma.	Smoking, industrial and environmental pollutants, respiratory infections, allergies.	Productive cough, shortness of breath that gradually gets worse; heart failure *(cor pulmonale)*.	No smoking; living and working environment as free from pollution as possible; treatment for allergy.
Treatment	No smoking; avoidance of air pollution; bronchodilators, nebulizers, diuretics, oxygen as needed.			

SUMMARY TABLE Chronic respiratory, digestive, and excretory diseases—cont'd				
Disease	**Special Characteristics**	**Predisposing Factors**	**Common Symptoms**	**Prevention**
Emphysema	Walls of alveoli destroyed; alveoli lose elasticity; chest becomes barrel shaped, with struggle for breath; victims do not die quickly.	Smoking, air pollution, and deficiency of alpha-antitrypsin (hereditary).	Labored breathing, gasping for breath; chronic cough, anorexia, weight loss, barrel chest, hypoxemia, heart failure *(cor pulmonale)*	No smoking, avoidance of environmental pollutants.
Treatment	Bronchodilators, mucolytic agents, normal weight, oxygen, no smoking, avoidance of air pollutants, chest physiotherapy.			
Digestive Disorders				
Peptic ulcer	May be in stomach (gastric) or duodenum; lesion in mucous membrane; 80% duodenal; more likely in males; acid may be dumped into duodenum through pyloric valve.	Cause of original lesion unknown; may be inherited factor; theories include bacterial infection, overactive vagus nerve, hyperacidity of gastric juice, inadequate mucosal blood flow, hormonal stimulation; duodenal ulcers more frequent with blood type O, gastric with blood type A.	Indigestion, heartburn, and pain in left epigastrium for gastric ulcer, midepigastrium for duodenal ulcer; feeling of fullness right after eating for gastric (weight loss); nausea, pain 2-4 hours after eating for duodenal (weight gain); if untreated, may rupture and hemorrhage or penetrate pancreas; can cause severe back pain.	Avoid nicotine, caffeine, alcohol, aspirin; manage stress.
Treatment	Antacids, drugs, surgery.			
Hiatal hernia	Defect in diaphragmatic hiatus allows part of stomach to protrude into chest cavity; may be sliding or rolling hernia or combination of the two.	More in women than men; results from muscle weakness, congenital or brought on by trauma; any condition producing intraabdominal pressure may cause; if reflux, heartburn present.	None; heartburn, chest pain 1 to 4 hours after eating.	Maintaining ideal weight to reduce risk of intraabdominal pressure.
Treatment	Antiemetics, cough suppressants; avoid movements straining intraabdominal area; no smoking; antacids, weight control; elevated head of bed; drugs to strengthen cardiac sphincter; surgery (hernia often returns).			

Continued.

SUMMARY TABLE   Chronic respiratory, digestive, and excretory diseases—cont'd

Disease	Special Characteristics	Predisposing Factors	Common Symptoms	Prevention
Cirrhosis of the liver	Destruction of cells, fibrotic regeneration lead to permanent loss of liver function; many complications.	Alcoholism (30%–50%), bile duct disease, hepatitis.	Anorexia, indigestion, nausea, vomiting, hepatomegaly; sometimes asymptomatic; liver enlarged; later symptoms: edema, splenomegaly, hemorrhoids, esophageal varices, jaundice.	Good nutrition; little or no alcohol.
Treatment	Removal or alleviation of underlying cause.			
Gallbladder disease	Caused by calculi (gallstones) that irritate gallbladder or clog bile duct. A common condition requiring surgery.	Sluggish gallbladder caused by pregnancy, oral contraceptives, diabetes mellitus, other conditions; may be hereditary; obesity, high levels of estrogen.	Asymptomatic; symptoms: mild abdominal discomfort, acute right-side pain radiating to back with nausea, vomiting.	Unknown.
Treatment	Laparoscopic surgery now used more than conventional surgery.			

Disorders of the Excretory Organs

Disease	Special Characteristics	Predisposing Factors	Common Symptoms	Prevention
Chronic renal failure	One or more kidney disorders cause progressive loss of renal function; 75% of glomerular function lost before most symptoms develop; if untreated, progresses until fatal.	Glomerulonephritis, chronic infections, congenital defects, vascular diseases, kidney stones, some systemic and endocrine diseases; arteriosclerosis.	All body systems in late-stage disease; early symptoms: nausea, drowsiness, vomiting, breathlessness, decrease in urine output; 75% loss of function.	Treatment for kidney infections, control of hypertension; proper nutrition; avoid drug abuse; healthful lifestyle.
Treatment	Dialysis; low-protein diet; maintenance of fluid balance, potassium levels; regular stool analysis; drugs; kidney transplant.			
Kidney stones	Usually consist of uric acid, oxalate, or calcium phosphate (2 or more).	Infections, irritation and disease of parathyroid glands, family history, dehydration, certain medications and diet.	Dull or severe pain in back, legs, or abdomen; nausea, vomiting, chills, fever, may accompany severe pain.	Attention to diet, medications if there is family history.
Treatment	Promotion of natural passage of stone if possible; laser, cystoscope, ultrasonic lithotripsy, analgesics, surgery.			

SUMMARY TABLE Chronic respiratory, digestive, and excretory diseases—cont'd				
Disease	**Special Characteristics**	**Predisposing Factors**	**Common Symptoms**	**Prevention**
Irritable bowel syndrome	Most common disorder of intestines; twice as common in women as in men.	Psychological stress, physical factors.	Abdominal pain, diarrhea, constipation; sometimes mucous in feces; sense of incomplete evacuation; gas.	None known.
Treatment	High-fiber diet, antispasmodic drugs, antidiarrheal drugs if necessary.			
Diverticular disease	Diverticulosis and diverticulitis: in United States, over half have it by age 80.	Pressure on weak areas in walls of intestines; lack of fiber.	Diverticulosis: if present, same as for irritable bowel syndrome; diverticulitis: fever, pain, tenderness; rigidity of abdomen over intestinal area involved.	High-fiber diet may lower risk.
Treatment	High-fiber diet, fiber supplements, antispasmodic drugs, bed rest, antibiotics; liquid diet, intravenous feeding, or surgery if severe.			

QUESTIONS FOR REVIEW

1. What are the differences between chronic bronchitis, asthma, and emphysema?
2. What are the possible causes for peptic ulcers?
3. What measures can be taken to prevent a gastric ulcer?
4. What conditions may predispose a person to hiatal hernia?
5. What happens to the liver in cirrhosis, and what are the consequences?
6. To what extent are alcoholism, hepatitis, and bile duct disease factors in cirrhosis of the liver?
7. What factors may determine whether or not a person gets gallbladder disease?
8. How do the symptoms of peptic ulcer, hiatal hernia, cirrhosis of the liver, and gallbladder disease differ?
9. What is the treatment for chronic bronchitis, asthma, and emphysema?
10. What is the treatment for peptic ulcer, hiatal hernia, cirrhosis of the liver, and gallbladder disease?
11. What conditions may lead to chronic renal failure?
12. What are the symptoms for chronic renal failure?
13. How can the risk of chronic renal failure be reduced?
14. What are the predisposing factors, symptoms, and prevention for kidney stones?

15. What factors are linked to irritable bowel syndrome?
16. How do the symptoms for irritable bowel syndrome and diverticular disease differ?
17. What is the difference between diverticulosis and diverticulitis?
18. What is the treatment for chronic renal failure, kidney stones, irritable bowel syndrome, and diverticular disease?

FURTHER READING

Respiratory.

"Chronic Obstructive Pulmonary Disease Mortality—United States, 1986." *Journal of the American Medical Association,* Sept. 8, '89, 262:1301-1302.

Culliton, Barbara J. "A Genetic Shield to Prevent Emphysema?" *Science,* Nov. 10, '89, 246:750-751.

Dalphin, J.C. et al. "Etiologic Factors of Chronic Bronchitis in Dairy Farmers. Case Control Study in the Doubs Region of France." *Chest,* Feb. '93, 103(2):417-421.

Eggland, Ellen Thomas. "Teaching the ABCs of C.O.P.D." *Nursing,* Jan. '87, 17:60-64.

Gibson, P.G. et al. "Chronic Cough: Eosinophilic Bronchitis without Asthma." *Lancet,* June 17, '89, 1:1346-1348.

McGowan, Stephen E. and Gary W. Hunninghake. "Neutrophils and Emphysema" (Editorial). *New England Journal of Medicine,* Oct. 5, '89, 321:968-970.

Pierce, John A. "Antitrypsin and Emphysema: Perspective and Prospects." *Journal of the American Medical Association,* May 20, '88, 259:2890-2895.

Snider, G.L. "Emphysema: The First Two Centuries—and Beyond. A Historical Overview, with Suggestions for Future Research: Part 2." *American Review of Respiratory Disease,* Dec. '92, 146(6):1615-1622.

Digestive.

Cotton, Paul. "Parents' Behavior May Lead Irritable Bowel Syndrome Patients into Physicians' Offices." *Journal of the American Medical Association,* July 17, '91, 266:317-318.

Dooley, Cornelius P. et al. "Prevalence of *Helicobacter Pylori* Infection and Histologic Gastritis in Asymptomatic Persons." *New England Journal of Medicine,* Dec. 7, '89, 321:1562-1566.

Goldsmith, Marsha F. "Biliary, as Well as Urinary, Calculi Become the Targets of New, Improved Shock Wave Lithotripsy." *Journal of the American Medical Association,* Sept. 11, '87, 258:1282-1284.

Goodwin, Stewart C. "Duodenal Ulcer, *Campylobacter Pylori,* and the 'Leaking Roof' Concept." *Lancet,* Dec. 24, '88, 2:1467-1469.

Hofmann, A.F. "Primary and Secondary Prevention of Gallstone Disease: Implications for Patient Management and Research Priorities." *American Journal of Surgery,* Apr. '93, 165(4):541-548.

Hood, Kathryn et al. "Prevention of Gallstone Recurrence by Non-Steroidal Anti-Inflammatory Drugs." *Lancet,* Nov. 26, '88, 2:1223-1225.

Kaplan, Marshall M. "Primary Biliary Cirrhosis." *New England Journal of Medicine,* Feb. 26, '87, 316:521-528.

Kerrigan, D.D. et al. "Duodenal Bulb Acidity and the Natural History of Duodenal Ulceration." *Lancet,* July 8, '89, 2:61-63.

Kershenobich, David et al. "Colchicine in the Treatment of Cirrhosis of the Liver." *New England Journal of Medicine,* June 30, '88, 318:1709-1713.

Laws, H.L. and J.B. McKernan. "Endoscopic Management of Peptic Ulcer Disease." *Annals of Surgery,* May '93, 217(5):548-555, discussion 555-556.

Levi, Sassoon et al. "*Campylobacter Pylori* and Duodenal Ulcers: The Gastrin Link." *Lancet,* May 27, '89, 1:1167-1168.

Lieber, Charles S. "Biochemical and Molecular Basis of Alcohol-Induced Injury to the Liver and Other Tissues." *New England Journal of Medicine,* Dec. 22, '88, 319:1639-1650.

McClure, Malcolm K., C. Hayes, Graham A. Colditz et al. "Weight, Diet, and the Risk of Symptomatic Gallstones in Middle-Aged Women." *New England Journal of Medicine,* Aug. 31, '89, 321:563-569.

McHenry, L., Jr., L. Vuyyuru, M.L. Schubert. "*Helicobacter Pylori* and Duodenal Ulcer Disease—the Somatostatin Link?" *Gastroenterology,* May '93, 104(5):1573-1575.

Petitti, D.B. and S. Sidney. "Obesity and Cholecystectomy among Women: Implications for Prevention." *American Journal of Preventive Medicine,* Nov./Dec. '88, 4:327-330.

Romelsjo, A. et al. "The Prevalence of Alcohol-related Mortality in Both Sexes: Variation between Indicators, Stockholm, 1987." *American Journal of Public Health,* June '93, 83(6): 838-844.

Salen, Gerald. "Nonsurgical Treatment of Gallstones" (Editorial). *New England Journal of Medicine,* Mar. 9, '89, 320:665-666.

Schubert, T.T. et al. "Ulcer Risk Factors: Interactions between *Helicobacter pylori* Infection, Nonsteroidal Use, and Age." *American Journal of Medicine,* Apr '93, 94(4):413-418.

Sidebotham, R.L. and J.H. Baron. "Hypothesis: *Helicobacter Pylori,* Urease, Mucus, and Gastric Ulcer." *Lancet,* Jan. 27, '90, 335:193-195.

Thomas, Patricia. "Top Ten Advances of 1991." *Harvard Health Letter,* Mar. '92, 17:1-4.

Van Deventer, Gary M. et al. "A Randomized Study of Maintenance Therapy with Ranitidine to Prevent the Recurrence of Duodenal Ulcer." *New England Journal of Medicine,* Apr. 27, '89, 320:1113-1119.

Weber, F.H. and R.W. McCallum. "Clinical Approaches to Irritable Bowel Syndrome." *Lancet,* Dec. 12, '92, 340(8833):1447-1452.

Whorwell, P.J., L.A. Houghton et al. "Physiological Effects of Emotion: Assessment via Hypnosis." *Lancet,* July 11, '92, 340:69-72.

Willis, Dawn A. "Gallstones: Alternatives to Surgery." *RN,* Apr. '90, 53:44-51.

Excretory.

Bayless, Theodore M. et al. "Managing Inflammatory Bowel Disease." *Patient Care,* Sept. 30, '88, 22:20-35.

Christensen, J. "Pathophysiology of the Irritable Bowel Syndrome." *Lancet,* Dec. 12, '92, 340(8833):1444-1447.

Coe, F.L., J.H. Parks, and J.R. Asplin. "The Pathogenesis and Treatment of Kidney Stones." *New England Journal of Medicine,* Oct. 15, '92, 327(16):1141-1152.

Deniston, O. Lynn et al. "Assessment of Quality of Life in End-Stage Renal Disease." *Health Services Research,* Oct. '89, 24:555-578.

Hahn, Karen. "The Many Signs of Renal Failure." *Nursing,* Aug. '87, 17:34-42.

"Irritable Bowel Syndrome—Can Medication Help?" *Harvard Medical School Health Letter,* Jan. '89, 14:7-8.

Nolph, Karl D., Anne S. Lindblad, and Joel W. Novak. "Continuous Ambulatory Peritoneal Dialysis." *New England Journal of Medicine,* June 16, '88, 318:1595-1600.

Perneger, T.V. et al. "Projections of Hypertension-related Renal Disease in Middle-aged Residents of the United States." *Journal of the American Medical Association,* Mar. 10, '93, 269(10):1272-1277.

"Prevention and Treatment of Kidney Stones." *Journal of the American Medical Association,* Aug. 19, '88, 260:977-981.

Rimmer, J. and F.J. Gennari. "Atherosclerotic Renovascular Disease and Progressive Renal Failure." *Annals of Internal Medicine,* May 1, '93, 118(9):712-719.

Sandler, Dale P. et al. "Analgesic Use and Chronic Renal Disease." *New England Journal of Medicine,* May 11, '89, 320:1238-1244.

Starr, Cynthia. "Tell Your Patients—There's Help for the Cranky Colon." *Drug Topics,* Mar. 7, '88, 132:32-33.

Thomas, Patricia. "Gut Feelings: How to Quit Your Bellyaching." *Health,* Apr. '90, 22: 76-78.

Chapter 16

Chronic Skin and Musculoskeletal Disorders

O B J E C T I V E S

1 Identify basic skin lesions.

2 Describe common disorders of the skin.

3 Evaluate treatments for acne.

4 Explain the reason for the symptoms of psoriasis.

5 Distinguish between osteoarthritis and rheumatoid arthritis (Chapter 2).

6 State the suspected cause of gout.

7 Explain what causes the symptoms of gout.

8 Identify the predisposing factors for fibromyalgia.

9 Explain how carpal tunnel syndrome occurs.

10 Distinguish between tendinitis and bursitis.

11 Discuss the symptoms of osteoporosis.

12 State the best treatment for osteoporosis.

13 Identify the best means of prevention for back problems.

14 Distinguish among lordosis, kyphosis, and scoliosis.

SKIN DISORDERS

The skin is the largest organ of the body. This tough, resilient, protective barrier against environmental threats contains body fluids, regulates body temperatures, and plays a part in the production of vitamin D. The skin also contains touch and pressure receptors that provide sensations. The functions of the skin can be seen in Figure 16-1.

The skin has three primary layers, the epidermis, dermis, and subcutaneous tissue (Figure 16-2). The epidermis is the thinnest layer, although it is thicker on some parts of the body where it is subjected to much "wear and tear," such as the soles of the feet and palms of the hand. The skin of men is generally thicker than that of women, and it becomes thinner with age.

The dermis contains the hair follicles, sweat glands, and sebaceous glands. There are also blood vessels, lymph vessels, and nerves in the dermis.

The subcutaneous tissue, or hypodermis, is mainly fat and provides heat, insulation, shock absorption, and a reserve of calories. It also has a nerve supply.

In addition to immune disorders, infectious diseases and cancer, disorders of the skin include those due to injury, hormonal disorders, poor nutrition, impaired blood supply, and drug reactions.

ACNE

Most adolescent boys and many adolescent girls experience acne vulgaris, which is the most common type of acne. It is a chronic disorder of the skin caused by inflammation of the hair follicles and sebaceous glands. It can appear as early as age 8 but most often begins at puberty.

**Predisposing
Factors** Acne spots occur when a hair follicle becomes obstructed by sebum. The follicle becomes inflamed when the sebum is trapped because bacteria are able to multiply, producing the inflammatory response. No one is sure why this happens at puberty, but it seems to be linked to the release of hormones. There may be a hereditary factor too.

FIGURE 16-1 Functions of the skin.

> **FUNCTIONS OF THE SKIN**
> Protects against infection
> Contains body fluids
> Regulates body temperature
> Produces vitamin D
> Provides sensations of touch and temperature

Other predisposing factors are drugs that increase oil production by the skin, barbiturates, isoniazid, rifampin, bromides, and iodides. Acne may also be caused by oil and grease, such as that at the hairline, or regular contact with mineral or cooking oil as in restaurant kitchens may make the condition worse. Cosmetics with an oil base are another risk factor.

Symptoms   The places where acne occurs have a high concentration of sebaceous glands. They are found mainly in the face, center of the chest, upper back, shoulders, and around the neck. The most common acne spots are blackheads, whiteheads, pustules, nodules, and cysts. Figure 16-3 shows an outbreak of acne on the face. Some spots, particularly if squeezed or irritated, leave scars, and the cystic spots may leave scars even without being touched. The scars tend to be small, depressed pits.

FIGURE 16-2 Structure of the skin.

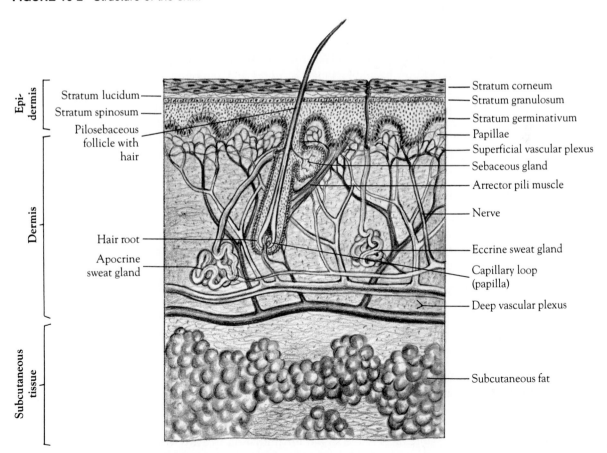

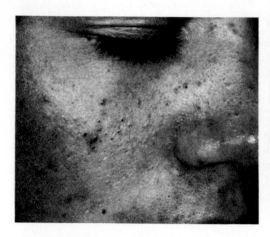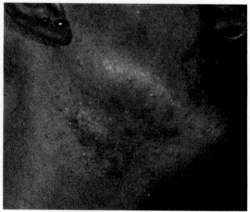

FIGURE 16-3   Acne on face.

Prevention   There is no known dietary substance that causes acne. However, each person may be sensitive to certain foods on an individual basis. Many myths have grown up around the disorder that is so disfiguring just when young people are becoming extremely sensitive about their appearance. No evidence shows that avoiding chocolate or any other dietary substance will help. Washing the affected areas twice daily will not prevent the disorder, but it may keep it from spreading. Washing simply removes surface oil.

Treatment   Many treatments are available for acne, but no cures. Topical treatments may relieve the condition by unblocking the pores and removing the sebum. They will also promote healing. If topical therapy is not effective, systemic drugs may be used. Antibiotics are sometimes used and can have a healing effect over a long period (up to 6 months). Recently, retinoid drugs have been prescribed to reduce oil secretions and facilitate drying on the skin, but they have dangerous side effects and cannot be used during pregnancy. Acne generally clears up by the end of the teenage years.

DERMATITIS

Some forms of dermatitis are due to disorders of the immune system and were discussed in Chapter 2. Others have no known cause. Seborrheic dermatitis and contact dermatitis are two of the most common. Sometimes, dermatitis is known as eczema.

SEBORRHEIC DERMATITIS

A common site for seborrheic dermatitis is the eyebrows (Figure 16-4), although it may occur at many places on the body.

Predisposing Factors   The exact cause is unknown, but stress and neurologic conditions may be predisposing factors.

Symptoms   There is itching, redness, and inflammation in areas with many sebaceous glands, usually the scalp, face, and trunk, and in skin folds. The lesions may appear greasy.

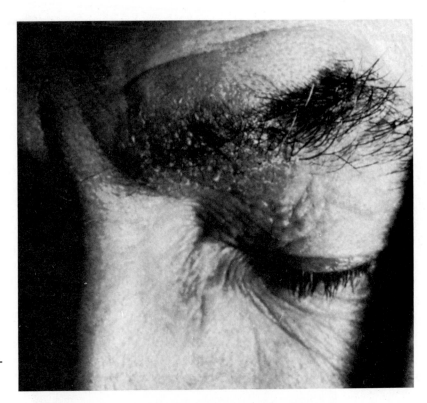

FIGURE 16-4 Seborrheic dermatitis of eyebrow.

The victim also may have yellowish, scaly patches, and dandruff may be caused by a mild seborrheic dermatitis.

Prevention   None known.

Treatment   The basic treatment is frequent washing and shampooing with a medicated soap to remove the scales. Topical corticosteroids and/or antibiotics may also be used. Skin should be handled gently; scratching and irritating substances, such as detergents, should be avoided.

CONTACT DERMATITIS

This kind of dermatitis is caused by something that has touched the skin.

Predisposing Factors   Contact dermatitis may be caused by an allergy to a substance such as poison ivy, or it may be due to a direct toxic effect of the substance. Common substances that cause the reaction are detergents, nickel, chemicals in rubber gloves and condoms, certain cosmetics, plants, and medications.

Symptoms   A rash occurs and varies considerably according to the substance that causes it. The skin is often itchy and may flake, or a blister may develop. The rash covers the area of skin that came in contact with the substance.

Prevention Identification of the causative substance and avoidance in the future is the best means of prevention.

Treatment Topical application of corticosteroids may be used for treatment of the rash.

PSORIASIS

Psoriasis is a common skin disease characterized by thickened patches of inflamed, red skin that is often covered by silvery scaling (Figure 16-5). Close to 2% of the people in the United States and Europe are affected by the disease, which is not as common among blacks and Asians. The affected areas may be so extensive that the individual is embarrassed to go out in public, particularly if the patches are on exposed surfaces. Common sites of the patches are the knees, elbows, scalp, trunk, and back. The disorder occurs when new skin cells are produced at 10 times the usual rate while the shedding of old cells does not change. The live cells accumulate, causing the thickened patches covered with dead, flaking skin. There are different forms of psoriasis; the most common form is discussed here.

FIGURE 16-5 Psoriasis.

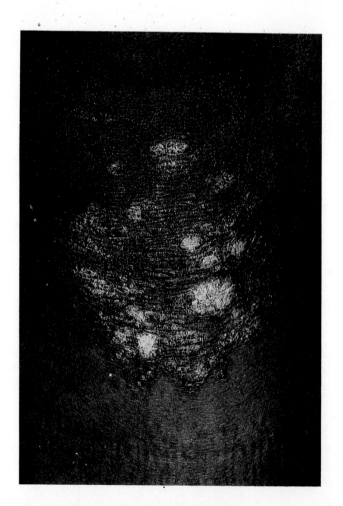

Predisposing Factors   A number of possible causes are being investigated, and there may be a genetic basis. Psoriasis tends to recur in attacks that may be triggered by emotional stress, skin damage, and physical illness.

Symptoms   In addition to the red skin and silvery patches, the most common symptom is itching. Because the patches tend to be dry and become cracked and encrusted, there may also be pain. The disease usually begins with small red papules that enlarge and join into larger inflamed lesions. When they develop in skin folds, the lesions are smooth and have a deep red color. There may be small bleeding points if the scales are removed. Many individuals with psoriasis also have arthritic symptoms.

Prevention   None known.

Treatment   Treatment depends upon the severity of the attack and form of the disease. Sunlight or ultraviolet lamps in small doses can be helpful, along with an emollient to help soften the affected area. The same therapies are used in moderate attacks, with the addition of an ointment containing coal tar. More severe attacks are treated with corticosteroids and other drugs. A nonsteroidal anti-inflammatory drug (NSAID), antirheumatic drug, or methotrexate may be used to treat the arthritis that accompanies psoriasis.

DISORDERS OF THE MUSCULOSKELETAL SYSTEM

Without the muscles, bones and joints, and connective tissue, activity as we know it would not exist. Moreover, disease or disorder in the parts of the musculoskeletal system can cripple and incapacitate until a normal life is impossible. It is easy to think of a bone as something nonliving. Those we generally see from the human skeleton are dry and lifeless. But bones are living, productive parts of the body in addition to giving support. The center of each bone is a cavity in which blood cells are manufactured. And each bone is composed of a supply of minerals and fibrous tissue that are also active in various growth processes. Figure 16-6 shows the basic structure of a bone. In most chronic disorders of the musculoskeletal system, it is not the bone shafts that sustain injury, but the joints, which are susceptible throughout life to the stresses and strains of activity. One exception in the diseases that follow is osteoporosis, which is a metabolic bone disease affecting the integrity of the bone itself. Another exception is fibromyalgia, a disease of the muscles, tendons, and ligaments. Some of the other diseases affecting the musculoskeletal system are known to be neurologically or genetically oriented and will be dealt with in Chapters 17 and 18.

DISORDERS OF THE JOINTS

OSTEOARTHRITIS

Osteoarthritis is the most common form of arthritis and is present to some extent in everyone over 60. It is a chronic, progressive disorder causing deterioration of joint cartilage and bone. The body's response to this deterioration is to produce excess bone, which eventually makes joint movement painful and difficult, if not impossible. Figure 16-7 shows a diseased hip joint.

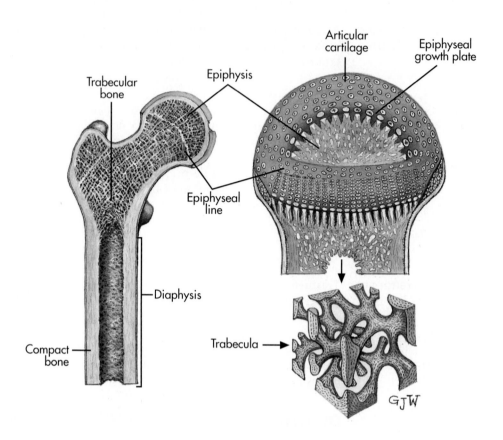

FIGURE 16-6 Structure of a bone.

FIGURE 16-7 Diseased hip joint.

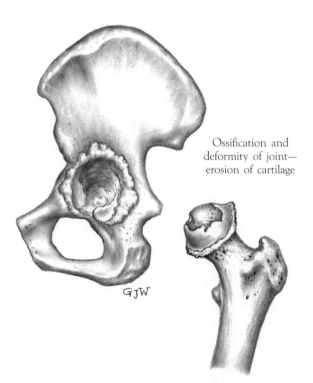

DID YOU KNOW?

For Osteoarthritis Pain Relief

Acetaminophen (Tylenol) was shown to be as effective as ibuprofen (Advil) in relieving some chronic pain caused by osteoarthritis. This surprising news was reported in *The New England Journal of Medicine* (July '91). Acetaminophen had been known to be effective as an analgesic, but aspirin, ibuprofen, and other nonsteroidal anti-inflammatory drugs (NSAIDs) are usually prescribed first for arthritic conditions. Now it seems that acetaminophen, which has fewer side effects than NSAIDs, might be a better choice.

Predisposing Factors   Continual exposure of the joint(s) to trauma such as in athletics or a professional trade, inherited predisposition, and normal aging processes all have been identified as predisposing factors.

Symptoms   In osteoarthritis, joint pain occurs, particularly after exercise or weight bearing, that is usually relieved by rest. There may also be stiffness in the morning, aching during changes in weather, limited movement, and fluid accumulation in the affected joint(s). Severity increases with poor posture, obesity, and occupational stress.

Prevention   Sensible exercise routines, but avoidance of athletic and occupational activities that cause constant stress to weight-bearing joints, may decrease the severity and deter the onset of osteoarthritis.

Treatment   The traditional treatment has been medication to relieve pain and surgery to replace joints that have been destroyed. Water exercise has been found to be helpful for many. Read the above Did You Know? for information on pain relievers.

DID YOU KNOW?

Meet Robodoc

Scientists have developed a robot to help surgeons in hip replacement. According to *The Journal of the American Medical Association* (Feb. 5, '92), the robot, nicknamed Robodoc, reams out the femur for placement of the prosthesis and does so with 40 times more accuracy than the surgeon is capable of. The surgeon still must guide the robot, but it is hoped that the more precise dimensions of the hole, allowing 95% of the implant to contact the bone rather than only 20% by the current method, will lead to more comfortable, more stable, and longer lasting replacements. The method has worked with dogs and has been approved for human trials.

GOUT

Gout is a painful arthritic disease that occurs most often in men. It involves a disruption of the body's control over uric acid production or excretion, resulting in high levels of uric acid in the blood. When the uric acid builds to a certain level in the blood, it crystalizes, and these crystals are deposited in connective tissue all over the body. When the crystals are deposited in the synovial fluid, they cause sudden sharp pain in the joint. Primary gout, which has a strong hereditary tendency, usually occurs in men over the age of 30 and in postmenopausal women. Secondary gout, which arises as a result of another disorder, occurs in the elderly. The disease follows an intermittent course and may disappear for years and then return.

Predisposing Factors

Although excess use of alcohol may cause an exacerbation of the symptoms of gout, diet and "high living" are no longer considered the major factors. It is known that ingestion of excess amounts of protein can lead to high uric acid levels. Some evidence points to an inherited metabolic defect. Secondary gout may result from leukemia, chronic renal diseases, lead poisoning, and drugs such as chlorothiazide.

Symptoms

Primary gout is an interesting disease that may affect any joint at any time. The most frequent site, for some unknown reason, is the big toe. The victim may wake suddenly in the middle of the night with such excruciating pain that he or she cannot tolerate the touch of even a sheet. In fact, the uric acid level in the blood may have been increasing for some time. As the disease moves into a more advanced stage, hypertension and kidney stones with severe back pain may occur. When the first arthritic attack occurs, affected joints appear hot, tender, and inflamed. A low-grade fever may be present. A mild attack may subside quickly. In the final stages there is unremitting pain, and deposits of urate called tophi cause swollen and deformed joints at many sites, including fingers, hands, knees, and feet. The skin is drawn taut over these tophaceous deposits and may ulcerate, releasing a chalky white substance or pus. Gout can lead to chronic disability and crippling in addition to renal dysfunction.

Prevention

Decreasing the amount of protein in the diet could be of some help.

Treatment

Treatment for acute gout consists of bed rest, immobilization of the painful joints, local application of heat or cold, some dietary restrictions, and drugs to adjust the level of uric acid in the blood. Colchicine, a drug that was used 1500 years ago in the treatment of gout, is still the most effective drug in reducing pain and inflammation. It is used concomitantly with other analgesics. In severe cases that do not respond to other therapy, corticosteroids may be used.

DISORDERS OF MUSCLE AND CONNECTIVE TISSUE

FIBROMYALGIA

Fibromyalgia is a very common disease of the muscles, ligaments, and tendons that has only recently been recognized by medical science. According to the Arthritis

Foundation, "There are, currently, millions of Americans who have been diagnosed with fibromyalgia" (Arthritis Foundation. Fibromyalgia Booklet. P. O. Box 1900, Atlanta, Georgia, 30326, 1991). In the past, it was called fibrositis, but since investigation has failed to show any inflammation in the muscles, the syndrome has been renamed. Fibromyalgia is more common in women than men, and those diagnosed with it are usually between the ages of 20 and 50.

Predisposing Factors

The exact cause of fibromyalgia is not yet known, but a number of factors have been associated with the disease. Individuals with the syndrome have unfit or poorly developed muscles. It is not known whether the unfit muscles are the cause or the result of fibromyalgia. A second factor linked to the disease is sleep disturbances. In sleep laboratory studies, people with fibromyalgia show an interruption or disturbance of stage IV sleep. This is the deepest and most restful stage of sleep and the time when the body repairs tissue damage. There is also evidence to show that loss of stage IV sleep can lead to muscle pain. The combination of pain and fatigue that results leads to lack of physical exercise, which can contribute to the overall symptoms of the disease. Stress is a third factor linked to fibromyalgia. Although it is not thought that stress causes the syndrome, it is known that it can make the symptoms worse.

Symptoms

There are two major symptoms: pain and fatigue. Pain in fibromyalgia is felt as an aching, stiffness, and tenderness around the joints. The pain may be general over much of the body or it may be localized. Extreme soreness is felt over points where muscles attach to bones (Figure 16-8). These sites are tender points or trigger points; they are the same for all people with fibromyalgia and are an important part of diagnosing the disease. The other major symptom, fatigue can be so severe that the individual must rest at 1-2 hour intervals each day. People with fibromyalgia also have other symptoms that are confusing to doctors, such as Raynaud's phenomenon, tension headaches, migraine, dizziness, tingling and numbness, irritable bowel syndrome, muscle tremors, bladder spasms, and blurred vision.

Prevention

None known.

Treatment

The only treatment for fibromyalgia now is to help individuals increase their physical fitness, improve their sleep, and ease the pain and fatigue. Exercise is recommended to improve muscular and general physical fitness. An antidepressant is prescribed at bedtime to promote stage IV sleep. NSAIDs do not seem to help the pain of fibromyalgia, which generally decreases as fitness and sleep improve. A hot bath may give temporary relief.

CARPAL TUNNEL SYNDROME

This syndrome occurs when the median nerve that passes through the carpal tunnel at the wrist is compressed, cutting down the circulation and sensation in the thumb and fingers (Figure 16-9). It usually occurs in women between the ages of 30 and

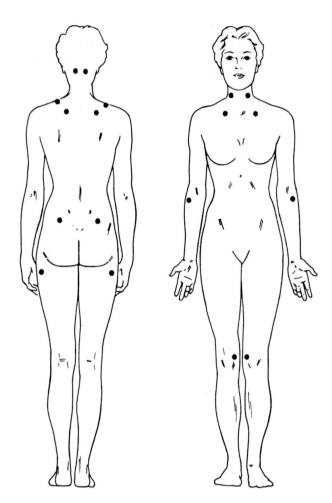

FIGURE 16-8 Tender points for fibromyalgia.

FIGURE 16-9 Carpal tunnel in wrist.

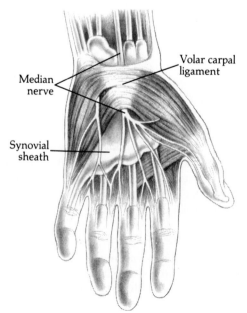

Median nerve

Volar carpal ligament

Synovial sheath

60. In recent years, the incidence has been increasing, possibly as a result of the computer age. Assembly line workers, packers, typists, guitar players, bakers, and computer operators are particularly susceptible.

Predisposing Factors — There are many conditions that can cause swelling in the carpal tunnel and, subsequently, pressure on the nerve. Included in these are pregnancy, diabetes mellitus, menopause, rheumatoid arthritis, tuberculosis, and hypothyroidism. Dislocation or an acute sprain of the wrist may also cause the syndrome.

Symptoms — Carpal tunnel syndrome produces weakness, burning, tingling, numbness and/or pain in one or both hands. The sensations are usually felt in the thumb, forefinger, middle finger, and part of the fourth finger. Individuals may be unable to clench their fist; the fingernails may be smaller than normal, and the skin dry and shiny. Symptoms are often worse at night and in the morning. Shaking the hands vigorously or dangling them at the sides may relieve the symptoms temporarily.

Prevention — For people who perform repetitive tasks, regular breaks from their work may help. Correct posture, good chair level, and correct height for worktables are also important.

Treatment — The first step is to splint the wrist in a neutral position for 1 to 2 weeks. If symptoms persist, a small quantity of corticosteroid may be injected to reduce inflammation. If these measures do not help, surgery is the only alternative. In some cases, it may be necessary to change occupations.

TENDINITIS AND BURSITIS

Tendinitis and bursitis are two different disorders, but the predisposing factors, symptoms, prevention, and treatment are often the same. Tendinitis is a painful inflammation of tendons or tendon-muscle attachments. Bursitis is a painful inflammation of one or more of the bursae, the small, fluid-filled sacs that facilitate the movement of muscles and tendons over bony parts of joints. Figures 16-10 and 16-11 show common sites of tendinitis and bursitis.

Predisposing Factors — Strain during sports activity, repetitive movements, rheumatic diseases, congenital defects, postural misalignment, and gout are among the causes of both disorders. Infection of the bursae may also be a cause of bursitis.

Symptoms — Tendinitis often occurs in the shoulder, producing pain on movement and also localized pain, which is most severe at night and interferes with sleep. If the tendinitis is due to calcium deposits, there may also be weakness. In bursitis, there are sudden or gradual pain and limitation of movement. Symptoms vary depending on the affected site.

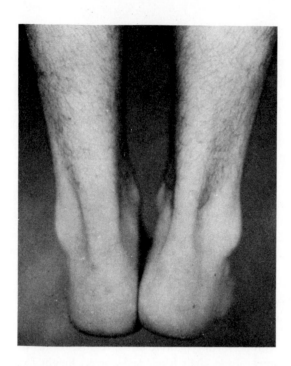

FIGURE 16-10 Common site of tendinitis.

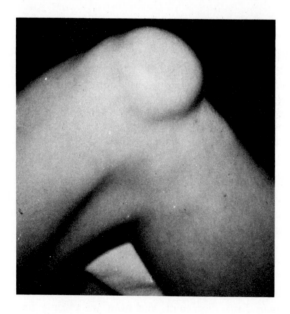

FIGURE 16-11 Common site of bursitis.

Prevention Maintaining adequate body strength and flexibility and avoiding stress and strain in sports activities are the principal preventive measures.

Treatment Resting the joint, analgesics, and application of cold, heat, and ultrasound are helpful. In severe cases, an injection of an analgesic and corticosteroids may be used to reduce inflammation.

DISORDERS OF THE BONE

OSTEOPOROSIS

Osteoporosis is a metabolic bone disorder resulting in resorption of calcium from the bone. More than 1.5 million Americans have fractures related to osteoporosis each year. Because this disorder affects so many of the elderly, Medicare pays their medical expenses, and the annual cost to the health care system is at least $10 billion.

Osteoporosis generally occurs after menopause and is linked to low levels of estrogen. It is estimated that half of the women over 60 in North America have osteoporosis, and some elderly men also have it. Osteoporosis may also be secondary to another primary disease.

Osteoporosis is known to occur in women with anorexia nervosa. These women experience amenorrhea, low estrogen levels, and loss of bone mass as do post-menopausal women. Highly trained women athletes also experience amenorrhea and reduced bone mass. Studies have shown that women athletes who are deficient in estrogen regain their bone mass after treatment, as well as resumption of menses, whereas anorectics who are treated and regain at least 80% of their ideal weight do not regain their bone mass.

Predisposing Factors

Factors that have been linked to osteoporosis are race (white), smoking, alcohol consumption, European nationality or descent, sedentary living, and inadequate estrogen in women.

Symptoms

Osteoporosis is often discovered only after an elderly person breaks a bone. Although in the past, broken hips were attributed to falls, it is known now that the bone generally breaks first and causes the fall. (For research on hip replacement surgery, see the Did You Know? section that follows.) The most common symptom is backache pain that radiates around the trunk. This is due to broken vertebrae that snap easily when osteoporosis is present. Another common sign is kyphosis, a humped back condition that occurs because of crushed vertebrae (Figure 16-12). Breakage of a bone with no unusual stress having been placed upon it is a common occurrence in those with osteoporosis.

Primary Prevention

Individuals who get regular exercise and have a balanced diet with adequate calcium throughout life have less risk of developing osteoporosis.

Secondary Prevention

High calcium intake plus exercise involving active weight-bearing movement have been found to slow the loss of bone in some and increase bone mass in others.

Treatment

A regular individualized activity program and increased dietary calcium are the best treatment. In severe cases, estrogen, fluoride, and supplemental calcium and vitamin D may be prescribed to decrease the rate of bone resorption.

HERNIATED DISK

Commonly called slipped disk, a herniated disk is the result when the soft central part of an intervertebral disk is forced through its outer covering (Figure 16-13).

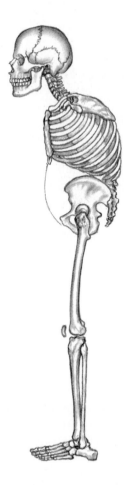

FIGURE 16-12 Kyphosis in aged skeleton.

When this happens, the disk may press on a nerve, causing lower back pain. The condition occurs more often in men, and usually in individuals under age 45.

Predisposing Factors Although herniated disks usually occur in those under the age of 45, in elderly people they may occur because of degeneration of the joints. In younger men and women, the disk may herniate because of strain or trauma. Incorrect lifting and carrying procedures, especially if required repeatedly because of occupation, can produce the condition. Some individuals may be more susceptible because of congenital spinal canal malformation.

Symptoms Pain in the lower back and radiating down the sciatic nerve on one side to the buttocks, legs, and feet is the common sign of a herniated disk. Depending on the location of the hernia and nerves affected, there may be other symptoms.

Prevention Good posture and proper lifting and carrying procedures can help prevent many back problems. Back exercises to strengthen those muscles that are subject to strain are very important.

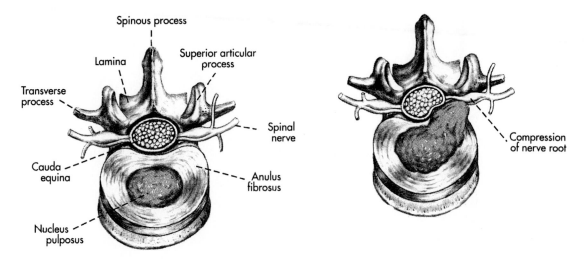

FIGURE 16-13   Herniated disk.

Treatment   Instruction on proper care of the back along with rest, heat applications, and therapeutic exercises are the usual treatment. Analgesics and muscle relaxants may give relief from the pain. If the condition does not improve, surgery may be necessary.

SCOLIOSIS

There are three common disorders having to do with the curve of the spine. Lordosis, commonly called swayback, is an accentuation of the normal curve that is present in the lower back and is generally the result of poor posture. Kyphosis is an exaggeration of the normal curve in the upper back and produces the disfigurement commonly called humpback or hunchback and will be discussed next. Scoliosis is a lateral curvature of the spine that generally affects the chest or lower back regions (Figure 16-14). It is often associated with lordosis and kyphosis. Scoliosis may begin in childhood or adolescence and progress until the age when growth stops, or it may begin in later life.

Predisposing Factors   Functional factors that lead to scoliosis are poor posture, a discrepancy in leg lengths, unfit muscles, and/or obesity. If it is structural, it may be congenital, caused by a disease that weakens muscles, such as polio; genes may also be a factor.

Symptoms   The most common curve is in an S shape. As the spine curves laterally, the body develops compensatory curves to maintain balance. Systemic symptoms do not occur until the curve becomes well established. When symptoms do occur, they include backache, fatigue, and dyspnea. If left untreated, there may be pulmonary insufficiency, back pain, degenerative arthritis of the spine, disk disease, and sciatica.

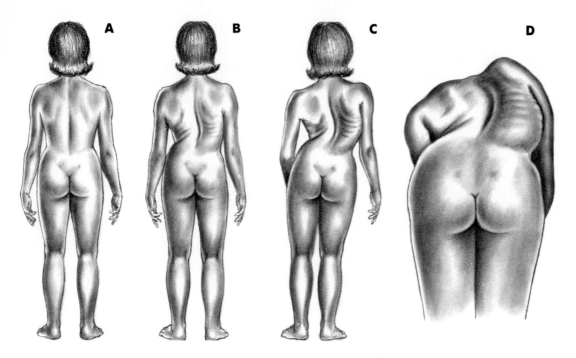

FIGURE 16-14 Scoliosis. **A,** Normal. **B,** Mild. **C,** Severe. **D,** Rotation and curvature of scoliosis.

Prevention   Children, and particularly teenagers, are shy about their bodies and may not notice or allow anyone else to see whether there is a deformity. Doctors should check routinely during physicals, and teachers should know what to look for and screen students for signs of scoliosis or other back problems in each grade. Parents need to be educated about the possibility that scoliosis may develop, particularly if anyone else in the family has had it.

Treatment   Treatment depends upon the age of the individual and the severity of the deformity. It may include exercise, a brace, surgery, or a combination of these. If obesity is a factor, then dieting is necessary, and if different leg lengths is a factor, then orthopedic shoes are recommended also.

KYPHOSIS

Kyphosis is the medical term for excessive backward curvature of the spine. It usually affects the spine at the top of the back, resulting in either a hump or a more gradually rounded back (Figure 16-15).

Predisposing Factors   Kyphosis may be caused by a number of disorders affecting the spine. In adolescents, the disorder may result from growth retardation or congenital causes. In adults, it may be a result of aging, osteoporosis, endocrine disorders, steroid therapy, arthritis, polio, metastatic tumor, tuberculosis, and many other diseases.

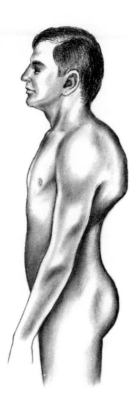

FIGURE 16-15 Kyphosis.

Symptoms In adolescents, there may be mild pain at the top of the curve, accompanied by fatigue, tenderness, or stiffness in the involved area or along the entire spine. Symptoms for adults with kyphosis may be pain, weakness of the back, and generalized fatigue.

Prevention Maintaining a correct posture, ideal weight, and good nutrition should help to reduce the risk factors.

Treatment Treatment is rarely successful but is aimed at the underlying disorder.

SUMMARY

The table on pages 426–429 summarizes the disorders of the skin and musculoskeletal system discussed in this chapter.

SUMMARY TABLE Chronic skin and musculoskeletal disorders				
Disease	**Special Characteristics**	**Predisposing Factors**	**Common Symptoms**	**Prevention**
Acne	Experienced by most teenage boys and some teenage girls; inflammation of hair follicles, sebaceous glands.	Obstruction of hair follicle by sebum, leading to infection; linked to hormone release; may be hereditary; perhaps drugs, oily skin, cosmetics.	Blackheads, whiteheads, pustules, nodules, cysts on face or other body parts with high concentration of sebaceous glands.	None known; no dietary connection; washing affected area twice daily may prevent spreading.
Treatment	Topical and systemic drugs, sometimes antibiotics; retinoid drugs to reduce oil secretions (but not during pregnancy); no cure; generally clears up at end of teens.			
Seborrheic dermatitis	Eyebrows are common site; may be cause of dandruff.	Unknown; perhaps stress, neurologic conditions.	Itching, redness, inflammation, usually on scalp, face, trunk, and in skin folds; greasy-looking, yellowish, scaly.	None known.
Treatment	Frequent washing, shampooing with medicated soap; topical corticosteroids and/or antibiotics.			
Contact dermatitis	Caused by something that touches the skin.	Allergic reaction or toxic substance.	Rash varies, depending on cause, covers area that had contact with substance; itchy skin may flake, blister.	Identify causative substance, avoid in future.
Treatment	Topical application of corticosteroids.			
Psoriasis	Nearly 2% affected in United States, Europe; not so common among blacks, Asians; may cause embarrassment; new skin cells produced at 10 times normal rate, but shedding rate of old cells unchanged.	May be triggered by emotional stress, skin damage, physical illness; initial cause unknown.	Thickened patches of inflamed skin often covered by silvery scaling; itching, pain; skin-fold lesions smooth, deep red; bleeding if scales removed.	None known.
Treatment	Sunlight or ultraviolet lamps, emollient, coal tar ointment, corticosteroids, other drugs, depending on severity of attack.			
Osteoarthritis	Present to some extent in everyone over 60; deterioration of joint cartilage and bone; ex-	Continual joint trauma, normal aging.	Joint pain after exercise, weight bearing, usually relieved by rest; morning stiffness, aching during	Avoidance of athletic, occupational activities placing constant stress on joints; sensible

SUMMARY TABLE Chronic skin and musculoskeletal disorders—cont'd				
Disease	**Special Characteristics**	**Predisposing Factors**	**Common Symptoms**	**Prevention**
Osteoarthritis cont'd	cess bone builds up, joint movement difficult.		weather changes, limited movement, fluid in joints; worsens with poor posture, obesity, occupational stress.	exercise routines may help.
Treatment	Medication for pain, surgery to replace joints, water exercise.			
Gout	Occurs most in men over 40; secondary gout in elderly; too much uric acid in blood.	Inherited metabolic disorder.	Severe pain in joints of big toe most frequent; sudden onset; hypertension, kidney stones, back pain develop; affected joints hot, tender, inflamed; low-grade fever possible; tophi in final stages with unremitting pain; taut skin over tophi may ulcerate; chronic disability, renal dysfunction.	None known; no verified connection with diet.
Treatment	Bed rest; immobilization of painful joints; local application of heat or cold; dietary restrictions; drugs: colchicine (most effective), analgesics, corticosteroids.			
Fibromyalgia	Disease of muscles, ligaments, tendons; afflicts women more than men; mostly ages 20-50.	Unfit muscles, unrestorative sleep, stress associated with disease (not known whether cause or result).	Pain, fatigue; tender points where muscles attach to bones; other unexplained symptoms: Raynaud's phenomenon, tension headaches, migraine, dizziness, tingling and numbness, irritable bowel syndrome, muscle tremors, bladder spasms, blurred vision.	Unknown.
Treatment	Exercise, antidepressant (to induce stage IV sleep), hot bath for temporary pain relief.			
Carpal tunnel syndrome	Median nerve compressed in carpal tunnel at wrist; usually in women 30-60; occupational hazard.	Anything that causes swelling in carpal tunnel.	Weakness, burning, tingling, numbness and/or pain in thumb, fingers; inability to clench fist; dry, shiny skin, fingernails smaller than usual.	Splinting wrist for 1-2 weeks; corticosteroids, surgery.

Continued.

SUMMARY TABLE Chronic skin and musculoskeletal disorders—cont'd				
Disease	**Special Characteristics**	**Predisposing Factors**	**Common Symptoms**	**Prevention**
Treatment	Wrist splint, corticosteroid injection, surgery, change of occupation.			
Tendinitis and bursitis	Tendinitis: inflammation of tendons/tendon-muscle attachments; bursitis: inflammation of bursae (fluid-filled sacs that facilitate joint movement).	Strain during sports activity; repetitive movements, rheumatic diseases, congenital defects, postural misalignment, gout; infected bursae.	Tendinitis: often in shoulder, producing pain that may interrupt sleep; bursitis: may be sudden, with limitation of movement.	Maintaining good body strength, posture, flexibility; avoiding physical stress, strain, repetitive movements.
Treatment	Resting joint; analgesics; application of cold, heat, ultrasound; analgesic injection; corticosteroids.			
Osteoporosis	Metabolic bone disorder resulting in resorption of calcium from bone; afflicts estimated over 50% of women over 60 in North America.	White race, smoking, drinking, European descent, sedentary living are links.	Easily broken bones, backache from snapped vertebrae, kyphosis.	Regular exercise, balanced diet throughout life; secondary: high calcium intake plus weight-bearing exercise.
Treatment	Individualized activity program; increased dietary calcium; estrogen; fluoride; supplemental calcium; vitamin D.			
Herniated disk	"Slipped disk"; soft central part of intervertebral disk forced through outer covering; usually in people under 45, more often in men.	Strain, trauma, or, in elderly, degenerative joints.	Pain in lower back, radiating down sciatic nerve on one side to buttocks, legs, and feet; other symptoms depend on location of hernia.	Good posture, lifting, and carrying procedures; exercises for muscles subject to strain.
Treatment	Rest, heat, therapeutic exercises, analgesics, muscle relaxants, surgery.			
Scoliosis	Lateral curvature of spine in chest or lower back; may begin in childhood, adolescence, or later life.	Poor posture, different leg lengths, unfit muscles, obesity, muscle-weakening disease; genetic or congenital.	Most common: S-shaped curve of spine; well-established: backache, fatigue, dyspnea; untreated: pulmonary insufficiency, back pain, degenerative arthritis of the spine, disk disease, sciatica.	Attention to underlying causes when possible, e.g. muscle fitness, posture.
Treatment	Exercise, a brace, surgery.			

SUMMARY TABLE Chronic skin and musculoskeletal disorders—cont'd				
Disease	**Special Characteristics**	**Predisposing Factors**	**Common Symptoms**	**Prevention**
Kyphosis	Excessive backward curvature of spine; usually at top of back, resulting in hump or rounded back.	Growth retardation, congenital defect, aging, osteoporosis, many other diseases, disorders.	Pain, fatigue, tenderness, stiffness along spine in children; pain, weakness of back, generalized fatigue.	Maintaining good posture, ideal weight, good nutrition will help, depending on cause.
Treatment	Aimed at underlying disorder.			

QUESTIONS FOR REVIEW

1. Describe the three layers of the skin.
2. What are the predisposing factors linked to acne?
3. What effect does diet have on acne?
4. What is the best treatment for acne?
5. What are the symptoms of seborrheic dermatitis?
6. What substances may cause contact dermatitis?
7. What process produces the symptoms of psoriasis?
8. What therapies are there for psoriasis?
9. How does osteoarthritis differ from rheumatoid arthritis?
10. What is the suspected cause of gout?
11. The symptoms of gout are a result of what process?
12. What predisposing factors have been linked to fibromyalgia?
13. How is fibromyalgia diagnosed?
14. What may be the cause of the recent increase of carpal tunnel syndrome?
15. What causes the symptoms of carpal tunnel syndrome?
16. Compare tendinitis and bursitis.
17. What is the cause of osteoporosis?
18. What is the best treatment for osteoporosis?
19. How can back problems be prevented?
20. How do lordosis, kyphosis, and scoliosis differ?

FURTHER READING

Disorders of the skin.

Abel, Elizabeth A. et al. "Insights into Psoriasis Management." *Patient Care,* Nov. 30, '89, 23:102-116.

Barker, Jonathan N.W.N. "The Pathophysiology of Psoriasis." *Lancet,* July 27, '91, 338:227-230.

Bencini, Pier Luca et al. "Creams for Treatment of Chronic Irritant Dermatitis." *Drug and Cosmetic Industry,* Feb. '90, 146:28-30.

Bos, J.D., Th. van Joost et al. "Use of Cyclosporin in Psoriasis." *Lancet,* Dec. 23, '89, 2:1500-1502.

Bruce, Suzanne. "Hand Dermatitis: Annoying and Persistent, but Treatable." *Consultant,* Dec. '90, 30:21-26.

Burns, M.K. et al. "Intralesional Cyclosporine for Psoriasis: Relationship of Dose, Tissue Levels, and Efficacy." *Archives of Dermatology,* June '92, 128(6):786-790.

Cinque, Chris. "Tennis Shoe Dermatitis: Making a Surefire Diagnosis." *Physician and Sportsmedicine,* Dec. '89, 17:123-126.

Coleman, Deborah Ann et al. "A Worst-Case Guide for Any Case of Psoriasis." *RN,* Mar. '88, 51:39-43.

Farnes, S.W. and P.A. Setness. "Retinoid Therapy for Aging Skin and Acne." *Postgraduate Medicine,* Nov. 1, '92, 92(6):191-196, 199-200.

Fisher, Alexander A. et al. "When to Suspect Cosmetic Dermatitis." *Patient Care,* June 15, '88, 22:29-40.

Klecz, R.J. and R.A. Schwartz. "Pruritus." *American Family Physician,* June '92, 45(6):2681-2686.

Kurban, R.S. and A.K. Kurban. "Common Skin Disorders of Aging: Diagnosis and Treatment." *Geriatrics,* Apr. '93, 48(4):30-31, 35-36, 39-42.

McCarthy, Laura Flynn. "Age Spot Overkill." *Health,* May '91, 23:20-21.

Menter, Alan et al. "Psoriasis in Practice." *Lancet,* July 27, '91, 338:231-234.

"Promise for Psoriasis: Vitamin D." *Harvard Medical School Health Letter,* Apr. '90, 15:2-4.

Disorders of the musculoskeletal system.

Boissevaine, Michael D. and Glenn A. McCain. "Toward an Integrated Understanding of Fibromyalgia Syndrome. Part I: Medical and Pathophysiological Aspects." *Pain,* June '91, 45:227-238.

Boissevaine, Michael D. and Glenn A. McCain. "Toward an Integrated Understanding of Fibromyalgia Syndrome. Part II: Psychological and Phenomenological Aspects." *Pain,* June '91, 45:239-248.

Cinque, Chris. "Fibromyalgia: Is Exercise the Cause or the Cure?" *Physician and Sportsmedicine,* Sept. '89, 17:180-183.

Cooper, Kenneth H. "The Basics of Bone: How to Keep Upright All Your Life." *Health,* Apr. '89, 21:80-82.

Cotton, Paul. "Symptoms May Return After Carpal Tunnel Surgery." *Journal of the American Medical Association,* Apr. 17, '91, 265:1922-1923.

De Krom, M.C.T.F.M. et al. "Risk Factors for Carpal Tunnel Syndrome." *American Journal of Epidemiology,* Dec. '90, 132:1102-1110.

Dickson, Robert A. "The Aetiology of Spinal Deformities." *Lancet,* May 21, '88, 1:1151-1155.

Eisenberg, David M. et al. "Unconventional Medicine in the United States: Prevalence, Cost, and Patterns of Use." *New England Journal of Medicine,* Jan. 28, '93, 328:246-252.

"Fibromyalgia." Atlanta, Arthritis Foundation, 1989. (16-page booklet)

"For Better Hip Replacement Results, Surgeon's Best Friend May Be a Robot." *Journal of the American Medical Association,* Feb. 5, '92, 267:613-614.

Franklin, Gary M, Joanna Haug et al. "Occupational Carpal Tunnel Syndrome in Washington State, 1984-1988." *American Journal of Public Health,* June '91, 81:741-746.

Glasser, R.S. et al. "The Perioperative Use of Corticosteroids and Bupivacaine in the Management of Lumbar Disc Disease." *Journal of Neurosurgery,* Mar. '93, 78(3):383-387.

Hamerman, David. "The Biology of Osteoarthritis." *New England Journal of Medicine,* May 18, '89, 320:1322-1330.

Harvey, Jack et al. "Tennis Elbow: What's the Best Treatment?" *Physician and Sportsmedicine,* June '90, 18:62-70.

Hasse, Gunter R. et al. "Coping with Carpal Tunnel Syndrome." *Patient Care,* July 15, '90, 24:127-130.

Jaret, Peter. "18 Points of Pain: Closing in on Barely Noticeable Tender Spots May Illuminate the Mystery of Fibromyalgia." *Health,* July / Aug. '90, 22:62-65.

Jilka, Robert L. and Giao Hangoc et al. "Increased Osteoclast Development after Estrogen Loss: Mediation by Interleukin-6." *Science,* July 3, '92, 257:88-91.

Kusack, James M. "The Light at the End of the Carpal Tunnel." *Library Journal,* July '90, 115:56-59.

Leach, Robert E. et al. "Achilles Tendinitis: Don't Let It Be an Athlete's Downfall." *Physician and Sportsmedicine,* Aug. '91, 19:87-91.

Ledingham, J., S. Doherty, and M. Doherty. "Primary Fibromyalgia Syndrome—An Outcome Study." *British Journal of Rheumatology,* Feb. '93, 32(2):139-142.

Leventhal, Larenence J. et al. "Fibromyalgia and Parvovirus Infection." *Arthritis and Rheumatism,* Oct. '91, 34:1319-1324.

Liang, Matthew H. "Osteoarthritis: A Joint Endeavor." *Harvard Health Letter,* Apr. '92, 17:1-4.

Lindsay, Robert. "Fluoride and Bone—Quantity versus Quality." *New England Journal of Medicine,* Mar. 22, '90, 322:845-846.

Lorig, K.R., P.D. Mazonson, and H.R. Holman. "Evidence Suggesting that Health Education for Self-management in Patients with Chronic Arthritis Has Sustained Health Benefits While Reducing Health Care Costs." *Arthritis and Rheumatism,* Apr. '93, 36(4):439-446.

Martell, J.M. et al. "Primary Total Hip Reconstruction with a Titanium Fiber-coated Prosthesis Inserted without Cement." *Journal of Bone and Joint Surgery Am,* Apr. '93, 75(4): 554-571.

McCarthy, Paul. "Managing Bursitis in the Athlete: An Overview." *Physician and Sportsmedicine,* Nov. '89, 17:115.

Millikan, L.E. and J.P. Shrum. "An Update on Common Skin Diseases: Acne, Psoriasis, Contact Dermatitis, and Warts." *Postgraduate Medicine,* May 1, '92, 91(6):96-98, 101-104, 107-110.

Munning, Frances. "Osteoporosis: What Is the Role of Exercise?" *Physician and Sportsmedicine,* June '92, 20:127-138.

Murray, P.M., S.L. Weinstein, and K.F. Spratt. "The Natural History and Long-term Follow-up of Scheuermann Kyphosis." *Journal of Bone and Joint Surgery Am,* Feb. '93, 75(2):236-248.

Pagnanelli, David M. "Hands On Approach to Avoiding Carpal Tunnel Syndrome." *Risk Management,* May '89, 36:20-23.

"Predicting Wrist Injury Risk." *USA Today,* Oct. '90, 119:7-8.

Preston, Diana S. "Nonmelanoma Cancers of the Skin." *New England Journal of Medicine,* Dec. 3, '92, 327(23):1649-1662.

Puig, J.G. et al. "Hereditary Nephropathy Associated with Hyperuricemia and Gout." *Archives of Internal Medicine,* Feb. 8, '93, 153(3):357-365.

Rashad, Shawky et al. "Effect of Non-Steroidal Anti-Inflammatory Drugs on the Course of Osteoarthritis." *Lancet,* Sept. 2, '89, 2:519-522.

Ray, Wayne A., Winanne Downey et al. "Long-Term Use of Thiazide Diuretics and Risk of Hip Fracture." *Lancet,* Apr. 1, '89, 1:687-690.

Resnick, Neil M. and Susan L. Greenspan. "'Senile' Osteoporosis Reconsidered." *Journal of the American Medical Association,* Feb. 17, '89, 261:1025-1029.

Riggs, B. Lawrence and L. Joseph Melton III. "The Prevention and Treatment of Osteoporosis." *New England Journal of Medicine,* Aug. 27, '92, 327:620-627.

Rigotti, Nancy A., Robert M. Neer et al. "The Clinical Course of Osteoporosis in Anorexia Nervosa." *Journal of the American Medical Association,* Mar. 6, '91, 265:1133-1138.

Roubenoff, Ronenn, Michael J. Klag et al. "Incidence and Risk Factors for Gout in White Men." *Journal of the American Medical Association,* Dec. 4, '91, 266:3004-3007.

Samanta, A. et al. "Is Osteoarthritis in Women Affected by Hormonal Changes or Smoking?" *British Journal of Rheumatology,* May '93, 32(5):366-370.

Seeman, Ego et al. "Reduced Bone Mass in Daughters of Women with Osteoporosis." *New England Journal of Medicine,* Mar. 2, '89, 320:554-558.

Shellenbarger, Teresa. "When You're Asked about Carpal Tunnel Syndrome." *RN,* July '91, 54:40-42.

Skolnick, Andrew. "It's Important, but Don't Bank on Exercise Alone to Prevent Osteoporosis, Experts Say." *Journal of the American Medical Association,* Apr. 4, '90, 263:1751-1752.

"Sleep and Scoliosis." *Lancet,* Feb. 13, '88, 1:336-337.

Spencer-Green, G. "Drug Treatment of Arthritis: Update on Conventional and Less Conventional Methods." *Postgraduate Medicine,* May 15, '93, 93(7):129-140.

Storti, Peter A. "Getting a Grasp on Carpal Tunnel Syndrome." *Risk Management,* Mar. '90, 37:40-44.

Chapter 17

Sensory, Nervous, and Endocrine Disorders

O B J E C T I V E S

1 Explain errors in refraction that make it necessary to wear glasses or contact lenses.

2 Describe the process that leads to a cataract.

3 Identify symptoms that may indicate the development of a cataract.

4 Explain why early detection of glaucoma is important.

5 Identify causes for hearing loss.

6 Compare the three types of cerebral palsy.

7 Describe the progression of symptoms for Parkinson's disease.

8 Explain the disease process in multiple sclerosis.

9 Identify the three stages of Alzheimer's disease.

10 Distinguish between type I and type II diabetes.

11 State characteristics, risk factors, symptoms, and prevention for the diseases in this chapter.

EYE DISORDERS

STRUCTURE OF THE EYE

The eye is composed of four different layers; they are the sclera and cornea, the uvea (choroid, ciliary body, and iris) and the retina (Figure 17-1).

The sclera is a dense, white, and fibrous protective coat covered by a thin layer of fine elastic tissue. Continuous with the sclera is the cornea, which is the transparent, avascular, curved layer of the eye. Aqueous humor bathes the surface of the cornea, maintaining intraocular pressure. The sole function of the cornea is to refract light rays.

The middle layer, or uvea, consisting of the iris, ciliary body, and choroid, is pigmented and vascular. The iris is suspended between the lens and cornea and perforated in the middle by the pupil. The ciliary body produces aqueous humor and controls the lens. The largest part of the uveal coat is the choroid, which is made up of blood vessels united by connective tissue containing pigmented cells.

The most essential structure of the eye is the retina, which receives the image formed by the lens. Light entering the eye passes through the cornea, then through the pupil, lens, and the jellylike vitreous body behind the lens, to the retina. Through changes in the curvature of the lens brought about by its elasticity and contraction of the ciliary muscles, light rays are focused on the retina, where they stimulate the rods and cones, the sensory receptors. Sensory impulses are relayed via the optic nerve to the brain, where they register as visual sensations. (For an insight into treatment for corneal abrasion, see the Did You Know? section that follows.)

REFRACTIVE ERRORS

When people have to wear glasses, it is generally for one or more refractive errors. The main types of refractive error are myopia (nearsightedness), hyperopia (far-sightedness), presbyopia (difficulty in focusing), and astigmatism (unequal curvature

DID YOU KNOW?

To Patch or Not to Patch

If you have an eye injury, a patch can cause more pain while the eye is healing than if it were to be left uncovered. A study reported in *The Lancet* used 30 patients with corneal scratches. Half were asked to wear eye patches while the eye was healing, but the control half were not. In both groups the scratch healed in just 2 days. However, a day after the injury, three quarters of the patients with a patch were experiencing pain, while only one quarter of those in the control group had pain. The best treatment for a scratched cornea may be antibiotic drops alone.

From *Lancet* 337(1991):643. In *The Edell Health Letter,* June/July '91, 10:4.

of cornea and/or lens). Figure 17-2 shows how myopia and hyperopia are corrected with lenses. Refractive errors occur because of a genetic predisposition, and about one third of the population wear glasses or contact lenses for them. Two other common disorders of the eye are cataract and glaucoma, which will be discussed next.

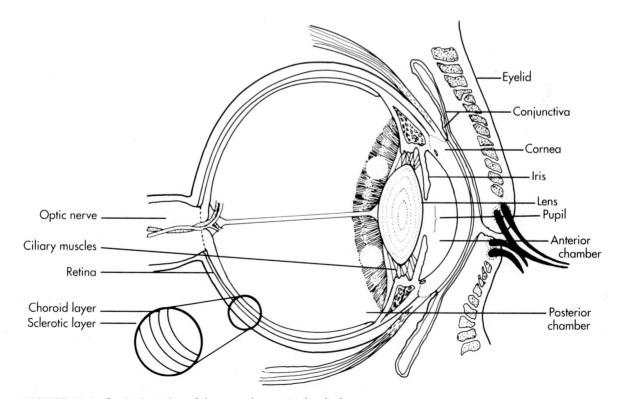

FIGURE 17-1   Sagittal section of the eye, demonstrating its layers.

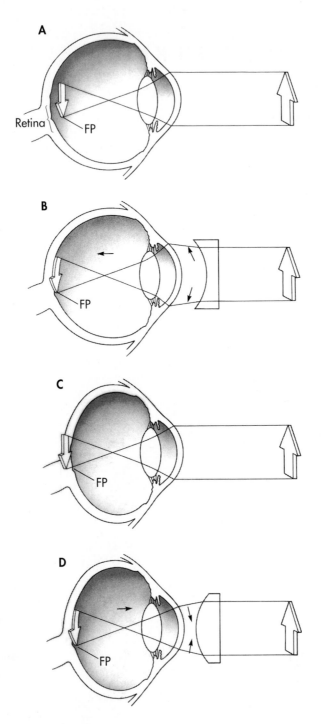

FIGURE 17-2 Visual disorders and their correction by various lenses.

CATARACT

There are a number of different types of cataract, but the most common are those that occur with aging. The lens gradually becomes opaque and the pupil turns white (Figure 17-3). Cataracts generally develop in both eyes at the same time but at different rates.

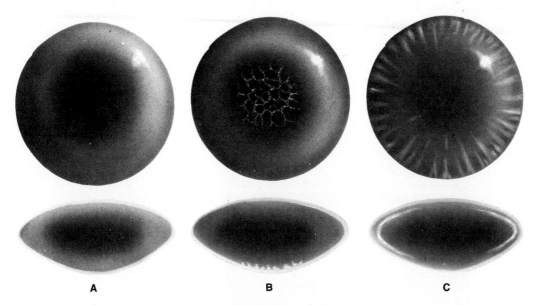

FIGURE 17-3   Drawing of an eye showing milky white cataract. **A,** Nuclear sclerosis, compression of lens fibers. **B,** Nuclear sclerosis subcapsular cataract in back of eye. **C,** Nuclear sclerosis cortical cataracts in front and back of eye.

Predisposing Factors   Most cataracts develop in persons over 70 and are considered to be a result of aging. Cataracts may be present in infants because of a genetic defect or because the mother contracted rubella during the first trimester of her pregnancy. Injury to the lens by a foreign body or toxic effects of drugs may also cause cataracts. Finally, cataracts may occur secondary to other disorders, such as glaucoma.

Symptoms   Blurring and loss of vision are generally the first signs of cataract. The patient may see halos around lights, and night driving may become more difficult because of the blinding glare of headlights. Sunlight may also cause an unpleasant glare and poor vision. Individuals with glaucoma often see better in dim light.

Prevention   No means of prevention is known for senile cataracts. Prepubertal vaccination for rubella is recommended to reduce the incidence of congenital cataracts. Proper safety measures during involvement in activities that have a possibility of eye damage, as well as use of drugs only under medical supervision, might prevent other types of cataracts.

Treatment   Surgery to remove cataracts has improved steadily, with new and better techniques for a 95% effectiveness rate.

GLAUCOMA

Glaucoma is due to an increase in intraocular pressure leading to atrophy of the optic nerve and blindness (Figure 17-4). The disease occurs in women more than in men and accounts for 15% of the blindness in the United States.

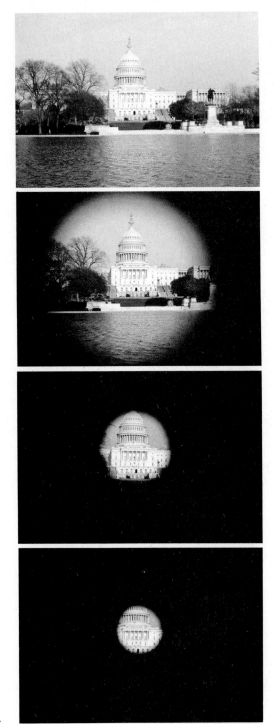

FIGURE 17-4 Progress in acute glaucoma.

Predisposing Factors Ninety percent of glaucoma cases result from an inherited predisposition to the disease, or it can occur as a result of other eye disease.

Symptoms Generally there are no symptoms until the disease is advanced. Late symptoms include mild aching in the eyes, halos around lights, loss of peripheral vision, and reduced visual acuity that cannot be corrected with glasses.

Prevention Everyone should have regular eye examinations. Individuals with a history of glaucoma should have yearly eye examinations, particularly after the age of 40. Screening for glaucoma is a routine practice in eye exams. Early detection can lead to good results with treatment.

Treatment Treatment involves using drugs and eye drops to reduce the pressure in the eyes. If the disease has been detected early enough, it can be arrested.

EAR DISORDERS
STRUCTURE OF THE EAR

Hearing begins when sound waves in the air go through the auditory canal and reach the tympanic membrane. The tympanic membrane vibrates the small bones in the middle ear (malleus, incus, and stapes), and the stapes sends these vibrations to the fluid in the inner ear by vibrating against the oval window. The fluid in the inner ear then conducts the sound across the hair cells of the organ of Corti (in the cochlea), which initiates auditory nerve impulses to the brain. An individual's balance is maintained by the fluid in the semicircular canals. Nerve cells line the canals and send messages to the brain by the acoustic nerve.

HEARING LOSS

All hearing loss or deafness is either conductive or sensorineural. If the passage of sound from the external ear to the place where the stapes meets the oval window is blocked, then it is referred to as conductive loss of hearing. When the hearing loss occurs because there is no transmission of sound impulses from the inner ear to the brain, then it is called sensorineural loss of hearing. Both conditions may exist in the same person, and the hearing loss is then referred to as mixed. Total deafness is rare and is usually congenital. One in 1000 babies has sensorineural deafness at birth that is incurable. When deafness develops in young children, it is usually conductive and curable. Almost 25% of children starting school have some hearing loss from otitis media (middle ear infection). About 25% of people over 65 need a hearing aid.

Predisposing Factors The causes of hearing loss are many and different for conductive and sensorineural deafness (Figure 17-5). Common causes for conductive hearing loss are
- Chronic middle ear infection (sticky fluid collects in the middle ear).
- Cerumen (earwax) blocking the outer ear canal.

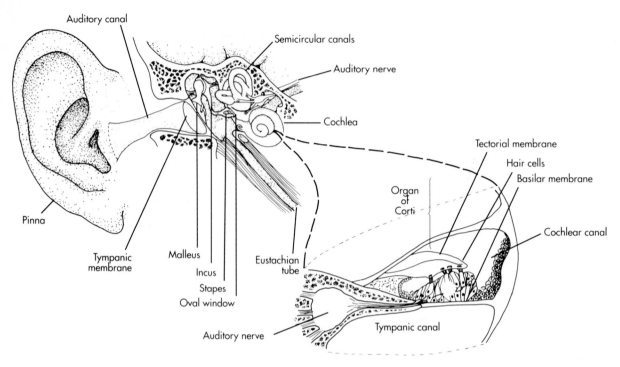

FIGURE 17-5 Drawing of ear showing sites of sensorineural and conductive deafness and causes.

- Loss of mobility in stapes.
- Damage to eardrum from sudden changes in air pressure, as in an airplane or underwater.
- Perforated eardrum.

Common causes for sensorineural hearing loss are:
- Birth injury or damage to developing fetus (measles, drugs or other factors affecting the mother during pregnancy that can affect the fetus).
- Prolonged exposure to loud noise.
- Ménière's disease.
- Use of certain drugs, such as streptomycin.
- Viral infections.
- Degeneration of cochlea or labyrinth with old age.
- Tumors on acoustic nerve.

Symptoms In young children, hearing loss may not become evident for a few days, when they do not turn their head at the sound of a voice. Although the hearing-compromised baby may cry as a hearing-normal child might, he or she will not make the babbling sounds that most children make preceding speech. Sometimes a child's seeming inattention to directions may be due to partial hearing loss. If the hearing loss is partial, there is generally difficulty in hearing very high or very low tones at first, which may not be noticed. This is the reason that early screening tests for hearing can be so beneficial. In older people whose hearing loss occurs because of a loss of hair cells in the organ of Corti, there may be tinnitus, or ringing in the ears; sounds become quieter, and some letter sounds (s, f, z) cannot be heard. Speech becomes harder to understand when there is background noise. When individuals are not aware that their hearing is impaired, they sometimes become paranoid, act confused, and have auditory hallucinations that can lead to withdrawal and depression if the problem is not diagnosed.

Prevention Early treatment for diseases that may affect hearing, as well as avoidance of constant loud noise, will reduce the risk of hearing loss. Individuals who work in a noisy environment should wear protective mechanisms to guard their hearing. Children should not be exposed to music that is above a safe level. Prolonged exposure to loud noise (85 to 90 decibels) or brief exposure to noise greater than 90 decibels can cause hearing loss. Pregnant women should be educated about the dangers to the fetus if they are exposed to drugs, chemicals, or infection. The best secondary prevention is periodic hearing tests after the child enters school. If there is any suspicion of a hearing loss, in a child or adult, a doctor should be consulted immediately.

Treatment In cases of hearing loss, the underlying cause must be identified first. Children who are born deaf must be taught sign language and speech. If a child becomes deaf from otitis media, then an operation is performed in which the eardrum is pierced in order to drain the fluid from the middle ear. If conductive hearing loss is caused by cerumen in the ear, a syringe is used to flush it out with warm water. A perforated eardrum will generally heal by itself. If it does not do so in 2 to 3 weeks, surgery may be necessary. The stapes can be replaced if conductive deafness occurs because of its lack of mobility. Hearing aids and training the individual to read lips are also part of treatment.

MÉNIÈRE'S DISEASE

Ménière's disease is a disorder of the inner ear. It occurs most often in adults between the ages of 30 and 60 and slightly more often in men. The symptoms are caused by an increase in the amount of fluid in the canals in the inner ear that control balance (Figure 17-6).

Predisposing Factors The cause of the increase in fluid is unknown.

Symptoms Tinnitus; dizziness that may be severe enough to cause the individual to fall to the ground. Victims may also experience nausea, vomiting, sweating, jerky eye movements, and a feeling of pressure or pain in the affected ear. If the condition continues, sensorineural hearing loss occurs and finally deafness.

Prevention None known.

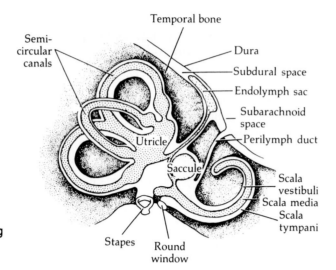

FIGURE 17-6   Drawing of semicircular canals and fluid levels.

Treatment   Atropine can stop an attack in 20 to 30 minutes. In a severe attack, other drugs may be used. The victim is put on diuretics or a vasodilator, and salt intake is restricted. Antihistamines and mild sedatives may also help.

NERVOUS SYSTEM DISORDERS
STRUCTURE OF THE NERVOUS SYSTEM

There are three main divisions to the nervous system, the central nervous system (CNS), which is composed of the brain and spinal cord, the peripheral nervous system, composed of the nerves that relay messages to and from all parts of the body to the CNS (Figure 17-7), and the autonomic nervous system, which regulates involuntary functioning of the internal organs (Figure 17-8).

The fundamental unit of the nervous system is the neuron, which consists of the cell body, axon, and dendrites (Figure 17-9). The axon carries messages away from the cell body, and the dendrites carry messages to the cell body. Thus, in the transmission of nerve impulses, the dendrites of one neuron receive a message from the axon of another neuron and transmit it through the cell body to another axon, which relays the message to other dendrites, and so on.

The minute space between the axon of one neuron and the dendrite of another neuron is called a synaptic gap. Special chemical substances called neurotransmitters diffuse across the gap and carry the message to the dendrites of the next neuron (Figure 17-10). A fatty substance called a myelin sheath envelops the axon and enables the impulse to pass at greater speed. Neurologic disorders occur when there is interference with the transmission of messages and can be crippling or life threatening, depending on what part of the system is involved.

CEREBRAL PALSY

In 1986 approximately one in every 200 children had cerebral palsy. The disorder can be very mild or severe enough to cause total disability. Cerebral palsy results from damage to the CNS that may occur before birth, at birth, or during infancy

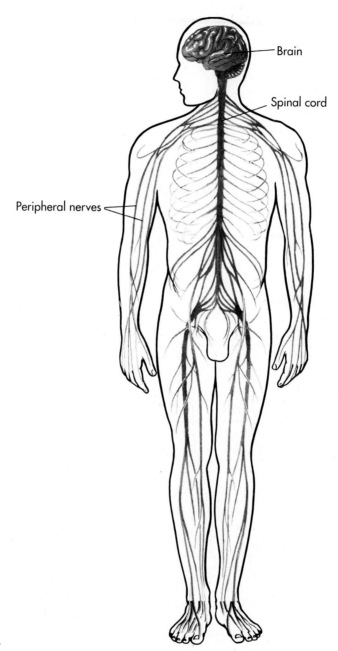

Brain

Spinal cord

Peripheral nerves

FIGURE 17-7 The central nervous system.

and childhood (Figure 17-11). The incidence is higher in whites and slightly higher in males. There are three forms of cerebral palsy: *spastic, athetoid,* and *ataxic.* Sometimes an individual has a mixture of the three. Many times other defects are present, such as mental retardation, disordered speech, and seizures.

Predisposing Factors   Any condition that results in damage to the brain may be a factor in cerebral palsy. During pregnancy, conditions in the mother such as German measles, diabetes, and

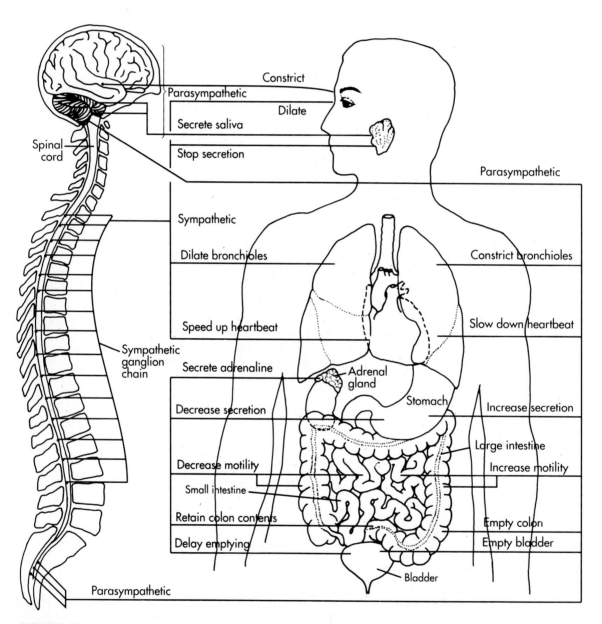

FIGURE 17-8 The autonomic nervous system and organs affected.

malnutrition may be responsible. These conditions are particularly dangerous to the fetus in the first trimester of pregnancy. Moreover, the earlier the condition occurs, the more severe the defect(s). In the birth process, a prolonged labor, forceps delivery, anesthetic, and other situations resulting in a reduced supply of oxygen to the baby could result in brain damage. Head trauma, brain infection, and brain tumor are also among the factors that might result in cerebral palsy for the infant or small child.

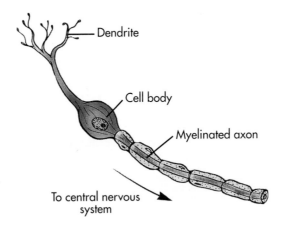

FIGURE 17-9 The neuron, showing transmission of a message and myelin sheath.

FIGURE 17-10 Synaptic gap and neurotransmitters.

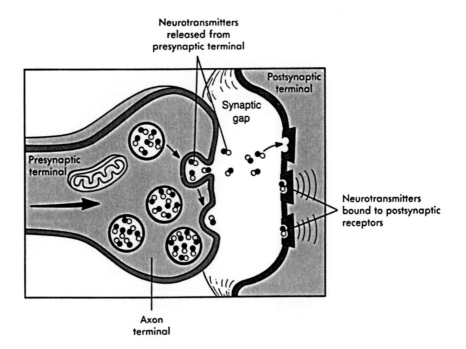

PRENATAL

Maternal metabolic disease
Maternal nutritional deficiency
Maternal bleeding, toxemia, exposure to radiation, infection
Multiple births
Blood incompatibilities
Prematurity (asphyxia leading to cerebral hemorrhage)
Genetic factors
Congenital brain abnormalities

PERINATAL FACTORS

Anesthesia, analgesia during labor and delivery
Mechanical trauma during delivery
Prematurity
Metabolic disorders
Electrolyte disturbances

POSTNATAL FACTORS

Head trauma
Infections such as meningitis, encephalitis
Cerebrovascular accidents
Toxicoses
Environmental toxins such as ingestion of lead or methyl mercury
from contaminated fish

Adapted from McCance and Huether, *Pathophysiology: The Biologic Basis for Disease in Adults and Children*. St. Louis: Mosby, 1990.

FIGURE 17-11 Predisposing factors and known causes of cerebral palsy

Symptoms   The spastic type of cerebral palsy is present in about 70% of the victims. Symptoms include excessive muscle contractions, muscle weakness, underdeveloped body parts (which are affected), and a tendency to walk on toes, with a scissorslike movement, crossing one foot in front of the other.

The athetoid form affects approximately 20% of the victims. These individuals have difficulty controlling the movements of their arms, legs, and/or facial muscles. The symptoms become more severe during stress, decrease when the individual is relaxed, and go away completely during sleep.

About 10% of cerebral palsy victims have the ataxic type of the disorder. Their major problem is with balance, and they fall frequently.

Some children have a combination of these types. Individuals with cerebral palsy may be average or above average in intelligence, but as many as 40% have mental retardation. About 80% have speech difficulties, and about 25% have seizure disorders.

Primary Prevention   Because the causative factors are linked to pregnancy and childbirth, there should be careful monitoring of the condition of the mother, particularly with respect to nutrition and drug use (including alcohol). Isolation from anyone who has rubella (vaccine should be given to girls before they reach puberty) is mandatory. Routine precautions must be taken in the use of forceps and anesthetic during childbirth. These procedures are all important in reducing the risk of cerebral palsy.

Secondary Prevention   Careful assessment and observation of infants for neurologic disorders by their doctor can lead to early detection, which results in more effective treatment. If infants have been premature or had a difficult birth, follow-up procedures to detect cerebral palsy or any other consequence of birth trauma are extremely important. A routine screening for cerebral palsy should be a part of every infant's 6-month checkup.

Treatment   There is no cure for cerebral palsy, but with proper treatment and cooperation between all the child's care givers, children can be helped to reach their full potential within the limits set by their disorder. For very mild cases, this may be near normal. Treatment may include anticonvulsants, braces, exercises that involve range of motion, muscle relaxants, speech therapy, and other measures to control symptoms.

EPILEPSY

Epilepsy is a seizure disorder related to disturbance of electrical patterns in the brain. Instead of firing in an ordered fashion, neurons discharge messages erratically, leading to an epileptic seizure. Epilepsy is in no way associated with lower intelligence or mental illness. One out of 200 in the population has the disorder. The seizures have different characteristics for different individuals and are identified by various terms.

Predisposing Factors   About half the cases of epilepsy are thought to be due to an abnormality in brain chemistry that is present at birth. Other factors include head injury, birth trauma, brain tumor, infectious diseases, and metabolic disorders.

Symptoms   Recurring seizures are the prevailing symptom in epilepsy. They range from the mild to severe and may be partial or generalized.

Prevention   None known.

Treatment   With drug therapy, an individual with epilepsy can now be stabilized and remain seizure free. The epileptic has to be monitored for side effects and to maintain the proper dosage. If drug treatment fails, there are surgical techniques that may help in some cases.

PARKINSON'S DISEASE

Parkinson's disease is characterized by fine muscle, slowly spreading progressive tremors, muscular weakness and rigidity, and a peculiar gait. It was first described by Dr. James Parkinson in 1817. The deterioration continues for an average of 10 years, at which time death usually occurs as a result of pneumonia or some other infection. The disease affects men more than women, with one in 100 over the age of 60 becoming a victim. Over 60,000 cases are diagnosed annually in the United States, and with our aging population, this figure will rise.

Predisposing Factors   The cause is unknown, but individuals with Parkinson's have been shown to have a dopamine deficiency. Dopamine is known to have an inhibitory effect on nerve transmissions within the CNS.

Symptoms   Muscle rigidity, inability to control muscle movement, and an insidious tremor that begins in the fingers are the first symptoms of Parkinson's. The symptoms increase during stress or anxiety and decrease when moving purposefully and sleeping. There is no intellectual impairment from Parkinson's, although a concomitant disease such as arteriosclerosis may cause it. Lack of muscle control can lead to change of voice pitch, drooling, unusual gait, and strange cries, with upward or closed position of the eyes.

Prevention   None known.

Treatment   There is no cure for Parkinson's at present. The primary aim of treatment is to keep the patient as comfortable and as functional as possible. Drugs, physical therapy, and surgery (in extreme cases) are used.

MULTIPLE SCLEROSIS

Multiple sclerosis (MS) is a chronic disease of the CNS that is a major cause of disability in young adults. Progressive demyelination of the nerve fibers of the brain and spinal cord leads to widely spread and varied neurologic dysfunction. It is a disease marked by remissions and exacerbations, and it may progress rapidly, causing death within months of the onset or, as in 70% of the cases, the patient may lead an active, productive life. The disease generally occurs between the ages of 20 and 40, with 27 being the average. It affects more women than men (3:2) and more whites than blacks (5:1). Japan has a low incidence of the disease, and it occurs more often in the cities and among upper income groups. In northern areas of the world, the incidence of the disease ranges from 50 to 80 per 100,000. It affects about 250,000 people in the United States.

Predisposing Factors   The exact cause of MS is unknown, but a family history of the disease and living in a cold, damp climate increase the risk. It is five times more common in temperate zones than in the tropics. There are many theories of causation, but one of the most widely held is that a slow-moving virus may be the disease agent. Other suspected factors include emotional stress, nutritional deficiencies, trauma, overwork, and acute respiratory infections.

Symptoms   For most patients, problems with the eyes and other sense organs are the first sign that anything is wrong. Numbness and tingling sensations, muscle weakness, urinary disturbances, and mood swings are included in the characteristic changes caused by the disease. Symptoms vary from being so mild that they are not noticed to being severe enough that the individual seems hysterical. Speech may be impaired also. As indicated before, remissions may occur and last for long periods, but then the disease may return with more severe symptoms than felt initially.

Prevention None known.

Treatment Various drugs are used to reduce the severity of the symptoms and the progression of the disease. Among these are adrenocorticotropic hormone (ACTH) and prednisone to reduce edema, and ACTH and corticosteroids to relieve symptoms and speed up remission. There is no cure for the disease.

ALZHEIMER'S DISEASE

This degenerative disease of the brain, Alzheimer's disease, which affects up to 30% of people over 85, is responsible for a great deal of suffering by the victims and their care givers. It is a progressive disease that rarely occurs in those under 60. There is no laboratory test to diagnose Alzheimer's disease, except an autopsy. If persons develop dementia (mental deterioration), and all other possible causes are ruled out, then they are diagnosed with Alzheimer's disease. For an idea of the chances of contracting Alzheimer's disease, see the Did You Know? section following.

Predisposing Factors Even though our aging population and subsequent increased incidence of the disease have resulted in increased research efforts to find a cause, none has been identified to date. The latest research indicates that neurotransmitters and acetylcholine may play a part. Although no one cause has been identified, there are three major theories:

DID YOU KNOW?

Odds for Alzheimer's

When studies are done to determine the chances of offspring inheriting a chronic disease, much depends upon the average lifespan assumed by investigators. In the case of Alzheimer's disease, some studies have indicated a 50-50 chance that children or siblings of Alzheimer's patients would develop the disease. However, this was based upon a lifespan of 90 to 95 years, which is not realistic at present for most people. If a lifespan of 70 years is assumed, the risk is much smaller—19% for children and siblings, 10% for nieces and neph-ews, and 5% for people without affected relatives. Alzheimer's does not appear in most people until they are in their sixties, seventies, or eighties. Most relatives of Alzheimer's patients will not live long enough to develop the disease. This observation is true for other chronic diseases that do not show up until later in life. For instance, if the chances for cancer of the prostate were figured on men reaching 100, almost 100% of men would develop cancer of the prostate.

From "Good News about Alzheimer's Odds." *Health*, Feb./March '92, p. 16. Statistics according to John Breitner of Duke University Medical Center.

(1) exposure to aluminum, (2) autoimmunity, and (3) slow viruses. The most popular is the third and holds that viruses with a 2-to-30-year incubation period cause the degenerative changes in the brain.

Symptoms   There are generally three stages of the disease: (1) the individual is aware of increasing forgetfulness and attempts to compensate by writing lists or by asking others for help; (2) there is severe memory loss, particularly for recent events, accompanied by disorientation, difficulty in finding the right words when speaking, sudden and unpredictable mood changes, and personality changes; (3) all the symptoms of the second stage become more severe, and the victim may revert to childhood behaviors. The people who have the disease may become violent and difficult to control, or they may become quiet and withdrawn. They neglect habits of personal cleanliness, may be incontinent or wander aimlessly, not knowing where they are. At this stage, they require around-the-clock care and usually must be institutionalized. These symptoms range over a 3-to-10-year period, and death is usually due to malnutrition or infection.

Prevention   None known.

Treatment   Tranquilizers and antidepressants can help control the behavior, but there is no real therapy available yet. Counseling the family to be sure they understand and can deal with the care of the person as long as possible is important. Adult day-care centers, home health aides, and extended-care facilities are all needed as the condition of the individual deteriorates.

ENDOCRINE DISORDERS
DISORDERS OF GLANDS AND HORMONES

The endocrine glands include the pituitary gland, thyroid gland, parathyroid glands, adrenal glands, islets of Langerhans of the pancreas, and the ovaries and testes. These are ductless glands that produce an internal secretion that is discharged into the blood or lymph and circulated to all parts of the body. The hormones secreted by these glands may have a specific effect on an organ or tissue or a general effect on the entire body. The secretions of the endocrine glands may be under nervous control, under the control of chemical substances in the blood, or under the control of other hormones. If the glands do not function as they should, many disease conditions can occur. Diabetes mellitus will be discussed in this chapter.

DIABETES MELLITUS

Diabetes mellitus is characterized by abnormal metabolism of carbohydrate, protein, and fat, resulting in increased levels of blood sugar. The adjective *mellitus* (for sweet) is used with diabetes to distinguish the disease from diabetes insipidus (tasteless), which is so rare that the word *diabetes* by itself generally refers to diabetes mellitus. The only thing that diabetes mellitus and diabetes insipidus have in common is polyuria, or frequent urination. There are two forms of diabetes mellitus: type I, or insulin-dependent diabetes mellitus (IDDM), and type II, or non–insulin-dependent diabetes (NIDDM).

Diabetes is one of the 10 leading causes of death from disease in the United States. It is the result of an insufficient supply of insulin or an inadequate use of the insulin that is supplied from the islets of Langerhans in the pancreas. In 1987, 5% of the population in the United States had a form of diabetes.

TYPE I

Type I was formerly known as "juvenile onset" diabetes, since it often begins in adolescence and usually before the age of 35. Type I is a more severe form than type II. It develops rapidly, the insulin-secreting cells in the pancreas are destroyed, and insulin production ceases almost completely. Without regular injections of insulin, the sufferer lapses into a coma and dies.

Predisposing Factors Type I was thought to be hereditary. However, recent studies of identical twins indicate that there are other factors involved, since in almost half of the cases, only one twin developed the disease. No theory has yet been accepted that identifies the factors involved.

Symptoms Type I has an abrupt onset, with dramatic weight loss, reversion to bedwetting, frequent urination, excessive thirst, and vaginal itching. It is often preceded by a flulike episode with slow recovery.

Prevention None known.

Treatment Diet, exercise, education, drugs (insulin), and self-testing are included in the treatment. Type I diabetes is not easily controlled, and because the victims are so young, it is difficult to keep them on a regular treatment schedule. Skipped insulin doses and neglect of self-testing can easily lead to diabetic coma and death.

TYPE II

Type II was formerly known as "adult onset," since it generally is not present until after the age of 40.

Predisposing Factors Type II diabetes mellitus may also have a hereditary factor, but it is most often found in obese, sedentary adults. Other factors include physiologic or emotional stress, pregnancy and oral contraceptives, and certain medications that are insulin antagonists. There is a high incidence among native Americans, blacks, and Hispanics.

Symptoms Type II has a gradual onset, with frequent urination, fatigue, and blurred vision. Since it may also be asymptomatic, about half of those with type II diabetes mellitus do not know they have it.

Prevention   Avoiding obesity, getting regular exercise, and learning to manage stress will reduce the risk.

Treatment   Type II may be managed by diet alone, which will mean a major change in eating habits. Exercise, education, a support group, and self-testing are also included. If the change in diet does not control the disease, then oral hypoglycemics (to stimulate insulin production) are used. It is not generally necessary for individuals with type II to have injections.

A number of complications may occur in diabetes. If the blood glucose goes too low, *insulin shock* is the result. The improper metabolism of fatty acids, generally from carbohydrate deficiency, or inadequate utilization, results in too many ketone bodies in the blood, leading to ketosis. If the blood glucose becomes too high, the patient will go into *diabetic coma,* which is life threatening. Diabetics generally carry sugar in some form to alleviate the former.

Other problems for the diabetic include low resistance to infections, especially those involving the extremities, ulceration of lower extremities, increase in incidence of toxemia in pregnancy, cardiovascular and renal disorders, and eye disorders such as blindness. Diabetes is one of the contributing factors in 50% of heart attacks and also a contributing factor in about 75% of strokes.

SUMMARY

The table summarizes relevant data on the sensory, nervous, and endocrine disorders discussed in this chapter.

SUMMARY TABLE Sensory, nervous, and endocrine disorders				
Disorder	**Special Characteristics**	**Predisposing Factors**	**Common Symptoms**	**Prevention/ Treatment**
Eye Refractive errors	Myopia (nearsightedness), hyperopia (farsightedness), presbyopia (difficulty focusing), astigmatism (unequal curvature of cornea and/or lens).	Mostly hereditary.	Difficulty in reading, recognizing people or objects at a distance or very close; difficulty focusing; astigmatism: variation in shades of print.	None known; glasses, contact lenses.
Cataract	Generally occurs with aging; individual can often see better in dim light.	Mostly hereditary; may be secondary to glaucoma or present in a baby because of rubella in mother during pregnancy; abuse of drugs, eye injuries.	Blurring of print, figures; halos around lights at night; headlights, sunlight decrease vision.	None for senile cataracts; prepubertal vaccination for rubella; protection of eyes in at-risk activities; medical supervision in drug use; laser surgery very successful.
Glaucoma	Increase in intraocular pressure leading to atrophy of optic nerve, blindness; occurs in women more than men; accounts for 15% of blindness in United States.	Inherited predisposition.	None until disease is far advanced; mild aching in eyes, halos around lights, loss of peripheral vision; reduced visual acuity not correctable with glasses.	Regular eye exams; yearly exams after 40 if family history of glaucoma; eye drops used early in disease will control.
Hearing Loss	Almost 25% of children entering school have some hearing loss; about 25% of people over 65 need a hearing aid.		Baby: cries but doesn't vocalize; doesn't respond to sound of voice; inattention; older people: tinnitus, loss of some letter sounds; speech harder to understand with background noise; may become withdrawn, depressed if not aware of problem.	Screening tests in school; protective equipment if exposed to long-term noise; education of pregnant women; treatment depends on cause; hearing aids help some; others may need to learn lip reading; some cleared up by surgery, other medical treatment.
Conductive	Passage of sound from the external ear to oval window blocked.	Otitis media, cerumen, immobile stapes, damaged eardrum, perforated eardrum.		
Sensorineural	No transmission of sound from inner ear to brain; one in 1000 babies at birth have this type; incurable.	Birth injury, fetus damage, loud noise, Ménière's disease, certain drugs, viral infections, degeneration of cochlea or labyrinth, tumors.		

Continued.

SUMMARY TABLE Sensory, nervous, and endocrine disorders—cont'd

Disorder	Special Characteristics	Predisposing Factors	Common Symptoms	Prevention/ Treatment
Ménière's disease	Caused by increase in inner ear fluid; may lead to sensorineural hearing loss, deafness.	Unknown.	Tinnitus, dizziness, nausea, vomiting, sweating, jerky eye movements, pressure or pain in ear.	Unknown; drugs used to stop an attack; vasodilators, diuretics, antihistamines, restricted salt intake may also be prescribed.
Nervous system Cerebral palsy	Three kinds: spastic, athetoid, ataxic; results from damage to CNS; about 70% spastic.	Many: any condition during pregnancy, birth, or childhood that results in brain damage; forceps delivery.	Spastic (70%): excessive muscle contractions, muscle weakness, underdeveloped body parts, unusual walk; athetoid (20%): difficulty controlling movement of body parts; more severe during stress; goes away during sleep; ataxic (10%): major problem is balance; frequent falling.	Monitoring of pregnant women; caution with forceps use in delivery; routine screening at 6 mos; treatment to help child reach full potential; anticonvulsants, braces, exercises, muscle relaxants, speech therapy.
Epilepsy	Seizure disorder related to disturbance of electrical patterns in brain, not associated with lowered intelligence, mental illness; 1 out of 200 has disorder.	About half due to abnormal brain chemistry at birth; also head injury, birth trauma, brain tumor, infectious disease, metabolic disorders.	Recurring seizures range from mild to severe.	None known; individual free of seizures with drug therapy.
Parkinson's disease	Fine muscle, slowly spreading, progressive tremors, muscular weakness, rigidity; usually lasts about 10 years before death from pneumonia, other infections; affects men (1 in 100 over age 60) more than women; increasing with aging population.	Unknown; possibly dopamine deficiency.	Muscle rigidity, inability to control muscle movement, tremor beginning slowly in fingers; increases during stress, decreases during sleep; no intellectual impairment; may be change of voice pitch, drooling, unusual walk, strange cries with upward or closed eyes.	None known; no cure; treatment to ease symptoms only.
MS	Chronic disease of CNS; major cause of disability in young adults; progressive	Family history of disease; cold, damp climate increases risk; possibly a slow-moving virus.	First: problems with eyes, sense organs; numbness, tingling, muscle weakness, urinary disturbances,	Symptom relief only: ACTH, prednisone, corticosteroids.

SUMMARY TABLE Sensory, nervous, and endocrine disorders—cont'd				
Disorder	**Special Characteristics**	**Predisposing Factors**	**Common Symptoms**	**Prevention/ Treatment**
	demyelination of nerve fibers; some die in months; others (70%) lead active, productive life; about 250,000 affected in United States.		mood swings as disease advances; possible speech impairment, and victim seems hysterical; sometimes remissions for long periods, more severe symptoms afterward.	
Alzheimer's disease	Affects up to 30% of people over 85; rare under age 60.	No cause identified, 3 major theories: aluminum; autoimmunity; slow viruses (most popular); 10%-30% have family history of disease.	Three stages: 1. increasing forgetfulness; 2. severe memory loss, disorientation, trouble finding right words when speaking, mood and personality changes; 3. all symptoms worsen; childish behaviors, aimless wandering; incontinence, personal cleanliness neglected; round-the-clock-care needed; usually institutionalized.	None known.
Diabetes mellitus	Abnormal metabolism of carbohydrate, protein, fat, resulting in increased blood sugar; leading cause of death in the United States; 5% of the population diabetic in 1987; low resistance to infection, especially in extremities; increased incidence of toxemia in pregnancy; cardiovascular, renal disorders; eye disorders often lead to blindness; cause of about 50% of myocardial infarcts, 75% of strokes.			
Type I	Insulin dependent; "juvenile onset"; usually begins before age 25.	Unknown; may be hereditary.	Abrupt onset, dramatic weight loss, bedwetting, frequent urination, vaginal itching, thirst; too much insulin can produce life-threatening insulin shock.	Unknown; diet, exercise, education, drugs, and self-testing part of treatment; adolescents not following treatment guidelines enter *diabetic coma,* die from high blood sugar.
Type II	"Adult onset," generally after age 40.	Possible hereditary factor; generally found in obese, sedentary adults; physiologic or emotional stress, pregnancy, oral contraceptives, certain drugs may all predispose.	Gradual onset, frequent urination, fatigue, blurred vision; asymptomatic too.	Avoiding obesity, regular exercise, managing stress reduce risk.

QUESTIONS FOR REVIEW

1. What refractive errors are discussed in the text, and why do they occur?
2. What is a cataract?
3. What causes cataracts?
4. What symptoms may be due to a cataract?
5. What is the treatment for cataracts?
6. What causes glaucoma?
7. Why should glaucoma tests be performed regularly after the age of 40?
8. Name and describe the two kinds of hearing loss.
9. Identify risk factors for conductive and sensorineural hearing loss.
10. Why are hearing tests for children important?
11. What is otitis media?
12. What symptoms occur in Ménière's disease?
13. What types of treatment may be used for Ménière's disease?
14. What are the predisposing factors for cerebral palsy?
15. Name the three types of cerebral palsy and the symptoms for each.
16. What is epilepsy?
17. What is the treatment for epilepsy?
18. How prevalent is Parkinson's disease?
19. What are the symptoms of Parkinson's disease?
20. How effective is the treatment for Parkinson's disease?
21. What is the physiologic process leading to MS?
22. What can be said about the incidence of MS?
23. What are the symptoms of MS?
24. What is the treatment for MS?
25. How is Alzheimer's disease diagnosed?
26. Describe the three stages of Alzheimer's.
27. What treatment is available for Alzheimer's?
28. What are the differences between type I and type II diabetes mellitus?
29. What complications may occur in diabetes?
30. What measures can be taken to avoid type II diabetes?

FURTHER READING

Disorders of the Senses

Alberti, P.W. et al. "Managing Adult Hearing Loss." *Patient Care,* Feb. 15, '88, 22:54-63.

Arenberg, I. Kaufman et al. "Van Gogh Had Ménière's Disease and Not Epilepsy." *Journal of the American Medical Association,* July 25, '90, 264:491-493.

Baloh, Robert W. et al. "Help for Ménière's Disease Patients." *Patient Care,* Sept. 30, '90, 24:80-89.

Christen, William G. et al. "A Prospective Study of Cigarette Smoking and Risk of Cataract in Men." *Journal of the American Medical Association,* Aug. 26, '92, 268:989-993.

Cinque, Chris. "Sunlight and Cataracts: Are Athletes at Risk?" *Physician and Sportsmedicine,* Mar. '89, 17:210-212.

Cleveland, Patricia J. et al. "Ménière's Disease: The Inner Ear Out of Balance." *RN,* Aug. '90, 53:28-32.

Collman, Gwen W. et al. "Sunlight and Other Risk Factors for Cataracts: An Epidemiologic Study." *American Journal of Public Health,* Nov. '88, 78:1459-1462.

Davies, Owen. "Glaucoma: RPh's Must Warn Patients That Failure to Follow a Regimen Leads to Blindness." *American Druggist,* Feb. '88, 197:68-71.

Donshik, Peter C. et al. "The Aging Eye: Thieves of Sight." *Patient Care,* Apr. 15, '89, 23: 38-48.

Freudenheim, Milt. "Laser Repair of Eyes Show Promise." *New York Times,* May 13, '92, sec D, p 1, col 3.

Gurwitz, J.S. et al. "Treatment for Glaucoma: Adherence by the Elderly." *American Journal of Public Health,* May '93, 83(5):711-716.

Hale, Ellen. "Lifting the Clouds of Cataracts." *FDA Consumer,* Jan. '89, 23:26-30.

Hankinson, Susan E. et al. "A Prospective Study of Cigarette Smoking and Risk of Cataract Surgery in Women." *Journal of the American Medical Association,* Aug. 26, '92, 268:994-998.

Hutchinson, B. Thomas. "Cataracts." *Harvard Medical School Health Letter,* Apr. '88, 13:6-8.

Kaufman, Laura. "A Diet to Prevent Cataracts." *American Health,* Oct. '91, 10:90.

Kirn, Timothy F. "Ophthalmologists Discuss Methods to Help Physicians See What Patients Can't See." *Journal of the American Medical Association,* Feb. 27, '87, 257:1025-1027.

"Laser Surgery: Too Much, Too Soon?" *Consumer Reports,* Aug. '91, 56:536-540.

"Noise and Hearing Loss." *Lancet,* July 6, '91, 338:21-22.

Seligson, Susan V. "Eyes on Blink." *In Health,* Mar. '91, 5:80-86.

"Senile Cataract and Vitamin Nutrition." *Nutrition Review,* Oct. '89, 47:326-328.

Strome, Marshall et al. "Hearing Loss and Hearing Aids." *Harvard Medical School Health Letter,* Apr. '89, 14:5-8.

"Sunrise Technologies Gets a U.S. Clearance for Laser." *New York Times,* July 16, '92, sec D, p 4, col 1.

Taylor, Allen. "Associations between Nutrition and Cataract." *Nutrition Reviews,* Aug. '89, 47:225-234.

Taylor, Hugh R. et al. "Effect of Ultraviolet Radiation on Cataract Formation." *New England Journal of Medicine,* Dec. 1, '88, 319:1429-1433.

Warren, Andrea. "Fix for Farsightedness." *American Health,* Jan. '92, 11:12-15.

Disorders of the Nervous System

Ahlskog, J.E. "Cerebral Transplantation for Parkinson's Disease: Current Progress and Future Prospects." *Mayo Clinic Proceedings,* June '93, 68(6):578-591.

Beardsley, Tim. "Multiple Choice: Viral Fingerprints Are Found in the Blood of MS Patients." *Scientific American,* Apr. '89, 260:34-35.

Crease, Robert P. "The Epilepsy 'Cure': Bold Claims, Weak Data." *Science,* Sept. 29, '89, 245:1444-1445.

Culliton, Barbara J. "Needed: Fetal Tissue Research." *Nature,* Jan. 23, '92, 355:295.

DeVore, Sheryl. "The Facts of Life with Epilepsy." *Current Health,* Jan. '89, 15:10-12.

Eicher, P.S. and M.L. Batshaw. "Cerebral Palsy." *Pediatric Clinics of North America,* June '93, 40(3):537-551.

Evans, Denis A. et al. "Prevalence of Alzheimer's Disease in a Community Population of Older Persons: Higher than Previously Reported." *Journal of the American Medical Association,* Nov. 10, '89, 262:2551-2556.

Fackelmann, Kathy A. "Myelin on the Mend: Can Antibodies Reverse the Ravages of Multiple Sclerosis?" *Science News,* Apr. 7, '90, 137:218-219.

Flieger, Ken. "Memories Are Made of This." *FDA Consumer,* Sept. '89, 23:14-19.

Ghanbari, Hossein A. et al. "Biochemical Assay of Alzheimer's Disease–Associated Protein(s) in Human Brain Tissue: a Clinical Study." *Journal of the American Medical Association,* June 6, '90, 263:2907-2910.

Goertz, Christopher G. et al. "Update on Parkinson's Disease." *Patient Care,* Apr. 15, '89, 23:124-140.

Grant, Adrian et al. "Cerebral Palsy among Children Born during the Dublin Randomized Trail of Intrapartum Monitoring." *Lancet,* Nov. 25, '89, 2:1233-1236.

Hardy, John A. and Gerald A. Higgins. "Alzheimer's Disease: The Amyloid Cascade Hypothesis." *Science,* Apr. 10, '92, 256:184-185.

Kosik, Kenneth S. "Alzheimer's Disease: A Cell Biological Perspective." *Science,* May 8, '92, 256:780-783.

Marx, Jean. "A New Link in the Brain's Defenses." *Science,* May 29, '92, 256:1278-1280.

Mitchell, G. "Update on Multiple Sclerosis Therapy." *Medical Clinics of North America,* Jan. '93, 77(1):231-249.

Nightingale, S.L. "From the Food and Drug Administration." (Multiple Sclerosis) *Journal of the American Medical Association,* Feb. 24, '93, 269(8):974.

"Parkinson's Disease: One Illness or Many Syndromes?" *Lancet,* May 23, '92, 339:1263-1264.

Patlak, Margie. "The Puzzling Picture of Multiple Sclerosis." *FDA Consumer,* July-Aug. '89, 23:17-21.

Paty, Donald W. et al. "The Challenge of Detecting MS." *Patient Care,* Sept. 30, '89, 23:62-69.

Paveza, Gregory J. and Donna Cohen. "Severe Family Violence and Alzheimer's Disease: Prevalence and Risk Factors." *Gerontologist,* Aug. '92, 32:493-497.

Poser, Charles M. and Michael Ronthal. "Exercise and Alzheimer's Disease, Parkinson's Disease, and Multiple Sclerosis." *Physician and Sportsmedicine,* Dec. '91, 19:85-92.

Pruchno, Rachel A. et al. "Husbands and Wives as Caregivers: Antecedents of Depression and Burden." *Gerontologist,* Apr. '89, 29:159-164.

Pugh, Carol B. "Treatment of Seizure Disorders." *American Druggist,* Mar. '88, 197:100-108.

Rao, Stephen M., Huber, Steven J., Bornstein, Robert A. "Emotional Changes in Multiple Sclerosis and Parkinson's Disease." *Journal of Consulting & Clinical Psychology,* June '92, 60:369-378.

Regland, Bjorn and Carl-Gerhard Gottfries. "The Role of Amyloid (Beta)-Protein in Alzheimer's Disease." *Lancet,* Aug. 22, '92, 340:467-469.

Rubin, E.H., D.A. Kinscherf, and J.C. Morris. "Psychopathology in Younger Versus Older Persons with Very Mild and Mild Dementia of the Alzheimer Type." *American Journal of Psychiatry,* Apr. '93, 150(4):639-642.

Ryan, C.A. and G. Dowling. "Drowning Deaths in People with Epilepsy." *Canadian Medical Association Journal,* Mar. 1, '93, 148(5):781-784.

Selkoe, Dennis J. "Aging Brain, Aging Mind." *Scientific American,* Sept. '92, 267:134-142.

Tanzillo, Kevin. "Fetal Tissue Implants: Therapy for Parkinson's Disease." *Geriatrics,* July '92, 47:70-76.

Thompson, Larry and David P. Hamilton. "Fetal Transplants Show Promise." *Science,* Aug. 14, '92, 257:868-870.

Weiss, Rick. "Toward a Future with Memory: Researchers Look High and Low for the Essence of Alzheimer's." *Science News,* Feb. 24, '90, 137:120-123.

Endocrine Disorders (Diabetes Mellitus)

Bock, Troels et al. "No Risk of Diabetes after Insulin-Shock Treatment." *Lancet,* June 20, '92, 339:1504-1506.

Bougneres, P.F. et al. "Factors Associated with Early Remission of Type I Diabetes in Children Treated with Cyclosporine." *New England Journal of Medicine,* Mar. 17, '88, 318:663-669.

Cahill, Jr., George F. "Beta-Cell Deficiency, Insulin Resistance, or Both?" *New England Journal of Medicine,* May 12, '88, 318:1268-1270.

Goodrich, Susan Williams et al. "Changing Roles and Challenges for Teachers of Students with Diabetes." *Journal of School Health*, Oct. '89, 59:341-345.

Healy, Bernadine. "From the National Institutes of Health: Research Offers New Hope for Young Persons with Diabetes." *Journal of the American Medical Association*, July 1, '92, 268:20.

Henry, Robert R. and Steven V. Edelman. "Advances in Treatment of Type II Diabetes Mellitus in the Elderly." *Geriatrics*, Apr. '92, 47:24-30.

Hirsch, I.B. and R. Frakas-Hirsch. "Type I Diabetes and Insulin Therapy." *Nursing Clinics of North America*, Mar. '93, 28(1):9-23.

Karjalainen, Jukka et al. "A Comparison of Childhood and Adult Type I Diabetes Mellitus." *New England Journal of Medicine*, Apr. 6, '89, 320:881-886.

Kurz, Zarrina. "Changing Prevalence of Juvenile-Onset Diabetes Mellitus." *Lancet*, July 9, '88, 2:88-90.

Leach, Deborah. "Children's Perspectives on Diabetes." *Journal of School Health*, Apr. '88, 58:159-161.

Maclaren, Noel and Mark Atlinson. "Is Insulin-Dependent Diabetes Mellitus Environmentally Induced?" *New England Journal of Medicine*, July 30, '92, 327:348-349.

Martin, Julio M. et al. "A Bovine Albumin Peptide as a Possible Trigger of Insulin-Dependent Diabetes Mellitus." *New England Journal of Medicine*, July 30, '92, 327:302-307.

Melkus, G.D. "Type II Non-Insulin-Dependent Diabetes Mellitus." *Nursing Clinics of North America*, Mar. 28, '93, 28(1):25-33.

Pydrowski, Kathryn L. et al. "Preserved Insulin Secretion and Insulin Independence in Recipients of Islet Autografts." *New England Journal of Medicine*, July 23, '92, 327:220-226.

Raloff, J. "Diabetes: Clarifying the Role of Obesity." *Science News*, Jan. 2, '93, 143:7.

Ritz, E. "Hypertension in Diabetic Nephropathy: Prevention and Treatment." *American Heart Journal*, May '93, 125(5 part 2):1514-1519.

Schmidt, Lois E. et al. "Compliance with Dietary Prescriptions in Children and Adolescents with Insulin-Dependent Diabetes Mellitus." *Journal of the American Dietetic Association*, May '92, 92:567-570.

Stehouwer, C.D.A. et al. "Urinary Albumin Excretion, Cardiovascular Disease, and Endothelial Dysfunction in Non–Insulin-Dependent Diabetes Mellitus." *Lancet*, Aug. 8, '92, 340:319-323.

Stern, M.P. et al. "Predicting Diabetes: Moving Beyond Impaired Glucose Tolerance." *Diabetes*, May '93, 42(5):706-714.

Tarn, Anne C. et al. "Predicting Insulin-Dependent Diabetes." *Lancet*, Apr. 16, '88, 1:845-850.

Velho, Gilberto et al. "Primary Pancreatic Beta-Cell Secretory Defect Caused by Mutations in Glucokinase Gene in Kindreds of Maturity Onset Diabetes of the Young." *Lancet*, Aug. 22, '92, 340:444-448.

Vikhanski, Luba. "Exercise Reduces Risk of Diabetes." *Medical World News*, July '92, 33:16-17.

General

Gilman, Sid. "Medical Progress: Advances in Neurology." *New England Journal of Medicine*, June 11, '92, 326:1608-1616.

Wallace, Douglas C. "Mitochondrial Genetics: A Paradigm for Aging and Degenerative Diseases?" *Science*, May 1, '92, 256:628-632.

Weiss, Rick. "Decade of Discovery." *American Health*, Mar. '92, 11:34-39.

Chapter 18

Genetic and Pediatric Disorders

O B J E C T I V E S

1 Distinguish between the terms *congenital* and *genetic*.

2 Explain how genetic disorders may occur.

3 State characteristics of at least one disease that occurs because of (1) a chromosome abnormality, (2) a unifactorial defect, and (3) a multifactorial defect.

4 Tell what is meant by autosomal dominant, autosomal recessive, and X-linked recessive.

5 Explain why a chorionic villus biopsy may be preferred over amniocentesis.

6 Explain why the transmission of Huntington's chorea may be difficult to prevent.

7 Distinguish between sickle cell trait and sickle cell anemia.

8 Identify a common risk factor for having a child with Down syndrome and other genetic diseases.

9 Explain when and why drinking alcohol is a high risk for a pregnant woman.

10 Compare respiratory distress syndrome and sudden infant death syndrome.

GENES AND GENETIC DISORDERS

Many theories have been developed over the years to explain how humans develop and why behavior differs from person to person. Early theorists believed the transmission of hereditary traits to be much simpler than we know it to be today. Knowledge in the field of genetics has grown at such a rapid pace that new findings outdate books on the subject before they are off the press. Nevertheless, it is important to have some knowledge of genetics to study genetic disorders.

Genetics now has three main branches: (1) Mendelian genetics, the study of the transmission of traits from one generation to the next; (2) molecular genetics, the study of the chemical structure of genes and how they operate at the molecular level; and (3) population genetics, the study of the variation of genes among and within populations. In this chapter, we will be most concerned with Mendelian and molecular genetics. The treatment will be necessarily brief, and students are urged to follow the literature in the field to increase their knowledge of genetics and keep up with new developments.

GENES

The essential ingredient of heredity is deoxyribonucleic acid (DNA). Along with some associated protein, DNA makes up the 23 pairs of chromosomes in the nuclei of all cells. A gene corresponds to a small section of DNA on a chromosome (Figure 18-1). Each gene has the responsibility for directing the creation of a specific human trait, such as hair color or the lining of the stomach. It is estimated that each human cell holds more than 50,000 genes within its nucleus. These genes direct the development and functioning of every organ and system within the body.

With the exception of the egg and sperm cells, each cell in a person's body contains an identical set of genes. However, in different locations in the body, some

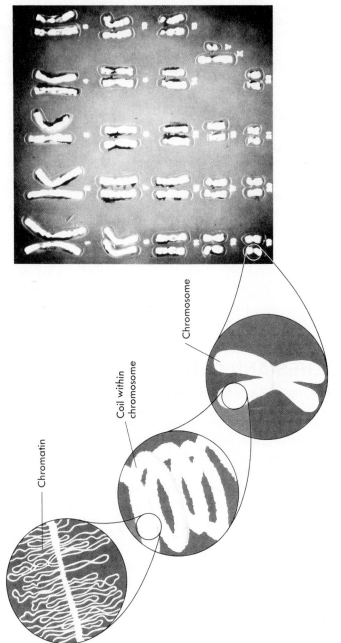

FIGURE 18-1   DNA, chromosomes, genes.

DID YOU KNOW?

A Wider Perspective

Marfan's syndrome is a rare disease, but famous people have been afflicted with the disorder. The sports world was shocked when Flo Hyman, a famous volleyball player, suddenly slipped off the bench on the sidelines of a game in Japan and was pronounced dead. Doctors suspected a heart attack, but an autopsy revealed that she had died of a ruptured aorta caused by Marfan's syndrome. People with the disorder are often taller than other family members and have arms that are disproportionately long. Defective genes are responsible for the syndrome, causing critical changes in the pro-

tein that gives connective tissue its strength. Marfan victims also tend to have long fingers, deformities of the breastbone, and nearsightedness. Some experts believe that Abraham Lincoln may have had Marfan's syndrome because of his long fingers and great height. It is a difficult disease to diagnose and many times remains hidden until sudden death occurs as it did with Hyman. Even with all the physicals that athletes are exposed to, a hint of Marfan's syndrome was not detected by physicians. Flo Hyman was considered to be in excellent health.

genes are active and others are idle, depending upon the location. (For example, different genes are active in stomach cells than in liver cells.) We know that our genes have an important role in the structure and function of the body, but their role in personality, behavior, and mental ability is not as clear.

Each body cell has 46 chromosomes (23 pairs), including two sex chromosomes. Females have a matched (homologous) pair, XX, whereas males have an unmatched (heterologous) pair, XY. Each gene occupies a specific place or locus on the chromosome. There are different loci for different traits, such as hair color, eye color, and so on. Genes are able to fulfill their function by directing the manufacture of proteins. The directions for making the necessary body proteins are encoded within the sequence of DNA that makes up the gene.

Whenever a cell divides, the DNA is first copied. This is an extremely complicated process and sometimes mistakes are made, resulting in mutant or defective genes that can lead to genetic disorders.

GENETIC DISORDERS

A genetic disorder is any disorder due to a defect or defects in the inherited genetic material. A genetic disorder may be congenital (with birth) or it may not appear for many years. There are many congenital disorders that are not genetic, and some of these will be discussed in this chapter also. See the box above.

With the exception of identical twins, every human being has a unique genetic makeup. Some of us have inherited a predisposition or susceptibility to certain diseases. If we do not come in contact with an initiating factor for a disease for which we are susceptible, we will never have it. For example, if a man has a genetic makeup that makes him susceptible to lung cancer, but never smokes and never is exposed to smoke or other carcinogenic substances in the air, lung cancer is not likely to develop. Or consider a woman who has inherited a tendency for skin cancer but spends most of her time indoors and little time in the sun—she is not likely to get skin cancer.

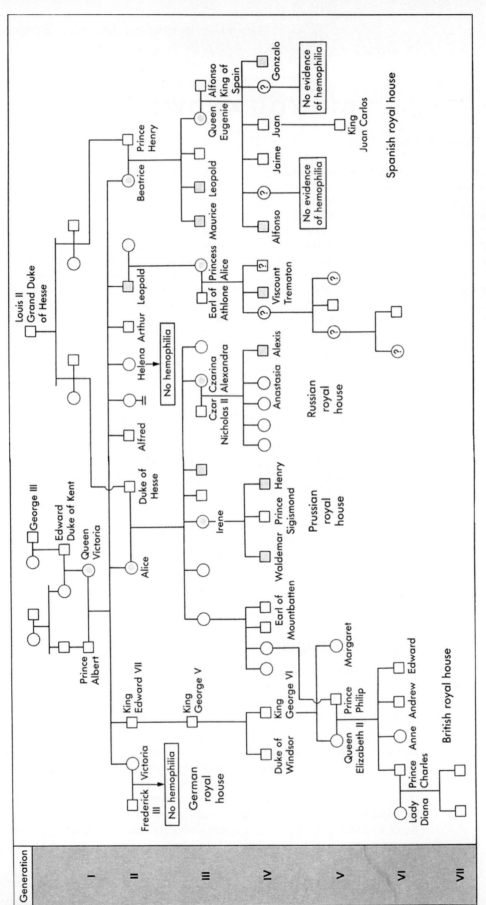

FIGURE 18-2 Partial pedigree for descendants of Queen Victoria showing the appearance of Hemophilia A in one of her sons and his descendants and the descendants of her daughters and granddaughters. Black squares indicate hemophiliacs; black spots indicate carriers.

For persons to have a genetic disorder, the genetic material that is abnormal must usually be present in each of their cells. For this to happen, the defect must be present in the egg or sperm cell (or both) from which the individuals were formed. This abnormal genetic material may have been present in the parent(s) at birth, or a mutation may have occurred during the formation of the egg or sperm cell. Because of mutations, a child with a genetic disorder may be born into a family that does not have a history of a known disorder. Figure 18-2 shows the pedigree of such a mutation in the royal family of England. One third of the cases of hemophilia, which will be discussed later, are due to new mutations.

CLASSIFICATIONS OF GENETIC DISEASE

Genetic diseases can be broadly classified as due to chromosome abnormalities, unifactorial defects, and multifactorial defects. Down syndrome is the best known example of a chromosome abnormality. Children born with this disorder have an extra chromosome. Unifactorial disorders occur rarely, but there are many of them. They are caused by a single defective gene or pair of genes. Unifactorial disorders can be divided into three groups:

Autosomal dominant disorders occur when a person carries only one defective gene, but because it is dominant, it overrides the normal gene and the individual can get the disease. Examples: Huntington's chorea, Marfan's syndrome.

Autosomal recessive disorders occur when a recessive defective gene is acquired from both parents who are carriers and have no apparent disease. With two recessive genes for the same disease, the child will get the disease. Examples: cystic fibrosis, sickle cell anemia.

X-linked recessive disorders occur when the defective gene is on the X chromosome. As has been stated earlier, women have two X chromosomes and men have one X and one Y. Men get the X chromosome from their mothers and pass it on to their daughters. When a woman inherits a defective single sex gene, it is masked by the gene on her other X chromosome, and she has no apparent disease. When a man inherits the defective gene, he has no normal X gene on another chromosome, and he will get the disease. Examples: color blindness, hemophilia, muscular dystrophy.

There are many disorders that fall into the category of multifactorial disorders. These disorders are thought to be determined by a number of different genes plus environmental influences. Examples of multifactorial disorders can be seen in Table 18-1.

RESEARCH IN AND DETERMINATION OF GENETIC DISEASE PREVENTION

Scientists have developed the capability of manipulating some genes before birth in order to prevent genetic diseases or provide each of us with the defenses to ward off disease. The procedures are still in the experimental stage for the most part, and there are hard ethical problems to be solved before these procedures can be used on humans. Tests have been used for some time that can detect genetic defects in the unborn fetus. Figure 18-3 shows one of these tests, amniocentesis. Another test used to identify genetic defects in the fetus is chorionic villus biopsy. This technique can be done earlier in the pregnancy (2 months) than amniocentesis (5 months), resulting in earlier diagnosis. However, there is more chance of miscarriage with chorionic villus biopsy. Both procedures have advantages and disadvantages.

TABLE 18-1 Noninfectious diseases thought to have genetic predispostions

Disease	Associated Pathophysiology or Hypothesis	Environmental Factors
Coronary heart disease (especially early disease)(several different syndromes)	Familial hypercholesterolemia LDL receptor defects Other high cholesterol? Low HDL Endothelial factors? Platelet factors? Diabetes I and II Hypertension (especially early onset) Multiplicative interactions of history and risk factors	Dietary fat, saturated fat, polyunsaturated fat, total fat intake Exercise, alcohol, diet Smoking
Stroke	Hypertension and diabetes	
Hypertension	Age at onset? Severity? Etiology?	Salt, stress, obesity Polyunsaturated fat, calcium, exercise
Type I diabetes	Islet cell destruction Immunologic cause	Viral infection Seasonal variation Complications a function of blood sugar control for years
Type II diabetes	Insulin resistance or decreased production	Obesity Dietary sugar and fiber Exercise protective Complications a function of blood sugar control and function
Breast cancer	Possibly estrogen related Certain benign tumor precursors	Age at first birth Alcohol? Female hormones
Colon cancer	Several different types of syndromes Often benign polyps are precursors	Fiber intake Dietary fat? (converted by bacteria to carcinogens)
Lung cancer	Chemical carcinogens from environment encounter enzymatically susceptible subjects	Cigarette smoke Environmental pollutants Radiation exposure
Rheumatic heart disease	Immunologic cross-reactivity to bacteria and heart valves	Strep bacterial infection
Asthma and other allergies	Immunologically reactive	Many possible allergens—fur, dust, pollen, mold, etc.
Autoimmune disorders	Autoantibodies to thyroid, adrenal, synovium, platelets	Viral infections trigger immune responses
Psychiatric disorders: manic-depressive, depression, schizophrenia	Neurochemical disorders in brain tissue	Uncertain influence Dramatic success with drug treatment for first two
Kidney stones	Mineral-acid-base imbalance	Milk? Soda pop? Other fluids?
Gallstones	Fat, cholesterol, bilirubin balance	Dietary fat Obesity?

TABLE 18-1 Noninfectious diseases thought to have genetic predispostions—cont'd

Disease	Associated Pathophysiology or Hypothesis	Environmental Factors
Obesity	Less energy wasted? Decreased thermogenesis in brown fat?	Dietary fat, sugar, and total calories Stress, etc., affecting appetite Exercise level Cultural perceptions attractive to be fat or thin
Gout	Several different enzyme defects found	Dietary intake of meat, etc.
Multiple sclerosis	Autoimmune demyelination of nerve fibers	Slow virus? Climate dependent
Peptic ulcer disease	Excess acid production and/or decreased mucosal resistance	Stress Diet Dramatic drug Rx
Lactose intolerance	Deficiency of lactase enzyme in intestinal mucosa	Milk products
Alcoholism	Possible neurochemical origin? Associated with other psychiatric disorders	Ethyl alcohol intake Social factors

FIGURE 18-3 Amniocentesis.

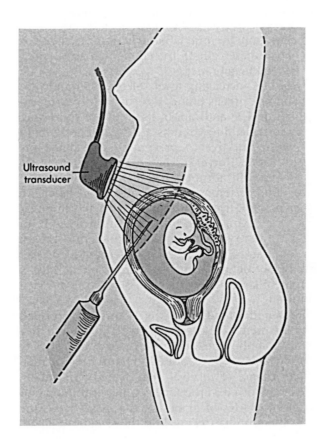

No matter which procedure is used to determine the health of the child, if a defect is found, parents must make the heart-rending choice of having a child with a serious disorder or terminating the pregnancy. The hope for the future is to make the decision unnecessary by genetic engineering that will correct defects before the baby is born. However, many moral and ethical problems must still be resolved before genetic engineering becomes a routine procedure. See the box below.

In this chapter, the more common genetic disorders will be discussed first; the second section will deal with the more common pediatric or developmental disorders, some of which are congenital and some of which appear sometime in the early life of the child.

AUTOSOMAL DOMINANT DISORDER
HUNTINGTON'S CHOREA

Huntington's chorea is an inherited disease of the central nervous system that usually has its onset between the ages of 30 and 50. Patients gradually lose their mental capabilities and musculoskeletal control. Death usually results 10 to 15 years after onset of the disease, from suicide, congestive heart failure, or pneumonia.

Because of the late onset of Huntington's, the victim has often had children before the disease becomes apparent. Because many families tend not to talk about any relative who has a neurologic disorder, there may be no record or recollection of anyone in the family having Huntington's. The stigma of "mental" disease has not yet been overcome, even with our increased understanding of the cause of these disorders. Therefore, this disease, which results in so much suffering and an early death, is unknowingly passed on from generation to generation.

Predisposing Factors   If a parent has had the disease, each child has a 50% chance of inheriting it.

DID YOU KNOW?

Determining Genetic Endowment

Scientists believe that within the next 20 years it will become possible to examine an individual's entire genetic endowment soon after conception. They expect to be able to determine whether the individual will become afflicted with glaucoma, schizophrenia, hypertension, coronary heart disease, some kind of cancer, and more. Parents will know before the baby is born whether it will have a serious disease or perhaps a number of minor diseases. Will they decide not to have a child who might develop cancer? We all carry genes that give us a predisposition to certain diseases. How will the "life or death" decisions be made?

Symptoms   The disease begins slowly with momentary loss of balance. Gradually, symptoms become more pronounced, with progressively severe uncontrolled movements. In the beginning, these movements are unilateral and occur more in the legs, arms, and face. As the chorea becomes more violent, the patient also loses mental competence, and personality changes such as obstinacy, untidiness, apathy, and paranoia take place.

Prevention   None known.

Treatment   There is no known cure for Huntington's, and treatment is aimed at relieving symptoms and providing support. Drugs can help control the involuntary movements and alleviate depression and discomfort. Emotional support and genetic counseling are needed for patient and family to help them understand the disease.

AUTOSOMAL RECESSIVE DISORDERS
CYSTIC FIBROSIS

Cystic fibrosis is an inherited disease of the exocrine glands, affecting the pancreas, respiratory system, and sweat glands. One gene for cystic fibrosis, located on the long arm of chromosome 7, must be inherited from each parent. Cystic fibrosis kills more children than any other genetic disease. Half of those afflicted with the disease die by age 16, and the rest do not live beyond age 30.

Predisposing Factors   The disease is more common in children of Central European ancestry and rare in blacks. In a family where both parents carry the defective gene, there is a 25% chance in every pregnancy that the baby will develop the disease.

Symptoms   In the newborn, intestinal mucus may be so sticky that it blocks the bowel, which leads to obstruction, rupture, and even death. The child does not gain weight, although a good appetite is present (Figure 18-4). The air passages in the lungs become blocked with mucous, leading to collapsed lungs and emphysema. Chronic respiratory infection and heat intolerance are also symptoms of the disease. If the child lives long enough, the bile ducts may become obstructed, leading to cirrhosis with portal hypertension. Many children with cystic fibrosis also have diabetes mellitus.

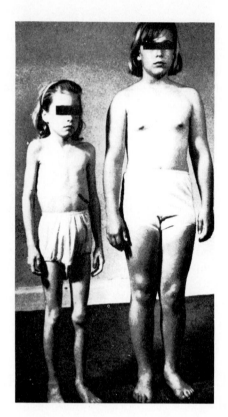

FIGURE 18-4 Child on left, with cystic fibrosis, is the same age as child on right.

Prevention   None known.

Treatment   Since there is no cure at present, the goal of treatment is to help the child live as normal a life as possible. Breathing exercises, physical therapy, and postural drainage help to manage the lung problems, and antibiotics can be used to hold off the threat of staphylococcal pneumonia. Oral pancreatic enzymes are used to offset the enzyme deficiencies. Extra salt on food and salt tablets in hot weather are used to combat electrolyte loss through sweating. Air conditioners and humidifiers help to decrease vulnerability to respiratory infections, and oxygen therapy is used as needed. The patient and the family need education about the disease and emotional support throughout the illness.

PHENYLKETONURIA

Phenylketonuria, or PKU, is an inherited disorder in which an enzyme that converts phenylalanine (an amino acid) into tyrosine (another amino acid) is defective. When phenylalanine builds up in the body, it causes severe mental retardation. About one baby in 12,000 is born with PKU in the United States.

Predisposing Factors

PKU is transmitted by a recessive gene. The incidence is higher among those of Celtic origin and Central Europeans.

Symptoms

Babies generally show no signs of PKU at birth, but by 4 months of age, neurologic disturbances, including epilepsy, become evident. PKU babies have an unpleasant musty, mousy smell about them caused by a breakdown product of phenylalanine excreted in their sweat and urine. Most of these children (90%) have blond hair and blue eyes that are effects of the condition. They may also have eczema, an abnormally large head, and a steep decline in IQ during the first year. They may be hyperactive, irritable, and display purposeless, repetitive motions.

Prevention

Early screening for PKU (by blood test) is now mandatory in most states and is the best means of prevention. Early detection and treatment of the disorder can minimize the damage to the central nervous system.

Treatment

PKU is treated with a diet free of phenylalanine, which is a natural constituent of most protein foods. Milk substitutes are given to babies, and after weaning they are given a very low-protein diet that is mainly vegetarian. Some physicians believe this diet should be followed throughout life, but others believe it can be discontinued by the age of 12.

SICKLE CELL ANEMIA

Individuals with sickle cell anemia have blood cells that are abnormal and become sickle shaped and thus unable to carry sufficient oxygen (Figures 18-5 and 18-6). The genetic defect is largely confined to blacks and is transmitted as a dominant characteristic by either sex. If both parents carry the defective gene, the child will have sickle cell anemia. If only one parent carries the gene, the child will have *sickle cell trait,* which means being a carrier of the disease. Approximately two out of every 25 black people carry the disease. The sickle cell trait may provide protection from malaria.

Predisposing Factors

Most of those with sickle cell anemia are members of the black race.

Symptoms

The symptoms, which usually do not occur until after 6 months, include heart problems, fatigue, breathlessness on exertion, joint swelling, and leg ulcers, especially around the ankles. Upon getting older, the child has acute crises when the anemia is intensified and suffers from severe abdominal pain and other symptoms, depending on the type of crisis.

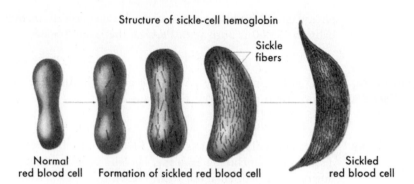

Structure of sickle-cell hemoglobin

Sickle fibers

FIGURE 18-5 A sickled cell.

Normal red blood cell   Formation of sickled red blood cell   Sickled red blood cell

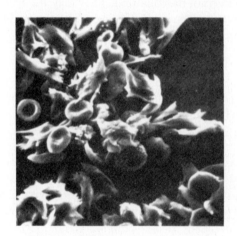

FIGURE 18-6 Normal and sickle-shaped blood cells from the same patient.

Prevention None known.

Treatment When an acute crisis occurs, the child is hospitalized for transfusions. At other times, the patient can stay at home and be treated for the symptoms.

X-LINKED RECESSIVE DISORDER
HEMOPHILIA A

Hemophilia is an inherited bleeding disorder that occurs because of a deficiency of certain clotting factors. There are several different forms of hemophilia, but A is the most common. Most hemophiliacs are male, since it is an X-linked recessive trait. Women who are carriers have a 50% chance of passing the disease on to their sons but transmit only the gene to their daughters (50% chance also). About one male in 10,000 is born with hemophilia. Affected males pass the gene on to none of their sons but to all of their daughters, who become carriers of the condition. In about one third of the cases, there is no family history of hemophilia. Since the advent of acquired immune deficiency syndrome (AIDS), the problems of hemophiliacs have increased because of the chance of transmission of AIDS through blood

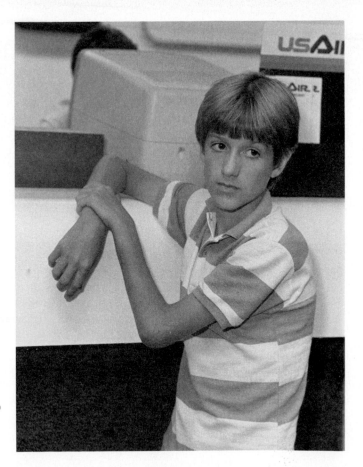

FIGURE 18-7 Ryan White, hemophiliac who contracted AIDS because of blood transfusions.

transfusions, which hemophiliacs must have to treat their condition (Figure 18-7). Blood screening has reduced the risk of transmission by transfusion until it is now estimated that chances of getting the human immunodeficiency virus (HIV) are one in several million.

Predisposing Factors   Hemophilia is passed on from mothers who are carriers to half of their sons, who are born with the condition, or to half of their daughters, who become carriers. All daughters of hemophiliac fathers are carriers. Rarely, the daughter of a father with hemophilia and a mother who is a carrier may have hemophilia.

Symptoms   There is great variation in symptoms among those who have hemophilia. Most bleeding episodes involve hemorrhage into joints and muscles. They often begin when an affected child begins to walk and becomes susceptible to falls. Pain accompanies the bleeding episodes, and if they are not treated, there may be crippling of the joints involved. If it is a mild case, it may not be diagnosed until surgery or some other major trauma causes bleeding. In addition to the pain, there may be other symptoms, depending upon the location of the bleeding, which may be internal as well as external.

Prevention   Children who have hemophilia need to avoid activities that expose them to risk of injury, such as contact sports. If a person who has hemophilia must have surgery, careful management is needed by a physician who has expertise in hemophilia care.

Treatment   Fifty years ago, most hemophiliacs did not survive to adulthood. Today, bleeding episodes can be controlled by a transfusion. Infusions of the missing clotting factor should be given as quickly as possible after the start of bleeding. Because of the threat of HIV in the blood supply, efforts are under way to develop a synthetic replacement for the clotting factor that hemophiliacs need.

CHROMOSOMAL ABNORMALITIES
DOWN SYNDROME

Down syndrome occurs in 1 per 650 births overall. A child with Down syndrome has 47 chromosomes instead of 46. This genetic disorder may be inherited from either of the two parents, who may have no physical or mental abnormalities themselves. Life expectancy for individuals with Down syndrome is short, with up to one third dying before age 10.

Predisposing Factors   The age of the mother at the time of birth seems to be a significant factor in the development of Down syndrome, since the incidence increases with mothers past 35 (Figure 18-8).

FIGURE 18-8 Rate of Down syndrome per 1000 live births related to maternal age.

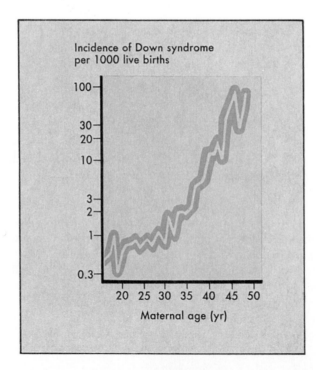

Incidence of Down syndrome per 1000 live births

Maternal age (yr)

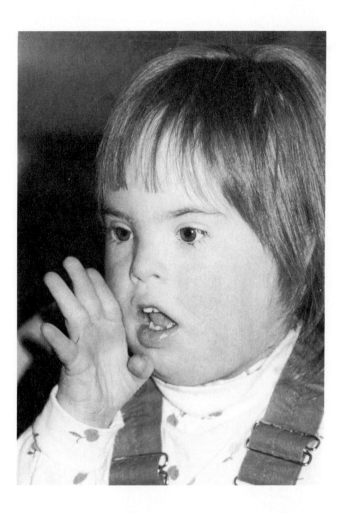

FIGURE 18-9 A child with Down syndrome.

Symptoms   Some typical signs and symptoms of the disorder are mental retardation; slanting, almond-shaped eyes; protruding tongue, small skull, abnormal dental development, small ears, and short neck (Figure 18-9). These persons often have heart disease, pelvic bone abnormalities, poorly developed genitalia, and delayed puberty. They are especially susceptible to leukemia and chronic infections.

Prevention   None known.

Treatment   Surgery to correct heart defects and antibiotics for chronic infections have helped to extend life for these individuals. They can be cared for at home or may be institutionalized. There is no cure.

KLINEFELTER'S SYNDROME

One in every 600 males has Klinefelter's syndrome, a genetic abnormality resulting from one or more extra X chromosomes. This disease is usually not apparent until puberty, when the secondary sex characteristics develop (Figure 18-10).

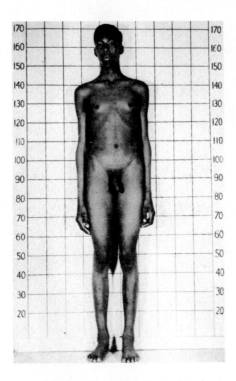

FIGURE 18-10 An individual with Klinefelter's syndrome.

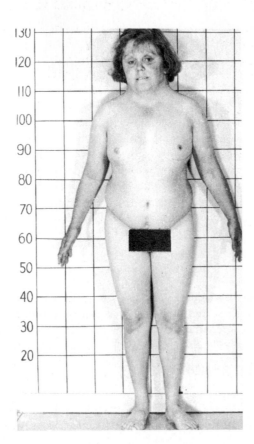

FIGURE 18-11 An individual with Turner's syndrome.

Although this genetic disorder occurs only in males, Turner's syndrome (Figure 18-11) is a similar disorder in females. Both syndromes result in sterility. However, Turner's syndrome occurs in only one out of 10,000 live female births.

Predisposing Factors   The disorder usually results from one extra chromosome. The possibility of this occurrence increases with the age of the mother, as with many other genetic disorders.

Symptoms   Mild cases may not have any apparent symptoms. The inability of a couple to conceive may be the first indication of the infertility of the male. Some of the characteristic features are a small penis and prostate; small, firm testicles; sparse facial and abdominal hair; impotence, and gynecomastia. The syndrome is also associated with mental retardation, osteoporosis, alcoholism, antisocial behavior, increased incidence of pulmonary disease, and breast cancer.

Prevention   None known.

Treatment   Hormonal treatment and psychotherapy to treat emotional problems, with acceptance of the disorder, are the best treatment, sometimes mastectomy in extreme cases. Nothing can be done to deter the changes that lead to infertility.

COMMON DISORDERS IN INFANTS AND CHILDREN

A number of disorders are present at birth that are not due to genetic abnormalities, but rather to unfavorable environmental factors for the fetus, or to lack of sufficient developmental time in the womb. The damage that can be caused to the baby by disease agents such as syphilis, gonorrhea, and rubella when they infect the mother during pregnancy has already been mentioned. In addition, some congenital disorders have been associated with the use of cocaine and other illegal drugs. Disorders that may occur because of prenatal drug use are spontaneous abortion, detached placentas, premature deliveries, sudden infant deaths, fetal urogenital tract malformations, and low birth weight. Women who smoke regularly during pregnancy also tend to have low-birth-weight babies, and those who drink may deliver a baby with fetal alcohol syndrome. Three of the most common of these disorders are discussed in the rest of this chapter.

FETAL ALCOHOL SYNDROME

Fetal alcohol syndrome (FAS) is a combination of birth defects found in a baby at birth. It is now thought that as little as one drink during pregnancy can produce fetal alcohol syndrome. Alcohol and tobacco both interfere with the growth of the fetus. Alcohol crosses the placenta in an amount equal to that in the mother's bloodstream. The fetal liver is underdeveloped and cannot oxidize the alcohol, and as a result the fetal brain is soaked in alcohol until the mother's blood alcohol count drops. Almost 20% of these babies die during the first few weeks of life.

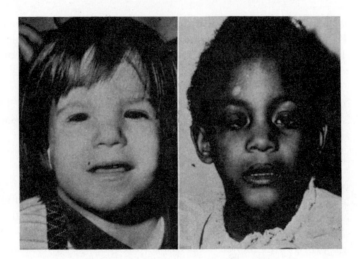

FIGURE 18-12 Children with fetal alcohol syndrome.

Predisposing Factors FAS results when a pregnant woman consumes alcohol. It is now thought that any amount of alcohol can cause difficulties for the fetus, but most cases of FAS occur in babies whose mothers were heavy drinkers during pregnancy. Alcohol consumed during the first 3 months is especially damaging to the fetus. Binge drinking is thought to be particularly harmful, since it produces high blood alcohol levels.

Symptoms Low birth weight, small head, mental retardation, learning disabilities, joint problems, and heart abnormalities are included in the signs and symptoms of FAS. FAS babies also tend to have distinctive facial features: small eyes that have vertical skin folds extending from the upper eyelid to the side of the nose, and a small jaw (Figure 18-12). The baby may also have a small brain, cleft palate, heart defects, a dislocated hip, and other joint deformities. As a newborn, the baby sleeps badly, sucks poorly, and is irritable because of alcohol withdrawal.

Prevention Most experts now believe that a woman should abstain from drinking if there is a chance she could be pregnant. Since the worst damage can occur in the first few months, any woman who has unprotected intercourse should not drink until she knows she did not conceive.

Treatment Treatment depends upon the type and extent of defects. Some defects can be corrected, but the mental and physical retardation will last for life.

RESPIRATORY DISTRESS SYNDROME

The most common cause of death of newborn babies, respiratory distress syndrome (RDS), results in 40,000 deaths every year. This lung disorder causes increasing difficulty in breathing, resulting in insufficient oxygen in the blood.

Predisposing Factors   A deficiency of surfactant, a chemical that keeps the alveoli open, is the cause of the syndrome in babies. It occurs most often in premature babies. About 3% of newborn babies die of RDS.

Symptoms   Babies make grunting noises and draw in the chest wall when they breathe. The baby will eventually turn blue as the condition worsens, and death may result if treatment is not given.

Prevention   Prenatal care to help the woman carry her baby to full term could reduce the risk of RDS in newborns.

Treatment   Babies who have the disorder are kept in an intensive care unit, where they can be given oxygen. If the condition worsens, they may need an endotracheal tube inserted through the nose or mouth, or a tracheostomy.

SUDDEN INFANT DEATH SYNDROME

When a baby is found dead in its crib and there is no known reason for its death, sudden infant death syndrome (SIDS) is suspected. SIDS is the most common cause of death for infants 1 month to 1 year in the United States and other developed countries. Three quarters of the time the baby is under 6 months of age. SIDS occurs slightly more frequently in boys, among second children, and in cold weather. For reasons unknown, more of these deaths occur between midnight and 9 a.m. and on weekends. Most experts believe there is no single cause of SIDS and that most deaths are caused by a respiratory or cardiac abnormality.

Predisposing Factors   Risk factors include prematurity, low birth weight, bottle feeding, and cold weather; young, single mothers; smoking, drug addiction, or anemia in the mother; poor socioeconomic background; the death of a brother or sister as a result of SIDS; and infants who have been discovered near death and were revived.

Symptoms   No symptoms have been identified for certain, but it is known that some of the babies have mild cold symptoms for several days previous to the death, and some have shown unexplained loss of weight.

Prevention   When the cause of a death cannot be identified, there is no way of being positive about preventive measures. It is possible that good prenatal care, avoidance of smoking, alcohol, and drugs during pregnancy, good obstetric care, breast-feeding, and close observation of any baby who has symptoms of being sick, no matter how minor, could help. Recently, studies have shown that infants who sleep on their backs are less likely to have SIDS. There is an alarm that can be used to detect if a baby stops breathing, but there is no evidence that use of this will prevent the disease.

Treatment   There is obviously no treatment for SIDS. However, it is such a shock to the family that it is important that they have help in working through their grief and probable feelings of guilt.

SUMMARY

Genetics is one of the most rapidly developing fields in science. Transmission of the genetic code is complicated, but scientists have deciphered much of it and are on the verge of being able to correct genetic defects before birth. Ethical problems will need to be addressed.

Genes direct the development and functioning of every organ and organ system in the body. We are not sure how much genes have to do with personality characteristics, but everyone inherits characteristics that might protect them from certain diseases, as well as predispositions to certain diseases that may be triggered by an initiating factor.

Genetic diseases may be due to chromosome abnormalities, unifactorial defects, or multifactorial defects. Unifactorial disorders may be autosomal dominant, autosomal recessive, or X-linked recessive. There are many multifactorial disorders, and some believe that a genetic factor may be present in every disease.

Tests have been used for some time to detect defects in the fetus. If defects are found, parents must make a difficult choice. It is hoped that genetic engineering may eventually make the choice unnecessary.

The table summarizes relevant data on genetic and pediatric disorders.

SUMMARY TABLE Genetic and pediatric disorders				
Disorder	**Special Characteristics**	**Predisposing Factors**	**Common Symptoms**	**Prevention/ Treatment**
Huntington's chorea	Onset between 30 and 50; death 10-15 years after onset from suicide, heart failure, or pneumonia.	Parent with disease—50% chance.	Begin slowly, become pronounced gradually; loss of mental capabilities, musculoskeletal control; personality changes, apathy, paranoia.	No known prevention; incurable; treatment to ease symptoms only.
Cystic fibrosis	Disease of the exocrine glands; half die by age 16, the rest by 30.	Genetic.	Sticky mucous blocking bowel in newborn may lead to rupture, death; child does not gain weight; air passages blocked with mucous lead to emphysema; respiratory infection, heat intolerance; eventually cirrhosis with portal hypertension.	No prevention or cure; palliative treatment.

Continued.

SUMMARY TABLE Genetic and pediatric disorders—cont'd				
Disorder	**Special Characteristics**	**Predisposing Factors**	**Common Symptoms**	**Prevention/ Treatment**
Sickle cell anemia	Red blood cells sickle shaped; mostly in blacks; carriers have sickle cell trait.	Parents with disorder; member of black race.	Heart problems, fatigue, joint swelling, leg ulcers, breathlessness on exertion; later, acute crises, anemia intensified.	No prevention or cure; hospitalized during acute crises.
Down syndrome	Child has extra chromosome, perhaps inherited from a parent; 1 per 650 births; short life expectancy.	Mother past 35 at time of birth.	Typical symptoms: mental retardation; slanting, almond-shaped eyes; protruding tongue, small skull, abnormal dental development, small ears, short neck, heart disease, delayed puberty; especially susceptible to leukemia, chronic infections.	No prevention or cure; treatment for defects when possible.
Klinefelter's syndrome	One in 600 males have one or more extra X chromosomes; usually not apparent until puberty; Turner's syndrome, among 1 in 10,000 women, is similar.	Possibility increases with age of mother.	Penis, testicles fail to develop; infertility; mental deficiency, gynecomastia; associated with some chronic diseases; may be no apparent symptoms.	No prevention; hormone treatment, psychotherapy; changes leading to infertility cannot be deterred.
Hemophilia A	Most common of several kinds; deficiency in clotting factor; passed from mother to sons; gene only passed to daughters, disease passed on to sons; one third of cases have no family history; some victims infected with HIV.	Fifty percent of sons of a carrier mother are born hemophiliacs.	Main symptom: uncontrollable bleeding accompanied by pain; degree varies; sometimes undiagnosed until surgery, major trauma.	Avoid activities that may cause injury; careful management of surgery; transfusion; synthetic clotting factor possible.
Phenylketonuria	Enzyme for amino acid conversion absent at birth; affects 1 in 12,000 born in the United States.	Recessive gene; Celtic or Central European descent.	Neurologic disturbances; musty, mousy smell; blond hair, blue eyes; eczema, large head, steep decline in IQ; may be hyperactive, irritable, display repetitive behavior.	Best prevention: early detection, treatment; very low-protein diet free of phenylalanine; milk substitutes; diet perhaps discontinued after age 12.

Continued.

	SUMMARY TABLE	Genetic and pediatric disorders—cont'd		
Disorder	**Special Characteristics**	**Predisposing Factors**	**Common Symptoms**	**Prevention/ Treatment**
Fetal alcohol syndrome	Alcohol passed through placental membrane not oxidized by underdeveloped fetal liver; baby's brain soaked in alcohol until mother's blood alcohol level drops; almost 20% die within first few weeks of life.	Alcohol in any amount during first 3 months of pregnancy; binge drinking any time especially endangers fetus.	Low birth weight, small head, mental retardation, joint problems, heart abnormalities; tendency to distinctive facial features; many other defects possible.	Any woman with chance of pregnancy should not drink any alcoholic beverage; some defects can be corrected; mental, physical retardation last for life.
Respiratory distress syndrome	Most common cause of death in newborns.	Deficiency of surfactant necessary to keep alveoli open; occurs mostly in prematures.	Grunting noises, chest wall drawn in during breathing; baby turns blue, dies without treatment.	Good prenatal care to ensure full-term babies; treatment: intensive care unit with oxygen; tracheostomy as necessary.
Sudden infant death syndrome	Baby dead in crib without apparent reason; most common cause of infant death in 1-month-to-1-year-olds (most under 6 months); more on weekends and between midnight and 9 a.m.	Prematurity, low birth weight; bottle feeding; cold weather; young, single mother; smoking, drug addiction, or anemia in mother; poor socioeconomic background; death of sibling from SIDS; infant discovered near death, revived.	A mild cold and/or unexplained weight loss; none identified for sure.	Have baby sleep on back; family counseling for grief, possible guilt feelings.

QUESTIONS FOR REVIEW

1. Where are genes located?
2. For what are genes responsible?
3. How do genes fulfill their function?
4. What is DNA?
5. What does an initiating factor have to do with disease?
6. How does a genetic disorder occur?
7. Define and give examples of the following: chromosome abnormality, unifactorial defect, multifactorial defect, autosomal dominant, autosomal recessive, X-linked recessive.
8. What is the difference between amniocentesis and chorionic villus biopsy?
9. What is genetic engineering?

10. Why is it difficult to keep the genetic defect that causes Huntington's chorea from being transmitted?
11. What is the progression of the symptoms for Huntington's chorea?
12. Why is cystic fibrosis such a devastating disease?
13. What physiologic problems can a child with cystic fibrosis have?
14. What are some of the therapies that may be used for cystic fibrosis?
15. What is the difference between sickle cell anemia and sickle cell trait?
16. Why can some individuals who are not black develop sickle cell anemia?
17. What are the symptoms of sickle cell anemia in the beginning stages and as the child gets older?
18. How often does Down syndrome occur?
19. What are the risk factors for Down syndrome?
20. What are the symptoms of Down syndrome?
21. What causes Klinefelter's syndrome?
22. What is the predisposing factor for Klinefelter's syndrome?
23. What are the chances that a baby will be born with hemophilia?
24. What are the chances of being infected with HIV through a blood transfusion?
25. What can be said about the symptoms of hemophilia?
26. How may it be possible for the person with hemophilia to avoid blood transfusions in the future?
27. What causes phenylketonuria?
28. What are the symptoms of PKU?
29. What is the best prevention for PKU?
30. How is PKU treated?
31. Why may one alcoholic drink be dangerous for the fetus?
32. What are the symptoms of fetal alcohol syndrome?
33. How can fetal alcohol syndrome be prevented?
34. What causes respiratory distress syndrome in babies?
35. What are the symptoms of RDS?
36. How is RDS treated?
37. What is the most common cause of death in infants in the United States?
38. What is thought to be the cause of sudden infant death syndrome?
39. What symptoms have been identified for SIDS?
40. What can be said about prevention and treatment for SIDS?

FURTHER READING

Ahmann, Elizabeth, Louise Wulff, Robert G. Meny. "Home Apnea Monitoring and Disruptions in Family Life: A Multidimensional Controlled Study." *American Journal of Public Health,* May '92, 82:719-722.

Baird, Patricia A. et al. "Life Expectancy in Down's Syndrome Adults." *Lancet,* Dec. 10, '88, 2:1354-1356.

Barinaga, Marcia. "Knockout Mice Offer First Animal Model for CF." *Science,* Aug. 21, '92, 257:1046-1047.

Benderly, Beryl Lieff. "Saving the Children (FAS)." *Health,* Dec. '89, 21:74-75.

Brady, Mary Sue et al. "Effectiveness of Enteric-Coated Pancreatic Enzymes Given before Meals in Reducing Steatorrhea in Children with Cystic Fibrosis." *American Dietetic Association,* July '92, 92:813-817.

Brock, David J.H. et al. "Predictive Testing for Huntington's Disease with Linked DNA Markers." *Lancet,* Aug. 26, '89, 2:463-466.

Carroll, Pat. "A Dim Prognosis on Bo's Return." *Sporting News,* Apr. 8, '91, 211:17.

"Chorion Villus Sampling: Valuable Addition or Dangerous Alternative?" *Lancet,* June 22, '91, 337:1513-1516.

Chua-Lim, C. et al. "Deficiencies in School Readiness Skills of Children with Sickle Cell Anemia: A Preliminary Report." *Southern Medical Journal,* Apr. '93, 86(4):397-402.

"Cot Deaths: Looking Up?" *Economist,* May 9, '92, 323:108-109.

"Cystic Fibrosis: Prospects for Screening and Therapy." *Lancet,* Jan. 13, '90, 335:79-80.

Davies, Kevin. "Slow Search for Huntington's Disease Gene." *Nature,* May 7, '92, 357:94.

Davies, Kevin. "The Search for the Cystic Fibrosis Gene." *New Scientist,* Oct. 21, '89, 124: 54-58.

Demak, Richard. "Marfan Syndrome: a Silent Killer." *Sports Illustrated,* Feb. 17, '86, 64:30-35.

Diamond, Jared. "The Cruel Logic of Our Genes." *Discover,* Nov. '89, 10:72-78.

Diamond, Jared. "Curse and Blessing of the Ghetto." *Discover,* Mar. '91, 12:60-65.

Dorris, Michael. "Fetal Alcohol Syndrome." *Parents' Magazine,* Nov. '90, 65:238-242.

Duimstra, C. et al "A Fetal Alcohol Syndrome Surveillance Pilot Project in American Indian Communities in the Northern Plains." *Public Health Reports,* Mar.-Apr. '93, 108(2): 225-229.

Fehrenbach, Annette M.B. et al. "Parental Problem-Solving Skills, Stress and Dietary Compliance in Phenylketonuria." *Journal of Consulting and Clinical Psychology,* Apr. '89, 57: 237-241.

Feldman, Miriam K. "Is the New Genetics Outpacing Primary Medicine?" *Minnesota Medicine,* May '92, 75:18-123.

Gil, Karen et al. "Sickle Cell Disease Pain: 2. Predicting Health Care Use and Activity Level at 9-Month Follow-Up." *Journal of Consulting & Clinical Psychology,* Apr. '92, 60:267-273.

Gordon, Hymie. "Examining the Past, Present, and Future of Clinical Genetics. " *Minnesota Medicine,* May '92, 75:11-14.

Gregg-Smith, S.J. et al. "Septic Arthritis in Haemophilia." *Journal of Bone and Joint Surgery in Britain,* May '93, 75(3):368-370.

Guntheroth, Warren G. and Philip S. Spiers. "Sleeping Prone and the Risk of Sudden Infant Death Syndrome." *Journal of the American Medical Association,* May 6, '92, 267:2359-2362.

Jackson, Laird G., Julia M. Zachary et al. "A Randomized Comparison of Transcervical and Transabdominal Chorionic-Villus Sampling." *New England Journal of Medicine,* Aug. 27, '92, 327:594-598.

Javitt, Jonathan E., A. Marshall McBean et al. "Undertreatment of Glaucoma among Black Americans." *New England Journal of Medicine,* Nov. 14, '91, 325:1418-1422.

Joachim, Hiroshi Mori et al. "Amyloid Beta-Protein Deposition in Tissues Other than Brain in Alzheimer's Disease." *Nature,* Sept. 21, '89, 341:226-230.

Karnes, Pamela S. "The Revolution in Clinical Genetics: Practical Applications." *Minnesota Medicine,* May '92, 75:35-37.

Kessler, Seymour. "Psychiatric Implications of Presymptomatic Testing for Huntington's Disease." *American Journal of Orthopsychiatry,* Apr. '87, 57:212-219.

Kiester, Edwin, Jr. "A Bug in the System." *Discover,* Feb. '91, 12:70-76.

"Klinefelter's Syndrome." *Lancet,* June 11, '88, 1:1316-1317.

Koch, C. and N. Hiby. "Pathogenesis of Cystic Fibrosis." *Lancet,* Apr. 24, '93, 341 (8852):1065-1069.

Kresevic, Denise. "Caring for Adults Who Have Cystic Fibrosis." *American Journal of Nursing,* Nov. '89, 89:1462-1465.

Kreuz, W. et al. "Incidence of Development of Factor VIII and Factor IX Inhibitors in Haemophiliacs." *Lancet,* Mar. 7, '92, 339:594-598.

Loupe, Diane E. "Breaking the Sickle Cycle: Potential Treatments Emerge for Sickle Cell Anemia." *Science News,* Dec. 2, '89, 136:360-362.

Luder, Elisabeth et al. "Teaching Self-Management Skills to Cystic Fibrosis Patients and Its Effect on Their Caloric Intake." *Journal of the American Dietetic Association,* Mar. '89, 89: 359-364.

Madden, B.P. et al. "Intermediate-Term Results of Heart-Lung Transplantation for Cystic Fibrosis." *Lancet,* June 27, '92, 339:1583-1587.

McCleary, Elliott H. "A Medical Breakthrough That Will Change Our Lives." *Consumer's Digest,* May '92, 31:28-31 +.

Meade, T.W., P. Ammala et al. "Medical Research Council European Trial of Chorion." *Lancet,* June 22, '91, 337:1491-1499.

Mennie, Moira E. et al. "Prenatal Screening for Cystic Fibrosis." *Lancet,* July 25, '92, 340: 214-216.

Merz, Beverly. "Capture of Elusive Cystic Fibrosis Gene Prompts New Approaches to Treatment." *Journal of the American Medical Association,* Sept. 22, '89, 262:1567-1568.

Mitchell, E.A. et al. "Smoking and the Sudden Infant Death Syndrome." *Pediatrics,* May '93, 91(5):893-896.

Mitchell, W.G. et al. "Effects of Human Immunodeficiency Virus and Immune Status on Magnetic Resonance Imaging of the Brain in Hemophilic Subjects: Results from the Hemophilia Growth and Development Study." *Pediatrics,* Apr. '93, 91(4):742-746.

Monahan, Terry. "Sickle Cell Trait: A Risk for Sudden Death During Physical Activity?" *Physician and Sportsmedicine,* Dec. '87, 15:143-145.

Morris, Michael J. et al. "Problems in Genetic Prediction for Huntington's Disease." *Lancet,* Sept. 9, '89, 2:60-62.

Mozer, Harold N. et al. "Perspectives on the Etiology of Alzheimer's Disease." *Journal of the American Medical Association,* Mar. 20, '87, 257:1503-1507.

Myerberg, D.Z. "Sleep Positioning and the Sudden Infant Death Syndrome." *Western Journal of Medicine,* Feb. '93, 158(2):181-182.

Okano, Yoshiyuki et al. "Molecular Basis of Phenotypic Heterogeneity in Phenylketonuria." *New England Journal of Medicine,* May 2, '91, 324:1232-1238.

Patlak, Margie. "Controlling Epilepsy: Science Replaces Superstition." *FDA Consumer,* May '92, 26:28-31.

Patterson, David. "The Causes of Down Syndrome." *Scientific American,* Aug. '87, 257: 52-58.

Platt, Orah S., Bruce D. Thorington et al. "Pain in Sickle Cell Disease." *New England Journal of Medicine,* July 4, '91, 325:11-16.

Post, Stephen G. "Huntington's Disease: Prenatal Screening for Late Onset Disease." *Journal of Medical Ethics,* June '92, 18:75-78.

Pueschel, Siegfried M. "Maternal Alpha-Fetoprotein Screening for Down's Syndrome." *New England Journal of Medicine,* Aug. 6, '87, 317:376-378.

Purvis, Andrew. "Laying Siege to a Deadly Gene (Cystic Fibrosis)." *Time,* Feb. 24, '92, 139:60-61.

Rabkin, Charles S. et al. "Incidence of Lymphomas and Other Cancers in HIV-Infected and HIV-Uninfected Patients with Hemophilia." *Journal of the American Medical Association,* Feb. 26, '92, 267:1090-1094.

Randall, Teri. "Gene Factor: Factor VIII Gene Explains Just Half of Severe Cases of Hemophilia A." *Journal of the American Medical Association,* Sept. 25, '91, 266:1612-1613.

Randall, Teri. "Pregnancy Hormone Levels Signal Trisomy 21, Improved Screening, Lower Costs Possible." *Journal of the American Medical Association,* Apr. 10, '91, 265(14):1797-1798.

Ransom, Lou. "Ali is Now 50! Won Title Three Times, Married Four Wives, Has 9 Children and Millions of Fans." *Jet,* Feb. 10, '92, 81:54-58.

Roberts, Harold R. "The Treatment of Hemophilia: Past Tragedy and Future Promise." *New England Journal of Medicine,* Oct. 26, '89, 321:1188-1191.

Roberts, Leslie. "Huntington's Gene: So Near, yet So Far." *Science,* Feb. 9, '90, 247:624-627.

Rothlind, J.C. et al. "Cognitive and Motor Correlates of Everyday Functioning in Early Huntington's Disease." *Journal of Nervous and Mental Disorders,* Mar. '93, 181(3):194-199.

"Safety of Therapeutic Products Used for Hemophilia Patients." *Journal of the American Medical Association,* Aug. 19, '88, 260:901-903.

Scriver, Charles R. "Phenylketonuria—Genotypes and Phenotypes." *New England Journal of Medicine,* May 2, '91, 324:1280-1281.

Seligson, Susan V. "Eyes on the Blink." *In Health,* Mar. '91, 5:80-86.

Shephard, R.W. et al. "Increased Energy Expenditure in Young Children with Cystic Fibrosis." *Lancet,* June 11, '88, 1:1300-1303.

Sinha, A. "Sudden Infant Death Syndrome—United States, 1980-1988." *Journal of the American Medical Association,* Aug. 19, '92, 268:856-858.

Spohr, H.L., J. Willms, and H.C. Steinhausen. "Prenatal Alcohol Exposure and Long-term Developmental Consequences." *Lancet,* Apr. 10, '93, 341(8850):907-910.

Sullivan, Louis. "The Risks of Sickle Cell Trait: Caution and Common Sense." *New England Journal of Medicine,* Jan. 26, '90, 263:490-491.

Thompson, Larry. "Mom and Pop Genes." *Discover,* Feb. '91, 12:20.

Thompson Jr., Robert J. et al. "Stress, Coping and Psychological Adjustment of Adults with Sickle Cell Disease." *Journal of Consulting Clinical Psychology,* June '92, 60:433-440.

Tizzano, E.F. and M. Buchwald. "Recent Advances in Cystic Fibrosis Research." *Journal of Pediatrics,* June '93, 122(6):985-986.

Unonu, Janet Ngozi and Allan A. Johnson. "Feeding Patterns, Food Energy, Nutrient Intakes, and Anthropometric Measurements of Selected Black Preschool Children with Down Syndrome." *American Dietetic Association,* July '92, 92:856-858.

Warren, Kenneth R. et al. "Alcohol-Related Birth Defects: An Update." *Public Health Reports,* Nov.-Dec. '88, 103:638-642.

Watson, Eila K. et al. "Psychological and Social Consequences of Community Carrier Screening Programme for Cystic Fibrosis." *Lancet,* July 25, '92, 340:217-220.

Weinberger, S.E. "Recent Advances in Pulmonary Medicine." *New England Journal of Medicine,* May 20, '93, 328(20):1462-1470.

Weiss, Rick. "Decade of Discovery." *American Health,* Mar. '92, 11:34-39.

Wilfond, Benjamin S. et al. "The Cystic Fibrosis Gene: Medical and Social Implications for Heterozygote Detection." *Journal of the American Medical Association,* May 23, '90, 263:2777-2783.

Wiswell, T.E. "Respiratory Distress Syndrome in the Newborn: Innovative Therapies." *American Family Physician,* Feb. 1, '93, 47(2):407-414.

Zamula, Evelyn. "Drugs and Pregnancy: Often the Two Don't Mix." *FDA Consumer,* June '89, 23:7-10.

GLOSSARY

ACE inhibitor Drug used to treat hypertension and heart failure

acetylcholine Type of neurotransmitter

ascites Excess of fluid in the peritoneal cavity—the space between the two layers of membrane that lines the inside of the abdominal wall and the outside of the abdominal organs

acromegaly Rare disease characterized by abnormal enlargement of bone; caused by a benign tumor of the pituitary gland in an adult

ACTH Adrenocorticotropic hormone that stimulates the adrenal cortex to release other hormones (corticosteroids)

active artificial immunity Acquired through vaccination with a weakened form of an active or disease-causing microorganism

active natural immunity Acquired through exposure to a disease-causing microorganism

acyclovir Antiviral drug used to treat herpes simplex infection

alimentary Referring to parts of the digestive system

allergen Agent that causes an allergic reaction

alveolar sacs Small saclike structures at the end of the bronchioles that contain the alveoli

alveoli Terminal saccules of the alveolar ducts where gases are exchanged in respiration

amantadine Antiviral drug sometimes used prophylactically for influenza

amniocentesis Test to identify genetic defects in a fetus as young as five months

anaerobic Lacking oxygen—some organisms multiply in anaerobic conditions

analgesic Agent that relieves pain without causing loss of consciousness

anaphylactic shock Rare, severe, life-threatening reaction to an allergen

aneurysm Weakened area of a blood vessel, usually an artery, which dilates (expands) with the pressure of blood flowing through it. May be caused by disease, injury, or a congenital defect. Usually results in severe pain; may rupture

angina pectoris Squeezing or crushing tightness in the chest; a symptom of coronary artery disease

angioplasty Insertion of a balloon into an artery; the balloon is inflated to widen the lumen, which has been narrowed by atherosclerotic plaques

angiotensin Vasopressant involved in regulating blood pressure

antibody-mediated immunity *See* humoral immunity

antiemetic Drug used to treat nausea and vomiting

antigen Any substance that can trigger the immune response resulting in the body's production of antibodies

antipyretic Relieving fever; agent that relieves or reduces fever

antisera *See* antitoxin

antitoxin Antibody produced in response to and capable of neutralizing a toxin

antrum Lower part of the stomach; churns food with enzymes and acids to produce chyme

aqueous humor Transparent liquid contained in the anterior and posterior chambers of the eye

arsphenamine Also called "606," first drug used to treat syphilis

arteriosclerosis Hardening of and loss of elasticity in the arteries

arthralgia Pain in a joint

arthropod vector Organism that transports a disease agent from infected to noninfected individuals

asymptomatic Without any apparent symptoms

atherogenesis Formation of masses of plaque in the arteries

atheroma Mass of plaque, formed of cholesterol and cellular debris

atherosclerosis Deposits of plaque formed within the arteries. A form of arteriosclerosis

atrophy Shrinkage or wasting away of a tissue or organ; a reduction in the number or size of cells

atropine Drug sometimes used to treat Menière's disease and other disorders

autoimmune disorder Misdirected immune response wherein the body's immune system attacks the body's own tissues

autoinfection Infection by an agent already present in or on the body

autonomic process Process controlled by the part of the nervous system that regulates the motor functions of body organs

avenue of escape *See* portal of exit

axon Part of a neuron that carries messages away from the cell body

azidothymidine (AZT) Drug that inhibits the human immunodeficiency virus that causes AIDS

bacilli Rod-shaped bacteria. Tuberculosis is caused by bacilli

bacteremia   Presence of bacteria in the blood

bacteria   Single-celled, plant-like organisms, some harmless, some beneficial, and a minority disease-causing. Common groups of bacteria are bacilli, cocci, and spirilla

BCG   Vaccination that provides immunity to tuberculosis

benign   Noncancerous, as a growth or tumor

beta blockers   Drugs prescribed mainly for heart disease

bile   Liquid secreted by liver which carries away waste products of the liver and helps break down fat in the small intestine

bilirubin   Bile pigment which, along with cholesterol and calcium, forms gallstones

biofeedback   Technique of furnishing an individual with auditory or sensory information that enables the individual to gain control over autonomic processes such as blood pressure or heart rate

bolus   Mass of chewed food that is ready to be swallowed

bradycardia   Slowness of the heart beat, as evidenced by slowing of the pulse rate to less than 60

bronchial tubes   Larger air passageways of the lungs

bronchiole   One of the finer subdivisions of the branched bronchial tree

bronchodilator   Drug used to relieve breathing difficulties such as those occurring in asthma

bubo   Tender, enlarged and inflamed lymph node, particularly in the axilla or groin and present in infections such as bubonic plague

bursa   Small, fluid-filled sac that facilitates the movement of muscles and tendons over body parts or joints

calcium channel blocker   Used in the treatment of angina pectoris, hypertension and certain types of arrhythmia

calculus   A hard, crystalline mass formed from precipitates of body fluids. Most often found in biliary or urinary tract

carcinogen   Cancer-causing substance

cardiac catheterization   Diagnostic test wherein a fine tube (catheter) is introduced into the heart, through a blood vessel, to investigate its condition

cardiovascular system   Composed of heart, blood vessels and lymphatics

carrier   Individual who, although infected with a disease, has no discernible symptoms, and is capable of spreading the disease to others

catarrhal stage   Stage of whooping cough marked by inflammation of the mucous membrane in the air passages of the head and throat

cell-mediated immunity   Involves the production of lymphocytes (T cells) in response to exposure to an antigen

cerebrovascular accident   Stroke

chancre   Characteristic sore and first apparent symptom of syphilis

chemotaxis   Movement of an organism or cells in response to a chemical attractant. In the inflammatory reaction, chemicals called mediators lure leukocytes to travel toward the site of an injury

chemotherapy   Use of drugs (chemicals) to treat disease

chest physiotherapy   Process of massaging and pressure applied to the chest

cholecystectomy   Surgery to remove the gallbladder

cholesterol   Lipid that plays an important part in the formation of atheromas in the arteries. Also important in normal body processes

chorea   Involuntary muscular twitching of face or limbs

chorionic villus biopsy   Test to identify genetic defects in a fetus as young as two months

choroid   Layer of blood vessels that lies at the back of the eye behind the retina

chylomicron   Lipoprotein composed primarily of triglycerides

chyme   Liquid produced in the antrum of the stomach during the digestive process and released gradually to the duodenum

cilia   Fine hairlike projections in the respiratory passages. Also found in other parts of the body

ciliary body   Membrane of the eye between the iris and front of the choroid

claw hand   Flexion and atrophy of the hand and fingers occurring in leprosy and other disorders

clinical   Stage of a disease when the characteristic symptoms appear

colchicine   Drug used 1500 years ago and still used today in the treatment of gout

COLD   Chronic Obstructive Lung Disease (see COPD)

collateral circulation   Side branches of blood vessels

complement   Contained in the plasma secreted by capillaries during the body's immune response; enhances the phagocytosis of the antigen by causing the destruction of its cell membrane

completed stroke   Maximal damage in the beginning

Computerized Axial Tomography (CAT scan)   Diagnostic technique using X-rays and a computer to produce clear, cross-sectional images of the tissue being examined

congenital disorder   Disorder present at birth

contact inhibition   Pertaining to the cancer cell's inability to know when to stop reproducing

contact investigation   Finding those known to have been exposed to a disease agent

convalescence   Recovery stage of a disease

COPD   Chronic Obstructive Pulmonary Disease - often a combination of chronic bronchitis and emphysema. Chronic asthma may also be present

cor pulmonale   Failure of right ventricle caused by disorders of the lungs, pulmonary vessels, or chest wall

cornea   Part of the eye that refracts light rays

corticosteroids   Drugs similar to the natural hormones produced by the adrenal glands that are prescribed in hormone replacement therapy

cruciferous vegetable   Vegetable such as cauliflower, broccoli, or brussels sprouts that contains nutrients and nonnutrients that protect against cancer

cryosurgery   Tissue destruction by freezing

cyanosis   Blueness caused by reduced oxygen in general circulation

cystectomy   Bladder removal

cystoscope   Tube with a light and various attachments. Used to examine and treat diseases of the bladder and urethra

debilitated   Weakened by some disease process

debridement   Removal of foreign material and dead, damaged, or infected tissue from a wound or burn until surrounding healthy tissue is exposed

decline   Stage of a disease when the symptoms begin to fade

defecation   Expulsion of feces via the anus

dementia   Mental deterioration

demyelination   Destruction or removal of myelin sheath of nerve tissue

dendrite   Part of neuron that carries messages to the cell body

deoxyribonucleic acid (DNA)   Principal carrier of genetic information in almost all organisms

dermis   Layer of skin containing hair follicles, sweat glands, sebaceous glands, blood vessels, lymph vessels, and nerves

desquamation   Shedding of epithelial elements, chiefly of the skin, in scales or small sheets

diabetic coma   Life-threatening condition in diabetics, occurring if blood glucose becomes too high

diastolic pressure   Resting period of the heart muscle. The second reading when blood pressure is taken

diethylstilbestrol (DES)   Synthetic estrogen used therapeutically to treat menopause and as a "morning after" pill until it was discovered that daughters of women who were given the drug during pregnancy, developed vaginal cancer later in life

differentiation   Term used in classifying cancer cells

dopamine   Neurotransmitter that is deficient in individuals with Parkinson's disease

duodenum   First section of the small intestine

dysentery   Diarrhea

dyspepsia   Indigestion

dyspnea   Difficult or labored breathing

ectopic pregnancy   Pregnancy that develops outside the womb, usually in a fallopian tube

edema   Presence of abnormally large amounts of fluid in the intercellular tissue spaces of the body

electrodesiccation   Tissue destruction by heat

electrolyte   Substance that plays an important part in regulation of heartbeat

embolus   Moving blood clot

emigration   During the inflammatory response, leukocyte movement along the endothelium and escape through the walls of blood vessels

emollient   Agent that softens skin or soothes irritated skin or mucous membrane

encapsulated   Enclosed in a sheath not normal to the part as in a benign tumor

endemic   Constantly present in a particular area or specific population

endocardium   Internal lining of the heart

endocrine gland   Ductless gland that discharges its secretions directly into the bloodstream

endogenous   Arising from causes on or within the organism

endometritis   Inflammation of the inner mucous membrane of the uterus

endometrium   Lining of the uterus

endothelium   Lining of the blood vessels and other body parts

enteritis   Inflammation of the intestine, applied chiefly to the small intestine

enterovirus   Genus of virus that includes the polio virus

epidemic   Disease occurring suddenly in numbers clearly in excess of normal expectancy

epidemiologic theory   Whether or not anyone gets a disease depends on the relationship among three factors: the disease, the host, and the environment

epidemiology   Science of studying the factors that determine and influence the frequency and distribution of disease

epidermis   Outermost and thinnest layer of the skin

erythema   Redness of the skin produced by congestion of the capillaries

erythema chronicum migrans (ECM)   Characteristic rash resulting from the bite of a tick carrying Lyme disease. The rash is a red spot that expands gradually, leaving a clear area in the middle

erythromycin   Drug used to treat infections of the skin, chest, throat, and ears

esophageal varices   Dilated, incompetent veins in the esophagus that are a result of liver disease

etiology   Study of the factors that cause disease

excise   To cut out diseased tissue

exocrine gland   Gland that discharges its secretions through a duct opening on an internal or external surface of the body

exogenous   Originating outside the organism

exotoxin   Toxic substance formed by species of certain bacteria that is found outside the bacterial cell

external barrier   Body's first line of defense against invaders

exudate   Material escaping from blood vessels that have increased permeability during the inflammatory responses

familial hyperlipoproteinemia   Increase in three fatty substances in the blood: cholesterol, phospholipid and triglyceride (lipoproteins) more common in some families

feces   Waste material of digestive tract, expelled through the anus. Consists of indigestible food residue (fiber), dead bacteria, dead cells shed from intestinal lining, secretions from intestines such as mucus, bile from the liver and water

fibrinous   Pertaining to an exudate containing fibrin, an aid to formation of a clot in the healing process; produced in a moderately severe wound

fibrotic regeneration   Repair of a wound with fibrous tissue

foamy macrophage   Macrophage containing lipids

fomite   Inanimate object capable of harboring pathogenic organisms and thus conveying an infection from one person to another. Respiratory infections such as colds and influenza are most commonly transmitted this way

fontanelle   One of two soft areas on a baby's scalp; a gap between the bones of the skull covered by a membrane

food poisoning   Term commonly used to denote any illness that seems to be the result of ingesting food

fundus   Upper part of the stomach that holds food as it is gradually delivered to the lower part

fungi   Single- or multi-celled plant-like organisms that release enzymes that digest cells

gangrene   Death of tissue, usually because of inadequate oxygen supply to the area

gastrin   Hormone secreted mainly by cells in the stomach to aid in digestion

gastroenterologist   Specialist in treating disorders of the digestive tract

glomerulus   Element in the nephron of the kidney that filters the blood

gold salts   Sometimes used to treat arthritis

grading   Classification of tumor cells by grades (I to IV) depending on their degree of difference from normal cells and their growth rate

griseofulvin   Drug prescribed to treat fungi orally when creams and lotions have not been effective

gumma   Advanced lesion of syphilis

gynecomastia   Excessive development of the male mammary glands

hajj   Pilgrimage to Mecca

heartburn   Burning pain in center of chest that may travel from tip of breastbone to throat. Generally a result of overeating, eating spicy foods or drinking alcohol

hemangioma   Birthmark caused by abnormal distribution or excess of blood vessels

hematuria   Blood in the urine

hemoccult test   Test to detect blood in the stool, a sign of colorectal cancer

hemorrhagic exudate   Exudate that appears in a severe injury, when a lesion is deep enough to penetrate blood vessels and allow red blood cells to escape

hemorrhoids   Varicose veins in the anal area

high-density lipoprotein (HDL)   Removes cholesterol from the blood and sends it to the liver to be processed and excreted (good cholesterol)

histamine   Substance released in an allergic reaction or as part of the inflammation response

human immunodeficiency virus (HIV)   Virus that causes AIDS

human T-cell lymphotrophic virus (HTLV)   Name once used for the virus which causes AIDS

humoral immunity   Protection against disease through B-lymphocytes, or B cells, which produce antibodies in the blood. Also called antibody-mediated immunity

hydrocephalus   An increased amount of fluid, usually under increased pressure within the skull

hypercalcemia   Abnormally high level of calcium in the blood

hypercholesterolemia   Excess of cholesterol in the blood

hyperesthesia   Increased sensitivity to sensory stimuli such as pain and touch

hyperlipidemia   Excess of fats in the blood

hypersensitivity disorder   Also called allergy, an inappropriate reaction of the immune system, e.g. allergic rhinitis, urticaria, angioedema, asthma

hypertension   High blood pressure

hypertrophy   Enlargement of an organ or tissue caused by increase in size, rather than number, of its cells

hyperuricemia   Excess uric acid in the blood

hypochondriac   Individual with an unreasonable belief or fear that he or she has a serious illness despite medical reassurance

hypodermis   Layer of skin consisting mainly of fat, which provides heat, insulation, shock absorption and a reserve of calories; also has a nerve supply

hypothermia   Significant loss of body heat

hypoxemia   Too little oxygen in the blood

I.M.   Intramuscular administration of a liquid form of a drug

I.V. Intravenous administration of a liquid form of a drug

idiopathic hypertension *See* primary hypertension

immunology Branch of biomedical science concerned with the response of the organism to antigenic challenge, the recognition of self and not-self, and all aspects of immune phenomena.

in situ Localized

incidence rate Number of new cases of a disease occurring during a specified time

incubation Period from the time when the agent enters the body to the appearance of the first symptoms

inflammation First response of the body when pathogenic agents penetrate external barriers

insidious Indicating the occurrence of a disease that comes on in such a way (no symptoms) that the individual is unaware of the onset

insulin shock State occurring in diabetics if blood glucose becomes too low

interferon Protein that protects the body against viral infection; released during the inflammatory response if the cell injury is due to a viral infection

intermediate-density lipoprotein (IDL) Lipid quickly removed from plasma or converted to LDL

ischemia Deficiency of blood in an area due to constriction or obstruction of a blood vessel

Islets of Langerhans Areas in the pancreas containing the beta cells that produce insulin

jaundice Yellowing of the skin and whites of the eyes; indicative of a liver and/or biliary system disorder

ketosis Potentially serious condition when chemical substances called ketones accumulate in the blood if there is not enough sugar available to use as energy. May be a result of untreated or inadequately controlled diabetes

Koplik's spots Small irregular, bright red spots on the inside of the mouth with a minute bluish-white speck in the center of each; seen in the prodromal stage of measles (rubeola)

laparoscopy Means of examining the abdominal cavity by means of a laparoscope (viewing tube)

laryngoscopy Means of examining the larynx with a laryngoscope (viewing tube)

leproma Superficial granulomatous nodule characteristic of lepromatous leprosy

Lindane Drug used for infestation with scabies or lice

lipid Fatty substance; includes triglycerides, phospholipids, and sterols such as cholesterol

lipoprotein Lipids in the plasma; they circulate attached to protein

lordosis Commonly called "swayback," an accentuation of the normal curve of the spine

low-density lipoprotein (LDL) Lipid strongly correlated with atherosclerosis

lumen Space in a tubular organ such as an artery

lymphadenopathy Swollen lymph glands

lymphadenopathy-associated virus (LAV) Name once used for the virus which causes AIDS

lymphokine Substance released by lymphocytes which have come in contact with an antigen; helps produce cellular immunity by stimulating macrophages and monocytes

macrophage Large cell that performs the final function of the body's immune response; i.e. "clean-ups" by killing and digesting antigens

macule Discolored spot on the skin that is not elevated above the surface

Magnetic Resonance Imaging (MRI) Provides high quality cross-sectional images of organs and structures within the body without the use of X rays or other ratiation

malaise Vague feeling of bodily discomfort

malignant Cancerous; used to describe neoplasm or tumor

malignant hypertension Severe form of high blood pressure in which blood pressure rises rapidly with possible injury to the arterioles

mediators Chemicals that lure leukocytes to an inflammatory site

Mendelian genetics Study of the transmission of traits from one generation to the next

menopause Time during which menstruation ceases and changes occur in a woman's body because of reduced hormone production

metastasize To spread, as a tumor, through the circulatory and lymphatic systems and to invade surrounding tissue

metazoon Multicellular parasitic animal (worm) that can cause disease

methotrexate Drug originally used in cancer chemotherapy

metronidazole An antibiotic effective against infections caused by anaerobic bacteria; also used to treat protozoan infections

miasma theory Theory that attributed disease to bad odors or emanations from the earth

mitral stenosis Narrowing of the mitral valve opening

mode of conveyance Means by which disease organisms pass from one host to another

molecular genetics Study of the chemical structure of genes and how they operate at the molecular level

monoclonal antibody therapy Experimental treatment for cancer whereby "clones" of antibodies carry substances to cancer cells and destroy them

mucolytic agent   Drug that makes mucus less sticky and easier to cough up

mucous membrane   Soft, pink, layer that lines many cavities and tubes of the body and secretes a fluid containing mucus to keep structures moist

myalgia   Muscle pain

myocardial infarct (MI)   Heart attack

myocarditis   Inflammation of the myocardium, the muscular walls of the heart

nebulizer   Device used to administer a drug in aerosol form through a face mask; often used for asthma attacks

necrosis   Death of tissue

neoplasm   New or abnormal growth

nephron   Anatomical and functional unit of the kidney providing the filtering, reabsorption and excretion functions

neuron   Fundamental unit of the nervous system consisting of the cell body, axon, and dendrites

neurotransmitter   Chemical substance that diffuses across the synaptic gap and carries a message from the axon of one neuron to the dendrite of another

nocturia   Increased urination at night

nodule   Small lump of tissue – hard or soft – usually more than one quarter of an inch in diameter

nonsteroidal anti-inflammatory drug (NSAID)   One of a number of drugs used to reduce inflammation and pain

occlusion   Blockage of any canal, opening, or vessel of the body

oncogene   Gene in tumor cells whose activation is associated with the conversion of normal cells into cancer cells

oncologist   Physician who specializes in treating cancer

oral hypoglycemic   Drug used to stimulate insulin production

orchitis   Inflammation of the testes

palliative   Affording relief but not cure

pallor   Paleness; absence of normal skin coloration

pandemic   Widespread epidemic of a disease

Pap smear   Test for cancer of the cervix

papule   Small circumscribed, superficial, solid elevation of the skin

parasitic   Pertaining to or caused by a parasite, a plant or animal which lives upon or within another living organism at whose expense it obtains some advantage

paresthesia   Abnormal sensation, as burning or prickling

parotid glands   Salivary glands located on either side of the face, above the jaw and in front of the ear

paroxysmal   Recurring sudden intensification of symptoms or spasms

passive artificial immunity   Acquired through inoculation with antibodies

passive natural immunity   Acquired through the transfer of antibodies from a mother to her baby through the placenta and, later, through breast milk

pathogenic   Disease-causing

pavementing   Adherence of leukocytes to the endothelium of venules after the immediate inflammatory response

pepsin   Chief digestive enzyme in the stomach

perianal   Around the anus

pericarditis   Inflammation of the membrane that surrounds the heart

peripheral neuritis   Inflammation of nerves in peripheral nervous system

peristalsis   Wave of contraction propelling contents through a tubular organ

phagocytes   Cells that attack and are capable of ingesting antigens that enter the body

phospholipid   Lipid that contains phosphorus

photophobia   Sensitivity to light

plaque   In the arteries; deposits containing cholesterol, foamy macrophages, smooth muscle cells and cellular debris

polyuria   Frequent urination

population genetics   Study of the variation of genes among and within populations

portal of entry   Avenue through which a pathogenic organism gets into a new host

portal of exit   Way for a pathogenic organism to leave the host

Positron Emission Tomography (PET)   Produces three-dimensional images that reflect the metabolic and chemical activity of tissues being studied

PPNG   Penicillinase-producing *N. gonorrhoeae*

predisposing factor   *See* risk factor

prednisone   Corticosteroid drug used to reduce inflammation and pain

prevalence rate   Number of cases of a particular disease in a community at a specified time

primary healing   *See* resolution

primary hypertension   Another name for essential hypertension, the most common form of high blood pressure

primary prevention   Measures taken before disease occurs to reduce susceptibility, such as a vaccination

prodromal   Second stage of a disease when nonspecific symptoms appear

progressive stroke   Stroke that starts with slight neurologic impairment that worsens in 24 to 48 hours

prophylactic   Drug, procedure, or equipment used to prevent disease

proteinuria   Passage of increased amounts of protein in the urine

protooncogene   Normal gene that with alteration becomes an oncogene

protozoon   Single-celled parasitic animal that may release toxins and enzymes that destroy cells or interfere with their functions

pruritic   Itching

pseudomembrane   False membrane

psychoneuroimmunology   New field of scientific inquiry that studies the system of communication between the mind and the body. The link between the nervous system and the immune system is of particular interest

psychosomatic factors   Mental and emotional processes that can originate or aggravate an actual physiological disease

purulent exudate   Also called pus, occurs in a severe injury

pustule   Visible collection of pus within or beneath the epidermis, often in a hair follicle or sweat pore

pyloric sphincter   Lower valve of the stomach

pyogenic   Pus producing

reflux   Abnormal backflow of fluid as when stomach acid flows back into the esophagus

regeneration   Natural renewal of lost tissue as it is replaced by tissue of the same type

rehydration   Administration of fluids to combat dehydration

repair   Replacement of lost tissue by granulation tissue, which becomes a fibrous connective tissue scar

reservoir   "Home" of pathogenic organisms. Humans, plants, animals, and organic matter are all reservoirs for various pathogenic organisms, allowing them to live and reproduce

resolution   When an injury is mild and heals without pus forming

respiratory system   The parts of the body involved in respiration, including the nose, pharynx, larynx, bronchial tubes, and lungs

retina   The most essential structure of the eye, which receives the image formed by the lens

rice water stools   White flecks in the stools, a symptom of cholera

rifampin   Antibacterial drug used to treat tuberculosis

risk factors   Or predisposing factors, the hereditary or lifestyle factors that help determine the likelihood of disease

risus sardonicus   A grinning expression caused by acute spasm of facial muscles as in tetanus

sclera   Dense white fibrous protective coat of the eye, connected to the cornea

sebaceous gland   Gland found mainly in the face, center of chest, upper back, shoulders and neck that secretes sebum

sebum   Fatty secretion of the sebaceous glands that can obstruct hair follicles causing acne spots

secondary healing   *See* repair

secondary prevention   Measures taken to diagnose a disease that may already be present

sequela   Condition following or caused by an attack of disease

serous   Watery, as exudate produced in the inflammation response

slow virus   Virus that may remain dormant for years before causing signs and symptoms of illness

sphygmomanometer   Instrument for measuring blood pressure consisting of an inflatable cuff, inflating bulb, and gauge

spirilla   Spiral-shaped bacteria, such as the spirillum that causes syphilis

splenomegaly   Enlargement of the spleen

staging   System used to quantify the extent of a cancer; allows for individualized therapy according to the characteristics of the patient and the case

stapes   Small bones in the middle ear vibrated by the tympanic membrane that relay these vibrations to the fluid in the inner ear

stoma   Mouth-like opening

streptomycin   The first effective drug treatment for tuberculosis

subcutaneous tissue   *See* hypodermis

sulfathiazole   Antibacterial drug

surfactant   Chemical that prevents alveoli from collapsing during exhalation

synaptic gap   Minute space between the axons of one neuron and the dendrites of another

systolic pressure   Maximum blood pressure resulting from contraction of the left ventricle

T cell   Cell produced in the thymus that is active in the immune response. Helper T cells enhance the production of antibodies. Killer T cells kill foreign cells. Suppressor T cells suppress the immune response

tachycardia   Excessive rapidity in the action of the heart, usually applied to a heart rate above 100 per minutes

tamoxifen   Anticancer drug

tender points   Areas of the body that are painful when pressure is applied; used in the diagnosis of fibromyalgia

tenesmus   Painful and often ineffectual straining at stool or in urination

tertiary prevention   Measures taken to return an individual to a healthy state or to keep the victim alive

tetanus immune globulin (TIG)   Specific immune globulin derived from blood of human donors hyperimmunized with tetanus toxoid and used prophylactically in treating tetanus

tetracycline Antibiotic used in the treatment of many bacterial diseases

thrombophlebitis Inflammation of a vein accompanied by the formation of a thrombus

thrombus Stationary clot, developed in a coronary artery or aorta because of plaque buildup

tinnitus Ringing in the ears

tophi Deposits of urate in the joints, as in gout

toxin Poison

toxoid Toxin that is no longer toxic but is still capable of inducing formation of antibodies upon injection

trachea The tube through which air passes from the larynx to the bronchial tubes

tracheostomy Operation in which an opening is made in the trachea and a tube is inserted to maintain an effective airway

transient ischemic attack (TIA) Decrease of blood flow in arteries supplying the brain; produces stroke-like symptoms lasting less than 24 hours and/or dizziness

triglyceride Fatty substance (lipid) circulating in the blood

TRNG Tetracycline resistant *Neisseria gonorrheae*

tumor Swelling

tympanic membrane Thin membrane inside the ear that vibrates when struck by sound waves

umbilicus Navel

ureter Fibromuscular tube conveying urine from kidney to bladder

uvea Middle pigmented and vascular layer of the eye, consisting of the iris, ciliary body and choroid

vaccine Suspension of attenuated or killed microorganisms (bacteria, viruses, rickettsiae) administered for the prevention, amelioration or treatment of infectious diseases

valvuloplasty Surgical reconstruction of a deformed cardiac valve

vector That which transports a pathogenic organism to a host

very-low-density lipoprotein (VLDL) Lipid with unknown atherogenic effects

vesicle Small bladder or sac containing liquid

virulent Exceedingly pathogenic, noxious or deleterious

virus Smallest disease-causing organism; made up of DNA or RNA; not technically alive but can penetrate cells and use the cells' nucleic acid to produce more viruses

zidovudine *See* azidothymidine (AZT)

zoonosis Disease of animals that may be transmitted to humans under natural conditions

CREDITS

Unit Opener 1, courtesy Graphics and Audiovisuals; World Health Organization.

Chapter 1 Figures 1.1, 1.6, 1.7, 1.16, 1.17, courtesy of World Health Organization; Figures 1.2, 1.8, 1.13, 1.14, 1.15, courtesy of Bettman Archives; Figure 1.3, courtesy of Underwood Photo Archives; Figure 1.4, courtesy of National Library of Medicine; Figures 1.11, 1.12 from Lyons, Harry N. Abrams, Inc. Publishers, NY, 1978; Figure 1.5 from Murray, *Medical Microbiology,* Mosby, 1990; Figure 1.9 courtesy of Jack Tandy, after Harvey, DeMotu Cordis; Figure 1.10 Templin, *Anatomy & Physiology Laboratory Manual,* ed 2, Mosby, 1992.

Timelines, p. 6 Marie Curie, Bettman Archives; streptococcus, Centers for Disease Control; p. 7 Jonas Salk, World Health Organization; HIV virus, Centers for Disease Control; p. 16 Leprosy, Centers for Disease Control; malaria, Science VU/Visuals Unlimited; p. 17 Diphtheria, Centers for Disease Control; yellow fever, Science VU/Visuals Unlimited.

Chapter 2 Figures 2.1, 2.2, 2.9, from Grimes, Infectious Diseases, Mosby—Year Book, Inc., 1991; Figure 2.3 from J.J. Canademse and B.C. Pugasheti/Tom Stack & Associates; Figures 2.4, 2.5 from Boyd, *General Microbiology,* ed 2, Mosby, 1988; Figure 2.6, from Schmidt/Roberts, *Foundations of Parasitology,* ed 4, Mosby, 1989; Figure 2.7, from Christiansen, *Biology of Aging,* Mosby, 1993; Figure 2.8, courtesy of Science VU/Visuals Unlimited.

Chapter 3 Figure 3.1, from Grimes, *Infectious Diseases,* Mosby—Year Book, Inc., 1991; Figure 3.2, from Seeley/Stephens/Tate, *Essentials of Anatomy & Physiology,* Mosby, 1991; Figures 3.3, 3.9, from McCance/Huether, *Pathophysiology,* Mosby, 1990; Figures 3.4, 3.5, 3.12, from Price-Wilson, *Pathophysiology,* ed 4, Mosby, 1992; Figures 3.10, 3.11, from Christiansen, *Biology of Aging,* Mosby, 1993.

Unit Opener 2, left, World Health Organization; right, Centers for Disease Control; unnumbered figure courtesy of Visuals Unlimited.

Chapter 4 Figure 4.1, from Christiansen, *Biology of Aging,* Mosby, 1993; Figures 4.2, 4.3, from Thibodeau/Patton, *Anatomy & Physiology Lab Manual,* ed 2, Mosby, 1993; Figures 4.5, 4.6, 4.7, Emond and Rowland, *A Color Atlas of Infectious Diseases,* ed 2, Mosby, 1987; Figure 4.8, from Murray, *Medical Microbiology,* Mosby, 1990; Figure 4.9, 4.10, courtesy Ernest W. Beck.

Chapter 6 Figures 6.1, 6.2, from Habif, *Clinical Dermatology,* Mosby, 1990; Figures 6.3, 6.14, from McCance/Huether, *Pathophysiology,* Mosby, 1990; Figures 6.4, 6.8, courtesy WM Meyers, CH Binford in Kissane, J.M., ed. *Anderson's Pathology,* Vol. I, ed. 9, St. Louis, Mosby, 1990; Figure 6.5, from Thibodeau/Patton, *Anatomy & Physiology Lab Manual,* ed 2, Mosby, 1993; Figure 6.6, from Murray, *Medical Microbiology,* Mosby, 1990; Figures 6.7, 6.9, 6.15, 6.16, 6.18, from Emond and Rowland, *A Color Atlas of Infectious Diseases,* ed 2, Mosby, 1987.

Chapter 7 Figures 7.2, 7.3, from Dutz, W., *Int. Patholo.,* 8:38, 1967, reprinted in Kissane, J.M., ed., *Anderson's Pathology,* Vol I ed. 9, Mosby, 1990; Figures 7.9, 7.10, from Lambert, H.P., Farrar, W.E., *Infectious Disease Illustrated,* London, 1982, Gower Medical Publishing; Figures 7.13, 7.14, 7.15, 7.19, from Habif, T.P., *Clinical Dermatology,* ed 2, Mosby, 1990; Figure 7.20, Binford, C.H., Connor, D.H. eds., *Pathology of Tropical and Extraordinary Diseases; An Atlas,* Washington D.C., 1976, Armed Forces Institute of Pathology.

Chapter 8 Figures 8.5, 8.6, 8.7, 8.9, from Habif, T.P., *Clinical Dermatology,* ed 2, Mosby, 1990; Figures 8.8, 8.12, 8.13, from Emond/Rowland, *A Color Atlas of Infectious Disease,* ed 2, Mosby, 1987; Figure 8.10, from Lambert, H.P., Farrar, W.E., *Infectious Disease Illustrated,* London, 1982, Gower Medical Publishing; Figure 8.14, courtesy Dr. Samuel Sweitzer, reprinted in Kissane, J.M. ed., *Anderson's Pathology,* Vol I, ed 9, Mosby, 1990.

Chapter 9 Figure 9.1, courtesy of Bettman Archives; Figures 9.12, 9.14, 9.21, from Habif, T.P., *Clinical Dermatology,* ed 2, Mosby, 1990; Figures 9.13, 9.15, from Price-Wilson, *Pathophysiology,* ed 4, Mosby, 1992; Figure 9.16, from McCance/Huether, *Pathophysiology,* Mosby, 1990.

Chapter 10 Figures 10.4, 10.5, 10.7, 10.8, from Habif, T.P., *Clinical Dermatology,* ed. 2, Mosby, 1990; Figure 10.6, from McCance/Huether, *Pathophysiology,* Mosby, 1990.

Chapter 11 Figures 11.1, 11.2, 11.5, 11.6, 11.7, 11.9, 11.10, 11.11, courtesy of Visuals Unlimited; Figure 11.12, from Price-Wilson, *Pathophysiology,* ed 4, Mosby, 1992; Figure 11.13, from Schmidt/Roberts, *Foundations of Parasitology,* ed 4, Mosby, 1989.

Unit Opener 3, Visuals Unlimited and Raven, Mosby, Understanding Biology.

Chapter 12 Figures 12.1, 12.6, from McCance/Huether, *Pathophysiology,* Mosby, 1990; Figures 12.2, 12.4, 12.5, 12.9B, from Canobbio, *Cardiovascular Disorders,* The C.V. Mosby Company, 1990; Figures 12.3, 12.7, 12.9A, 12.10, 12.12, from Christiansen, *Biology of Aging,* Mosby, 1993; Figure 12.11, from Thompson, *Mosby's Clinical Nursing,* ed 3., Mosby, 1993.

Chapter 13 Figure 13.1, from Price-Wilson, *Pathophysiology,* ed 4, Mosby, 1992; Figures 13.6, 13.9, 13.12, from McCance/Huether, *Pathophysiology,* Mosby, 1990; Figure 13.10, from Christiansen, *Biology of Aging,* Mosby, 1993; Figure 13.13, courtesy of American Cancer Society; Figure 13.14, from Thibodeau/Patton, *The Human Body in Health Disease,* courtesy of A.L. LeTreut, Mammography, Mosby, 1991; Figures

13.16, 13.19, 13.21, from McCance/Huether, *Pathophysiology,* Mosby, 1990.

Chapter 14 Figure 14.16, Courtesy of American Cancer Society.

Chapter 15 Figures 15.1, 15.2, 15.3, 15.5, 15.6, 15.7, 15.8, 15.9, 15.10, 15.11, from McCance/Huether, *Pathophysiology,* Mosby, 1990; Figures 15.4, 15.12, from Christiansen, *Biology of Aging,* Mosby, 1993.

Chapter 16 Figures 16.2, 16.3, 16.4, 16.5, 16.14, from McCance/Huether, *Pathophysiology,* Mosby, 1990; Figures 16.6, 16.12, 16.13, from Christiansen, *Biology of Aging,* Mosby, 1993; Figures 16.7, 16.9, 16.15, from Thompson, *Mosby's Clinical Nursing,* ed 3, Mosby, 1993; Figure 16.8, courtesy of Arthritis Foundation; Figures 16.10, 16.11, from Booher, *Athletic Injury Assessment,* ed 2, Mosby, 1989; Figure 16.13, from Christiansen, *Biology of Aging,* Mosby, 1993.

Chapter 17 Figures 17.1, 17.2, 17.4,

17.5, 17.7, 17.8, 17.9, from Christiansen, *Biology of Aging,* Mosby, 1993; Figure 17.10, from Seeley/Stephens/Tate, *Essentials of Anatomy & Physiology,* p. 190, Mosby, 1991; Figure 17.3, 17.6, from Thompson, *Mosby's Clinical Nursing,* ed 3, Mosby, 1993; Figure 17.11, adapted from McCance/Huether, *Pathophysiology,* Mosby, 1990.

Chapter 18 Figures 18.1, 18.4, from Thibodeau/Patton, *Anatomy & Physiology,* ed 2, Mosby, 1993; Figures 18.2, 18.3, from Moffett, *Human Physiology,* ed. 2, Mosby, 1993; Figures 18.5, 18.6, 18.8, 18.10, 18.11, from McCance/Huether, *Pathophysiology,* Mosby, 1990; Figure 18.7 courtesy of Bettman Archives; Figure 18.9, courtesy of March of Dimes Birth Defects Foundation; Figure 18.12, from Payne/Hahn, *Understanding Your Health,* Mosby, ed 3, 1992.